KU-446-804

Analgesia, Anaesthesia and Pregnancy

A Practical Guide

Second Edition

Edited by

STEVE YENTIS,
ANNE MAY and
SURBHI MALHOTRA

With David Bogod, Diana Brighouse and Chris Elton

CAMBRIDGE
UNIVERSITY PRESS

CAMBRIDGE UNIVERSITY PRESS
Cambridge, New York, Melbourne, Madrid, Cape Town, Singapore, São Paulo

Cambridge University Press
The Edinburgh Building, Cambridge CB2 8RU, UK
Published in the United States of America by Cambridge University Press, New York

www.cambridge.org
Information on this title: www.cambridge.org/9780521694742

© Cambridge University Press 2007

This publication is in copyright. Subject to statutory exception
and to the provisions of relevant collective licensing agreements,
no reproduction of any part may take place without
the written permission of Cambridge University Press.

First published 2007

Printed in the United Kingdom at the University Press, Cambridge

A catalogue record for this publication is available from the British Library

Library of Congress Cataloguing in Publication data
Analgesia, anaesthesia, and pregnancy: a practical guide / [edited by] Steve Yentis, Anne May,
and Surbhi Malhotra ; with David Bogod, Diana Brighouse and Chris Elton. – 2nd ed.
   p. ; cm.
   Includes bibliographical references and index.
   ISBN-13 978-0-521-69474-2 paperback
   ISBN-10 0-521-69474-4 paperback
   Anesthesia in obstetrics. I. Yentis, Steve II. May, Anne. III. Malhotra, Surbhi.
   [DNLM: 1. Analgesia, Obstetrical. 2. Anesthesia, Obstetrical. WO 450 A5328 2007]
   RG732.A5378 2007
   617.9′682--dc22

                                                                   2006102401

ISBN-13 978-0-521-69474-2 paperback

Cambridge University Press has no responsibility for the persistence or accuracy of URLs for
external or third-party internet websites referred to in this publication, and does not guarantee
that any content on such websites is, or will remain, accurate or appropriate.

Every effort has been made in preparing this publication to provide accurate and up-to-date
information which is in accord with accepted standards and practice at the time of
publication. Although case histories are drawn from actual cases, every effort has been made
to disguise the identities of the individuals involved. Nevertheless, the authors, editors and
publishers can make no warranties that the information contained herein is totally free from
error, not least because clinical standards are constantly changing through research and
regulation. The authors, editors and publishers therefore disclaim all liability for direct
or consequential damages resulting from the use of material contained in this publication.
Readers are strongly advised to pay careful attention to information provided by the
manufacturer of any drugs or equipment that they plan to use.

617.4682 4C

Analgesia, Anaesthesia and Pregnancy

A practical guide

A thoroughly updated edition of this well-established practical guide to obstetric analgesia and anaesthesia. All aspects of obstetric medicine relevant to the anaesthetist are covered, from conception, throughout pregnancy, to after-birth care.

The emphasis is on pre-empting problems and maximising quality of care. The authors have identified over 150 potential complications each covered in two sections: issues raised and management options, with key points extracted into boxes for quick reference. A section on organisational aspects such as record keeping, training, protocols and guidelines makes this an important resource for any labour ward or hospital dealing with pregnant women. Presented in a clear, structured format, this book will be invaluable to trainee anaesthetists at all levels and to experienced anaesthetists who encounter obstetric patients. Obstetricians, neonatologists, midwives, nurses and operating department practitioners wishing to extend or update their knowledge will also find it highly beneficial.

Steve Yentis is a Consultant Anesthetist at Chelsea and Westminster Hospital, London and Honorary Senior Lecturer at Imperial College, London.

Anne May is a Consultant Obstetric Anaesthetist at Leicester Royal Infirmary NHS Trust and Honorary Senior Lecturer at the University of Leicester.

Surbhi Malhotra is a Consultant Anaesthetist at St Mary's Hospital, London.

From reviews of the First Edition:

'This is a book that openly professes to be a ''short practical text'' – and it has achieved its objective very successfully indeed. Clearly set out with discrete well-organized chapters, the text is easy to read and presents a comprehensive overview of a difficult field in a ''user-friendly'' form.'

European Journal of Anaesthesiology

'The diversity of topics and their limited analysis makes it easy to read the text quickly and pick up key points. At the end of each topic is a bullet point synopsis... It is these characteristics of the book that create the practical approach...The book...is certain to be popular given its broad authorship and succinct style.'

British Journal of Anaesthesia

'The authors have succeeded in producing an excellent book in a style that sets it apart from, and possibly above, recent similar publications . . . . The book achieves its aim of targeting anaesthetists in training at all levels, and would provide a useful handbook for both the experienced and the occasional consultant obstetric anaesthetist.'

International Journal of Obstetric Anesthesia

Contents

Contributors

Dr Steve Yentis
Magill Dept of Anaesthesia, Intensive Care & Pain Management
Chelsea & Westminster Hospital
London, UK

Dr Anne May
Department of Anaesthesia
Leicester Royal Infirmary
Leicester, UK

Dr Surbhi Malhotra
Department of Anaesthesia
St Mary's Hospital
London, UK

Dr David Bogod
Department of Anaesthesia
City Hospital
Nottingham, UK

Dr Diana Brighouse
Department of Anaesthesia
Southampton General Hospital
Southampton, UK

Dr Chris Elton
Department of Anaesthesia
Leicester Royal Infirmary
Leicester, UK

Preface

There are now many large and authoritative texts on obstetric anaesthesia and analgesia available to the anaesthetic trainee. With reduced time available for obstetric anaesthetic training, we feel there is a need for a shorter, more practically based text, suitable for both the trainee starting in the maternity suite and the more experienced trainee preparing for anaesthetic examinations. Similarly, such a book may be of use to anaesthetists involved in teaching obstetric anaesthesia. In addition, obstetric anaesthetists of all grades are increasingly involved in the management of sick obstetric patients, and few manuals or handbooks bridge the gap between routine obstetric anaesthesia and analgesia and this challenging area of practice. Finally, the boundaries between obstetric anaesthesia and anaesthesia for certain gynaecological procedures are becoming increasingly blurred as women present for anaesthesia (or anaesthetic advice) before pregnancy as well as throughout pregnancy itself.

We hope this book fulfils these needs and provides useful, practical information and advice to obstetric anaesthetists. Whilst aimed primarily at trainees, we hope it will also be useful to more senior anaesthetists as a ready guide to be supplemented by larger and more comprehensive texts. Other specialties and disciplines are also involved in the care of pregnant women, and they too may find the book helpful. Indeed, we wish to stress the importance of a team approach to maternity care, particularly in the care of complex cases.

We have assumed basic anaesthetic knowledge and thus do not include topics such as anaesthetic equipment and drugs, etc. except where there are areas of specific obstetric relevance. We have tried to base the advice given on our own practice, supported by evidence wherever possible, although we accept that opinions differ amongst obstetric anaesthetists (including amongst ourselves!). Despite this, we hope that we have presented a consistent guide to anaesthesia and analgesia in pregnancy.

We hope the layout of the book is easy to follow and the difficulties we have had classifying some of the topics are not too apparent. There will inevitably be some repetition but we believe this is not necessarily a bad thing.

We have tried to provide a brief list of pertinent further reading where possible; often this has meant that very large topics have been left relatively unreferenced since there are few journal reviews broad enough in scope. The standard, more comprehensive texts, of which there are several excellent examples, would be good starting points for more comprehensive lists of references.

Section 1 – Preconception and Conception

1 ASSISTED CONCEPTION

There have been rapid developments in the treatment of infertility. The anaesthetist may be involved in many aspects of the patient's treatment, which may be complex. The harvesting of oocytes needs to take place within a defined period of time, or ovulation will have occurred and oocytes will be lost. Couples presenting for infertility treatment are generally anxious and often the women are emotional at the time of oocyte retrieval. It is therefore particularly important for the anaesthetist to understand the couple's anxieties and to be able to explain the effects of the anaesthetic technique that is to be used.

Problems/special considerations

All of the techniques involve extraction of oocytes from the follicles, either laparoscopically or, with the development of transvaginal ultrasonography, via the transvaginal route (ultrasound directed oocyte retrieval, UDOR). The techniques differ in the site of fertilisation and/or replacement of the gamete/zygote:

- *In vitro fertilisation (IVF):* fertilisation occurs in the laboratory and the developing embryo is transferred into the uterus via the cervix, usually 48 hours after oocyte retrieval. Embryo transfer is performed with the patient awake, although there are occasions when the help of the anaesthetist may be required to provide sedation. The success rate is approximately 15–25%.
- *Gamete intrafallopian transfer (GIFT):* the oocytes and sperm are placed together in the Fallopian tube, usually laparoscopically although an ultrasound-guided transvaginal procedure may also be used. The success rate is approximately 35%.
- *Zygote intrafallopian tube transfer (ZIFT):* fertilisation occurs in the laboratory and, before cell division occurs, the zygote is placed in the Fallopian tube as for GIFT. The success rate is approximately 28%.
- *Intracytoplasmic sperm injection (ICSI):* fertilisation occurs in the laboratory via injection of sperm into the oocytes, and the developing embryo is transferred into the uterus as for IVF. This technique is used for male infertility. The success rate is approximately 28%.

Analgesia, Anaesthesia and Pregnancy: A Practical Guide Second Edition, ed. Steve Yentis, Anne May and Surbhi Malhotra. Published by Cambridge University Press. © Cambridge University Press 2007.

The main considerations for laparoscopy are the type of anaesthesia, the pneumo-peritoneum and the effects of the anaesthetic agents on fertilisation and cell cleavage. The length of exposure to the drugs is also important. The effects of nitrous oxide and volatile anaesthetic agents on fertilisation and cleavage rates have been extensively examined. It is generally recognised that all the volatile agents and nitrous oxide have a deleterious effect, although opinion is divided as to the extent of the problem. It is also recognised that the carbon dioxide used for the pneumoperitoneum causes a similar effect, and it is difficult to separate the effects of the anaesthetic agents from those of the carbon dioxide.

Of the intravenous agents, the effect of propofol on fertilisation and cleavage appears to be minimal. Propofol accumulates in the follicular fluid, and the amount in the follicular fluid may become significant if there are a large number of oocytes to retrieve. Propofol decreases the fertilisation rates but there is no significant effect on the cell division rates.

All assisted conception techniques carry the risk of ovarian hyperstimulation (see Chapter 2, Ovarian hyperstimulation, p. 3), and multiple or ectopic pregnancy.

Management options

It would be logical to use regional anaesthesia wherever possible, although this is often not well suited for laparoscopy. The development of the transvaginal route for oocyte retrieval has increased the possibility of using regional anaesthesia.

For patients requiring laparoscopy, it would seem sensible to minimise the use of drugs. This has led to the increased use of propofol as the main agent in total intravenous anaesthesia.

For UDOR, which has become the most common method used for oocyte retrieval, the main anaesthetic techniques are intravenous sedation and regional anaesthesia. It is important to remember that patients requiring UDOR are day cases and the basic principles of day-case anaesthesia apply. There has been a considerable amount of work to date on the use of propofol with alfentanil, and this drug combination would appear to be the technique of choice for intravenous sedation. The propofol may be administered by intermittent boluses or by con-tinuous infusion, with the patient breathing oxygen via a Hudson mask. Many anaesthetists find that they are using levels of sedation close to anaesthesia. It is essential that the sedation is administered in a suitable environment with resusci-tation facilities and anaesthetic monitoring. Often the assisted conception unit is some distance from the main theatre suite; therefore it is important for the staff working in an isolated environment to maintain their skills in resuscitation.

The aim of minimising the drugs administered to women undergoing ultrasound-guided techniques has led to the use of regional anaesthesia. The main problem lay in developing techniques that allow the woman to go home the same day. Epidural and spinal anaesthesia have both been used with success, particularly where early ambulation is not essential. The low-dose spinal technique that is used for labour analgesia has been shown to give good operating conditions and to satisfy the criteria needed for day-case anaesthesia; it may be some way to achieving an ideal in this difficult group of patients.

Post-procedure analgesia may be provided with non-steroidal anti-inflammatory drugs such as diclofenac.

Key points

- Oocyte retrieval may involve laparoscopy requiring general anaesthesia, although intravenous sedation and regional anaesthesia are suitable for transvaginal ultrasound-directed techniques.
- Couples are usually very anxious and require constant reassurance.

FURTHER READING

Tidmarsh MD, May AE. Spinal analgesia for transvaginal oocyte retrieval. *Int J Obstet Anesth* 1998; **7**: 157–60.

Viscomi CM, Hill K, Johnson J, Sites C. Spinal anaesthesia versus sedation for transvaginal oocyte retrieval: reproductive outcome, side effects and recovery profiles. *Int J Obstet Anesth* 1997; **6**: 49–51.

Yasmin E, Dresner M, Balen A. Sedation and anaesthesia for transvaginal oocyte collection: an evaluation of practice in the UK. *Hum Reprod* 2004; **19**: 2942–5.

2   OVARIAN HYPERSTIMULATION SYNDROME

Ovarian hyperstimulation syndrome is associated with the medical stimulation of ovulation necessary for in vitro fertilisation. It occurs 3–8 days after treatment with human chorionic gonadotrophin (hCG), and the effects continue throughout the luteal phase. The active ingredient causing the syndrome via increased capillary permeability is thought to be secreted from the ovaries, and both histamine and prostaglandins have been implicated.

Problems/special considerations

Clinical manifestations of the syndrome are:
- Enlargement of the ovaries
- Pleural effusion
- Ascites.

Additional complications that may occur are:
- Hypovolaemic shock
- Renal failure
- Acute lung injury
- Thromboembolism
- Cerebrovascular disorders.

Table 2.1. Grading of ovarian hyperstimulation syndrome

Grade	Features		Incidence
1	Abdominal distension and discomfort	}	8–23%
2	Grade 1 plus nausea, vomiting and diarrhoea		
3	Grade 2 plus ascites (detected by ultrasonography)		1–8%
4	Grade 3 plus clinical ascites and shortness of breath		1–1.8%
5	Grade 4 plus clinical hypovolaemia, haemoconcentration, coagulation defects, decreased renal perfusion – therefore urea and electrolyte disturbance, thromboembolic phenomena	}	

Women undergoing ovarian stimulation who develop ovarian hyperstimulation syndrome can be assessed by placing them in one of five grades according to presenting symptoms and signs (Table 2.1).

Management options

When a large number of eggs (>20) have been retrieved, ovarian hyperstimulation should be suspected and the patient monitored. This may involve hospital admission.

Once suspected, the diagnosis of ovarian hyperstimulation syndrome can be confirmed by:
• A rapid increase in plasma oestradiol concentration
• The presence of multiple ovarian follicles on ultrasound examination
• An increase in body weight.

Immediate treatment is to stop hCG administration and to aspirate the enlarged follicles. Mild forms of ovarian hyperstimulation syndrome will be self-limiting, but those women graded 3 or worse will require intravenous fluids to correct the hypovolaemia and haemoconcentration. The intravenous administration of 1000 ml of human albumin is recommended at the time of oocyte retrieval if hyperstimulation is suspected.

In women graded 4 and 5, dopamine has been given to improve renal perfusion. In addition, it may be advisable to drain the ascitic fluid and to consider anti-coagulation. Ultrafiltration and intravenous reinfusion of ascitic fluid has been used in severe cases.

Monitoring is tailored to the severity of the syndrome, and the following progression is recommended:
• Urea and electrolytes
• Full blood count and packed cell volume
• Plasma/urine osmolality
• Clotting screen
• Chest radiography

- Central venous pressure if large volumes of fluids are needed
- Pulmonary artery catheter if the woman is severely affected.

Key points

- Hyperstimulation comprises ovarian enlargement, pleural effusion and ascites, which may be relentless.
- Severe protein loss may result in shock and renal failure.
- The most severe form occurs in 1–2% of cases treated with human chorionic gonadotrophin.

FURTHER READING

Shanbhag S, Bhattacharya S. Current management of ovarian hyperstimulation syndrome. *Hosp Med* 2002; **63**: 528–32.

Whelan JG 3rd, Vlahos NF. The ovarian hyperstimulation syndrome. *Fertil Steril* 2000; **73**: 883–96.

3 ANAESTHESIA BEFORE CONCEPTION OR CONFIRMATION OF PREGNANCY

Many women will require anaesthesia when they are pregnant and many will be unaware that they are pregnant at the time of the anaesthetic, especially in the first 2–3 months of their pregnancy. The thalidomide catastrophe initiated the licensing arrangements for new drugs and their use in pregnancy; the current cautious stance of the pharmaceutical industry is reflected in the *British National Formulary*'s statement that no drug is safe beyond all doubt in early pregnancy. The anaesthetist should have a clear knowledge of the time scale of the developing fetus in order to balance the risks and benefits of any drug given to the mother. A *teratogen* is a substance that causes structural or functional abnormality in a fetus exposed to that substance.

Problems/special considerations

The possible effect of a drug can be considered against the stage of the developing fetus:

- *Pre-embryonic phase (0–14 days post-conception):* the fertilised egg is transported down the Fallopian tube and implantation occurs at around 7 days post-conception. The conceptus is a ball of undifferentiated dividing cells during this time and the effect of drugs on it appears to be an all-or-none phenomenon. Cell division may be slowed with no lasting effects or the conceptus will die, depending on the severity of the cell damage.
- *Embryonic phase (3–8 weeks post-conception):* differentiation of cells into the organs and tissues occurs during this phase and drugs administered to the

mother may cause considerable harm. The type of abnormality that is produced depends on the exact stage of organ and tissue development when the drug is given.

- *Fetal phase (9 weeks to birth):* at this stage, most organs are fully formed, although the cerebral cortex, cerebellum and urogenital tract are still developing. Drugs administered during this time may affect the growth of the fetus or the functional development within specific organs.

Management options

The anaesthetist should always consider the possibility of pregnancy in any woman of child-bearing age who presents for surgery, whether elective or emergency, and should specifically enquire in such cases. If there is doubt, a pregnancy test should be offered. If pregnancy is suspected, the use of nitrous oxide is now generally considered acceptable, despite its effects on methionine synthase and DNA metabolism, as there is little evidence that it is harmful clinically. Similarly, although the volatile agents have been implicated in impairing embryonic development, clinical evidence is lacking. Some drugs cross the placenta and exert their effect on the fetus, e.g. warfarin, which may cause bleeding in the fetus.

Key points

- The possibility of pregnancy should be considered in any woman of child-bearing age.
- No drug is safe beyond all doubt in pregnancy.

FURTHER READING

Koren G, Pastuszak A, Ito S. Drugs in pregnancy. *N Engl J Med* 1998; **338**: 1128–37.

Section 2 – Pregnancy

■ Procedures in early/mid-pregnancy

4 CERVICAL SUTURE (CERCLAGE)

Cervical suture (Shirodkar or McDonald cerclage) is performed to reduce the incidence of spontaneous miscarriage when there is cervical incompetence. Although it can be done before conception or as an emergency during pregnancy, the procedure is usually performed electively at 12–16 weeks' gestation; it generally takes 10–20 minutes and is performed transvaginally on a day-case basis. A non-absorbable stitch or tape is sutured in a purse-string around the cervical neck at the level of the internal os; this requires anaesthesia since the procedure is at best uncomfortable, although the suture can usually be removed easily without undue discomfort (usually at 37–38 weeks' gestation unless in preterm labour); spontaneous labour usually soon follows.

In patients with a grossly disrupted cervix, e.g. following surgery, placement of the suture via an abdominal approach may be required. Delivery is usually by elective Caesarean section in these cases.

Problems/special considerations

Women undergoing cervical suturing may be especially anxious since previous pregnancies have ended in miscarriage. Otherwise anaesthesia is along standard lines, bearing in mind the risks of anaesthesia in the pregnant woman and monitoring of, and possible effects of drugs on, the fetus (see Chapter 7, Incidental surgery in the pregnant patient, p. 12).

Cerclage may be difficult if the membranes are bulging; the head-down position and/or tocolysis may be requested to counter this.

Management options

Many authorities advocate spinal anaesthesia as the technique of choice since only a small amount of a single drug is administered, although epidural anaesthesia is also acceptable. If spinal or epidural anaesthesia is chosen, standard techniques are used. The procedure itself requires a less extensive block than Caesarean section

Analgesia, Anaesthesia and Pregnancy: A Practical Guide Second Edition, ed. Steve Yentis, Anne May and Surbhi Malhotra. Published by Cambridge University Press. © Cambridge University Press 2007.

(from T8–10 down to and including the sacral roots) and thus smaller doses are required; however, the reduction is offset by the greater requirements at this early stage of pregnancy compared with the term parturient. Thus the doses required for regional anaesthesia are in the order of 75% of those used for Caesarean section. Low-dose techniques have also been used, as for Caesarean section; the women have more sensation (though painless) but have less motor block.

General anaesthesia may also be used; an advantage is the relaxing effect of volatile agents on the uterus, but it does usually involve administration of more than one drug, and the effects on the fetus of many agents in current use are not clear. There may also be an increased risk of regurgitation and aspiration of gastric contents, depending on the gestation and severity of symptoms (see Chapter 56, Aspiration of gastric contents; p. 138).

Paracervical and pudendal block and/or intravenous analgesia/sedation may also be used, but most authorities would recommend avoiding paracervical block because of the potential adverse effects on uteroplacental perfusion.

Key points

- Cervical suture is usually performed at 12–16 weeks' gestation.
- Patients may be especially anxious because of previous miscarriage.
- Standard techniques are used; spinal anaesthesia may be preferable.

FURTHER READING

Drakeley AJ, Roberts D, Alfirevic Z. Cervical stitch (cerclage) for preventing pregnancy loss in women (Cochrane Review). In: *The Cochrane Library*, Issue 4, 2003. Chichester, UK: John Wiley & Sons, Ltd.

5 ECTOPIC PREGNANCY

There are approximately 11 000 ectopic pregnancies per year in the UK (just over 1% of all pregnancies), and the incidence is thought to be increasing as a result of pelvic inflammatory disease. There are many risk factors, with tubal pathology or surgery and use of an intrauterine device the most important; others are infertility, increased maternal age and smoking. About 3–5 women die as a consequence in the UK per year, representing about 3–6% of all direct maternal deaths (~1 per 2500 ectopics). Most ectopic pregnancies occur in the Fallopian tube, but up to 5% occur elsewhere within the genital tract or abdomen. Typically, the tube initially expands to accommodate the growing zygote but when unable to do so any more, there may be bleeding from the site of implantation or even rupture of the tube. Thus the classic presentation is with abdominal pain, which may be sudden in onset, accompanied by a history of amenorrhoea (although there is vaginal bleeding at presentation in ~80% of cases). There may be sudden collapse if the tube ruptures, caused by reflex vagal activity or hypovolaemia if bleeding is severe, or both.

Problems/special considerations

The main risk of ectopic pregnancy is sudden severe haemorrhage, which may be intra-abdominal and thus concealed until rapid decompensation and collapse occur. A common theme in deaths associated with ectopic pregnancy is the failure to consider the diagnosis before collapse. Ectopic pregnancy may present with non-specific abdominal signs including diarrhoea or constipation, thus mimicking other intra-abdominal conditions (e.g. appendicitis), although with serial measurement of plasma human chorionic gonadotrophin (hCG; doubles every 2–3 days in normal pregnancy) and use of pelvic ultrasonography this should be unusual. The potential severity of the condition is not always appreciated by other hospital staff, the patient herself or her relatives. Ectopics outside the Fallopian tubes are more likely to be associated with massive haemorrhage, with abdominal pregnancies the most hazardous, especially when the placenta is removed.

Most ectopic pregnancies present early in pregnancy and thus many of the physiological changes of pregnancy are absent or mild – the patient may even be unaware that she is pregnant. However, even at this early stage there may be features of the physiological changes of pregnancy.

The implications for the current and future pregnancies pose a great psychological stress on the patient and her partner. There may be a previous history of ectopic pregnancy since its occurrence is itself a risk factor for subsequent ectopics.

Management options

Initial management is directed at treating and preventing massive haemorrhage; thus the patient requires at least one large-bore intravenous cannula and careful observation at least until the diagnosis has been excluded. Similarly, once the decision to operate has been made it needs to occur as soon as possible, since the risk of rupture is always present.

Operative management usually involves laparoscopy unless there is severe haemodynamic instability, in which case laparotomy is performed. Traditionally, laparoscopy was performed purely for diagnostic purposes, but laparoscopic removal of the zygote with or without tubal resection has become routine in many units. Anaesthetic aspects of the procedure itself are as for any laparoscopic operation.

Anaesthetic management is as for any emergency surgery, given the above considerations. Haematological assistance and admission to the intensive care unit should be available if required. In severe cases, anaesthesia must proceed as for a ruptured aortic aneurysm: full preoperative resuscitation may be impossible and the patient is prepared and draped before induction of anaesthesia, which may be followed by profound hypotension.

In some countries, medical management is increasingly used as the first-line treatment of early ectopic pregnancies, with intramuscular methotrexate. The drug antagonises folic acid and prevents further growth of the trophoblast, which is especially vulnerable at this early stage. Similar outcome to that following surgical management has been claimed. Local injection of hyperosmolar glucose, prostaglandin and potassium chloride have also been used. Finally, expectant management has been used in selected patients, although women whose pregnancies are self-limiting cannot yet be identified reliably.

Key points

- Ectopic pregnancy accounts for 3–6% of all direct maternal deaths in the UK.
- Severe haemorrhage and/or cardiovascular collapse is always a risk.

FURTHER READING

Pisarska MD, Carson SA, Buster JE. Ectopic pregnancy. *Lancet* 1998; **351**: 1115–20.
Tay JI, Moore J, Walker JJ. Ectopic pregnancy. *BMJ* 2000; **320**: 916–19.

6   EVACUATION OF RETAINED PRODUCTS OF CONCEPTION

Evacuation of retained products of conception (ERPC) may be required at any stage of pregnancy, but it occurs most commonly in early pregnancy following incomplete miscarriage or early fetal demise. It is also required during the puerperium following retention of placental tissue (see Chapter 41, Removal of retained placenta, p. 107).

Problems/special considerations

- ERPC following spontaneous abortion at 8 weeks' gestation may be a minor routine gynaecological emergency for the anaesthetist, but the mother may have lost a much-wanted baby.
- The urgency of the procedure varies greatly. The majority of ERPCs are performed as scheduled emergencies in fit young women, and this may lull the inexperienced anaesthetist into a false sense of security. Death may occur from spontaneous abortion; blood loss may be heavy and is frequently underestimated.
- The possibility of coexisting uterine or systemic sepsis must always be considered, especially in postpartum ERPC or in a repeat procedure following incomplete evacuation.

Management options

- Diagnostic ultrasound scanning is frequently used to confirm a non-viable early pregnancy or the presence of retained placental tissue. Transabdominal ultrasonography is facilitated by a full bladder, which is often achieved by asking the mother to drink large volumes of water. Most units now operate a policy of fully assessing mothers on the day of admission in an early pregnancy advisory unit (EPAU), allowing them home and readmitting them the following day for planned ERPC. This facilitates planning of medical and nursing staffing levels, reduces prolonged periods of waiting and starvation for the mother, and can be economically advantageous.
- Medical treatment is increasingly used and this enables women to be allowed home, after treatment with prostaglandin analogues, to await events. Some of these women will need surgical management if the products of conception are not fully expelled.
- Preoperatively, a full assessment is required. Assessment of blood loss may be difficult; fit young women may lose a significant proportion of their blood volume without becoming hypotensive. Tachycardia should alert the anaesthetist to possible hypovolaemia. Signs of sepsis should be sought, and prophylactic antibiotics may be considered.
- General anaesthesia is acceptable although in the absence of uncorrected hypovolaemia or other contraindications, regional anaesthesia is entirely suitable. The puerperal mother in particular may wish to stay awake if offered a choice, and she should be advised to do so if at risk of regurgitation.
- Rapid sequence induction of general anaesthesia is indicated for the non-fasting mother requiring urgent surgery (uncommon) and for the mother who is at risk of regurgitation (see Chapter 56, Aspiration of gastric contents; p. 138). Anaesthesia using a laryngeal mask airway or facemask using any standard day-case anaesthetic technique is appropriate for the majority of women needing ERPC. Sedative premedication is rarely needed. Intravenous anaesthesia e.g. with propofol or inhalational anaesthesia is acceptable, though if the latter is used high concentrations of volatile anaesthetic agents (>1 minimum alveloar concentration) should be avoided because of the uterine relaxation that may ensue.
- Oxytocic drugs may be requested by the surgeon, although there is little evidence for their efficacy at gestations of less than 15 weeks. A single intravenous bolus of 5 U Syntocinon usually suffices. Ergometrine causes increased intracranial and systemic pressure, and nausea and vomiting, and should not be used routinely.
- Spinal anaesthesia produces more rapid and dense anaesthesia than epidural and an anaesthetic level of at least T8 is recommended. Clinical experience shows that the traditionally taught anaesthetic level of T10 is insufficient to prevent pain occurring when the uterine fundus is manipulated or curetted.
- Postoperatively, the aim is rapid recovery and discharge home. Requirement for postoperative analgesia rarely exceeds simple non-opioid drugs. Non-steroidal anti-inflammatory agents may be beneficial in relieving uterine cramps.

Routine administration of antiemetics should be considered since these women are at risk of postoperative nausea and vomiting.

> **Key points**
>
> - A sensitive and sympathetic approach to the mother is necessary.
> - Prolonged preoperative waiting and starvation reflect poor communication and inefficiency.

FURTHER READING

Royal College of Obstetricians and Gynaecologists. *The management of early pregnancy loss.* London: RCOG, 2000.

7   INCIDENTAL SURGERY IN THE PREGNANT PATIENT

Pregnant women may present with the same surgical conditions as the non-pregnant population, or with problems related to their pregnancy. Most pregnant women are relatively young and fit, although there are an increasing number of women with systemic disease who are becoming pregnant because of advances in medical or surgical management of their condition. Points of particular relevance to anaesthetists are therefore any underlying condition in addition to the reason for surgery, the effects of pregnancy on its management and the effect upon the fetus.

Problems/special considerations

- Surgical diagnosis of the acute abdomen may be difficult because of the physical presence of the gravid uterus. Non-specific signs such as white cell count may be unreliable (up to $15\,000 \times 10^6$/l in normal pregnancy). The differential diagnosis may also include obstetric conditions such as placental abruption and HELLP (haemolysis, elevated liver enzymes and low platelets) syndrome. Surgical technique may be hindered by the pregnancy, and the operation itself may be more difficult than in the non-pregnant patient; e.g. laparoscopic procedures may be impossible.
- The risks of aortocaval compression, difficulties with airway management and aspiration of gastric contents are present as for any pregnant woman, and depend to a certain extent on the stage of pregnancy and the reason for surgery (see Chapter 56, Aspiration of gastric contents, p. 138).
- Surgery that normally requires the non-supine position, e.g. back surgery, may pose particular problems.
- Since surgery is generally withheld during pregnancy unless absolutely necessary, patients who do present for surgery tend to be more severely affected; thus careful

preoperative assessment and management are especially important. Problems of emergency surgery include inadequate preparation and investigation and an increased incidence of vomiting and dehydration.

- The fetus is at risk from the primary effects of the mother's illness (e.g. dehydration, sepsis), the possible teratogenic effects of any drugs that are given to the mother, especially during the first trimester (see Chapter 3, Anaesthesia before conception or confirmation of pregnancy, p. 5), alterations in uteroplacental blood flow or oxygenation during anaesthesia and surgery, and possible premature onset of labour provoked by the illness, drugs or surgery itself.

Management options

In general, surgery is delayed until the second trimester if possible, because the major fetal organs will have already developed; in addition, the risk of premature labour is lower and the surgery easier than in the third trimester.

Perioperative management requires attendance by senior surgical and obstetric staff, with investigations and scans as required.

Anaesthetic management includes preoperative assessment of the airway and antacid pretreatment. The supine position should be avoided at all times, although the efficacy of lateral tilt when the uterus is still small is uncertain. Particular attention should be paid to general assessment as for emergency surgery in any patient. The disadvantages of regional anaesthesia (e.g. hypotension, increased peristalsis, problems with managing the block during difficult or prolonged surgery) must be weighed against those of general anaesthesia (airway problems, risk of awareness, etc.). Although general anaesthesia involves administration of more drugs with possible effects on the fetus, it also allows administration of volatile agents that relax the uterus. In general, drugs with good safety records during pregnancy should be used; most anaesthetic drugs do not have licences for use in pregnancy (mainly because of the costs involved in extending their licences), but newer drugs should probably be avoided until more is known about their actions. The only standard anaesthetic drug that has excited controversy in recent years is nitrous oxide, because of its effects on methionine synthase and DNA metabolism. Although there is a theoretical risk of its affecting the fetus, there is no evidence to support this clinically and many, if not most, authorities would now consider its use acceptable. General anaesthetic management would thus usually consist of rapid sequence induction with standard agents, tracheal intubation and ventilation of the lungs with a volatile agent, as for any emergency general anaesthetic. Other drugs would be used as standard, but those that might increase uterine tone (e.g. ketamine, β-blockers) or vasoconstriction should be avoided if possible. Many obstetricians would request prophylactic administration of tocolytic drugs perioperatively. β-Adrenergic agonists are commonly used for this purpose, although their efficacy in this situation is uncertain and they may cause maternal tachycardia and pulmonary oedema; recent evidence suggests that calcium-channel blockers such as nifed-ipine may be at least equally effective with a better safety profile. In general, probably the fewer drugs used overall the better. Certain drugs given near to delivery may cross the placenta and affect the fetus, e.g. non-steroidal anti-inflammatory drugs (which can prevent the ductus arteriosus from closing).

Traditional fears about the detrimental effects of high levels of maternal oxygen by causing uteroplacental vasoconstriction are now known to be unfounded, and fetal arterial partial pressure of oxygen increases (up to a maximum of about 8 kPa (60 mmHg)) as maternal arterial oxygen content increases, so long as maternal hypotension is avoided. Maternal arterial partial pressure of carbon dioxide should be kept in the normal (pregnant) range during controlled ventilation.

The fetus must be monitored preoperatively and postoperatively. Intraoperative monitoring is controversial and may be difficult if the surgery is abdominal; it may be possible to use a sterile sleeve over an ultrasonic/Doppler probe. It may be difficult to arrange appropriate midwifery and surgical nursing care both before and after surgery, and the most appropriate area for the mother's postoperative care needs careful consideration.

Key points

- Surgical diagnosis and management may be difficult.
- Maternal risks are those of anaesthesia in the pregnant state.
- Fetal risks are related to the mother's condition, maternal drugs, and the premature onset of labour.

FURTHER READING

Melnick DM, Wahl WL, Dalton VK. Management of general surgical problems in the pregnant patient. *Am J Surg* 2004; **187**: 170–80.

Mhuireachtaigh RN, O'Gorman DA. Anesthesia in pregnant patients for nonobstetric surgery. *J. Clin. Anesth* 2006; **18**: 60–6.

Rosen M. Management of anesthesia for the pregnant surgical patient. *Anesthesiology* 1999; **91**: 1159–63.

8   INTRAUTERINE SURGERY

Fetal surgery is an option in cases where an isolated abnormality would be otherwise fatal to the fetus or neonate, and is clearly amenable to correction, e.g. neck tumours with airway obstruction, sacrococcygeal teratomas, obstructive uropathy and diaphragmatic hernia. However, results of intrauterine surgery have been conflicting and there is no clear consensus on its place. Simpler measures, e.g. intrauterine blood transfusion in haemolytic disease, are more widely accepted.

Problems/special considerations

Each procedure must be assessed on a risk–benefit basis, since there is a risk of up to 50% fetal loss associated with premature labour, haemorrhage, abruption and infection. For open procedures, vertical uterine incision is required, with Caesarean section to deliver the baby if pregnancy proceeds. Maternal thromboembolism has been reported. Thus each lesion must be carefully defined and a chromosomal abnormality or other malformation excluded. For example, intrauterine placement of intraventricular shunts is no longer considered suitable for treatment of hydrocephalus, since the risk–benefit ratio cannot be calculated for individual fetuses because of the difficulty in predicting outcome antenatally. Since most conditions that might be amenable to intrauterine surgery are rare or uncommon and already associated with poor outcome, it is difficult to demonstrate that outcome after fetal surgery is better than that after conventional postpartum therapy, because any expected improvement will be small.

Surgery is technically difficult because of the small size of the fetus and its mobility when small, but leaving the surgery until later may result in increased end-organ damage caused by the malformation. The optimal timing for most procedures is uncertain, although most open ones have been performed at around 18–24 weeks. Percutaneous procedures, e.g. transfusions, may be performed later or at intervals. The EXIT procedure (ex utero intrapartum therapy), for airway obstruction, is also done later and involves delivery of the fetal head through an open hysterotomy and tracheal intubation or tracheostomy while the fetus is oxygenated by the placenta. The fetus may then be delivered and undergo corrective surgery.

After intrauterine surgery, the mother may be confined to bed and receive β_2-agonists, with the risks of deep vein thrombosis and pulmonary oedema respectively.

Management options

Anaesthetic management is along the lines of that for incidental surgery during pregnancy. Local anaesthetic infiltration of the abdominal wall may be adequate for percutaneous procedures, although there may be a need for emergency Caesarean section if fetal bradycardia occurs, and so adequate preparation and facilities are required for this. Regional anaesthesia is a suitable alternative if extensive percutaneous procedures are required.

Fetal and maternal general anaesthesia for corrective surgery is administered by using standard techniques. Fetal injection of a neuromuscular blocking drug may be required to stop fetal movement. Analgesics may also be injected into the fetus – there is increasing evidence that the fetus can 'experience' pain, although the significance of this is disputed. Uterine relaxation has been achieved by using one or more of volatile agents, magnesium sulphate or glyceryl trinitrate. Fetal monitoring may be difficult but pulse oximetry, ultrasonography and cardiotocography have been used. Bleeding may be excessive in prolonged open procedures.

Key points

- The place of intrauterine surgery is uncertain.
- To be suitable, malformations must be clearly defined, fatal if untreated and amenable to corrective surgery.
- General principles of anaesthesia are as for incidental surgery during pregnancy.

FURTHER READING

Farmer D. Fetal surgery. *BMJ* 2003; **326**: 461–2.

Kimber C, Spitz L, Cuschieri A. Current state of antenatal in-utero surgical interventions. *Arch Dis Child* 1997; **76**: F134–9.

Myers LB, Cohen D, Galinkin J, Gaiser RC, Kurth D. Anaesthesia for fetal surgery. *Paediatric Anaesthesia* 2002; **12**: 569–78.

9 TERMINATION OF PREGNANCY

Termination of pregnancy in the UK is undertaken under the terms and conditions of the Abortion Act 1967. For the consideration of anaesthetic procedures and potential problems, patients presenting for a termination of pregnancy broadly fall into two groups:

1. The presence of a maternal problem, the most commonly stated reason being danger to the mental or physical health of the mother
2. Severe fetal congenital abnormality or early fetal death.

Problems/special considerations

When caring for women who are to undergo a termination of pregnancy, it is important to consider the physiological changes of pregnancy, the psychological state of the woman and the need for routine preoperative assessment of the patient.

Those women in the first group above are usually scheduled to have termination of pregnancy on a gynaecological operating list. The second group of patients are often looked after in the maternity unit.

Some members of staff may express conscientious objection to performing or being involved in termination of pregnancy and this must be respected. They cannot be made to participate in such procedures, although they do have a duty to find other staff who will, if that is the patient's wish.

Management options

Termination for maternal indications

Termination of pregnancy is usually a day-case procedure, and routine preoperative assessment is undertaken immediately preoperatively. Assessment should be conducted sympathetically as these women are often very distressed.

Gestation is usually less than 15 weeks and these women can usually be regarded as non-pregnant with respect to gastric emptying and acid aspiration unless they have symptoms of reflux.

An anaesthetic technique suitable for day-case anaesthesia should be employed, e.g. induction with propofol followed by nitrous oxide/oxygen and maintenance with propofol or a volatile anaesthetic agent. There has been concern about concentrations of volatile anaesthetic agents greater than one minimum alveolar concentration causing uterine relaxation unresponsive to oxytocics. For a termination of pregnancy at less than 15 weeks, standard concentrations of volatile anaesthetic agents do not appear to pose a risk and may be used to maintain anaesthesia. Analgesia may be provided by intravenous fentanyl or alfentanil with rectal diclofenac 100 mg.

The gynaecologist may request that 5–10 U Syntocinon is administered to aid uterine contraction. There is no clear evidence that this is helpful at this stage of pregnancy.

Termination for fetal abnormality or death

Women who present for termination of pregnancy because of fetal abnormality or intrauterine death present a difficult clinical problem. Induction of labour is usually required and this may be a long and tedious process involving the use of prostaglandin pessaries and Syntocinon infusion (see Chapter 71, Intrauterine death, p. 170).

Termination of a pregnancy at less than 28 weeks is often associated with the retention of products of conception, for which surgical evacuation and anaesthesia are required. Either regional or general anaesthesia may be offered to the woman, balancing the risks and benefits of each depending on the clinical condition and whether epidural analgesia is already in place. Rapid sequence induction and tracheal intubation may be appropriate.

Key points

- Women may present for termination of pregnancy because of maternal reasons or fetal abnormality/death.
- Such women are distressed and should be dealt with sympathetically.
- Early termination is usually performed as a day-case general anaesthetic procedure.
- Issues surrounding late terminations are as for intrauterine death.

II   Normal pregnancy and delivery

10   ANATOMY OF THE SPINE AND PERIPHERAL NERVES

Although not exclusive to obstetric anaesthesia, a sound knowledge of the anatomy pertinent to epidural and spinal anaesthesia is fundamental to obstetric anaesthetists because of the importance of these techniques in this field. In addition, knowledge of the relevant peripheral nerves is important in order to differentiate central from peripheral causes of neurological impairment.

The structures involved in obstetric neuraxial anaesthesia comprise the vertebrae and sacral canal, vertebral ligaments, epidural space, meninges and spinal cord. The important peripheral aspects are the lumbar and sacral plexi and the muscular and cutaneous supply of the lower part of the body.

Vertebrae (Fig. 10.1)

The vertebral column has two curves, with the cervical and lumbar regions convex anteriorly and the thoracic and sacral regions concave. Traditionally, T4 is described as the most posterior part (most dependent in the supine position), although T8 has been suggested by recent imaging studies. L3–4 is the most anterior part (uppermost in the supine position), although this curve may be flattened by flexing the hips. In the lateral position, the greater width of women's hips compared with their shoulders imparts a downward slope from the caudal end of the vertebral column to the cranial end.

There are seven cervical vertebrae, twelve thoracic, five lumbar, five fused sacral and three to five fused coccygeal. A number of ligaments connect them (see below). Vertebrae have the following components:

- *Body:* this lies anteriorly, with the vertebral arch behind. It is kidney-shaped in the lumbar region. Fibrocartilaginous vertebral discs, accounting for about 25% of the spine's total length, separate the bodies of C2 to L5. Each disc has an outer fibrous annulus fibrosus and a more fluid inner nucleus pulposus (the latter may prolapse through the former: a 'slipped disc'). The bodies of the thoracic vertebrae are heart-shaped and articulate with the ribs via superior and inferior costal facets at their rear. The bodies of the sacral vertebrae are fused to form the

Analgesia, Anaesthesia and Pregnancy: A Practical Guide Second Edition, ed. Steve Yentis, Anne May and Surbhi Malhotra. Published by Cambridge University Press. © Cambridge University Press 2007.

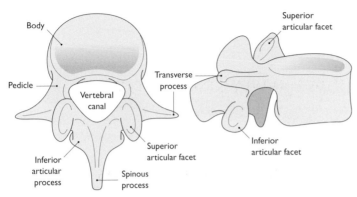

Fig. 10.1 A lumbar vertebra, seen from superior and lateral aspects. Reproduced with permission from Yentis, Hirsch & Smith: Anaesthesia and intensive care A-Z, 2nd edn, Butterworth Heinemann, 2000.

sacrum, which encloses the sacral canal; the coccygeal vertebral bodies are fused to form the triangular coccyx, the base of which articulates with the sacrum.

- *Pedicles:* these are round in cross-section. They project posteriorly from the body and join the laminae. Each intervertebral foramen is formed by the pedicles of the vertebra above and below.
- *Laminae:* these are flattened in cross-section. They complete the vertebral arch by meeting in the midline at the spinous process. The superior and inferior articular processes bear facets for articulation with adjacent vertebrae; those of the thoracic vertebrae are flatter and aligned in the coronal plane, whereas those of the lumbar vertebrae are nearer the sagittal plane.
- *Transverse processes:* in the lumbar region they are thick and pass laterally. The transverse processes of L5 are particularly massive but short. The transverse processes of thoracic vertebrae are large and pass backwards and laterally; they bear facets that articulate with the ribs' tubercles (except T11 and T12).
- *Spinous process:* these project horizontally backwards in the lumbar region; in the thoracic region they are longer and inclined at about 60° to the horizontal. The spinous process of T12 has a notched lower edge.

The cervical vertebrae have a number of features which distinguish them from the others, including the foramen transverarium in the transverse processes, bifid spinous processes and the particular characteristics of C1 and C2.

A line drawn between the iliac crests (Tuffier's line) usually crosses the L3–4 interspace (slightly higher than in the non-pregnant state because of rotation of the pelvis), although this is unreliable, and it has been shown that even experienced anaesthetists can be one or more interspaces lower (or more commonly, higher) than that intended.

Sacral canal (Fig. 10.2)

The sacral canal is 10–15 cm long, triangular in cross-section, runs the length of the sacrum and is continuous cranially with the lumbar vertebral canal. The fused

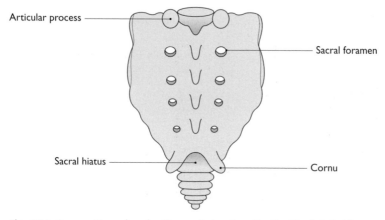

Articular process

Sacral foramen

Sacral hiatus

Cornu

Fig. 10.2 Sacrum. Reproduced with permission from Yentis, Hirsch & Smith: Anaesthesia and intensive care A-Z, 2nd edn, Butterworth Heinemann, 2000.

bodies of the sacral vertebrae form the anterior wall, and the fused sacral laminae form the posterior wall. The sacral hiatus is a deficiency in the fifth laminar arch, has the cornua laterally and is covered by the sacrococcygeal membrane. Congenital variants are common, possibly contributing to unreliable caudal analgesia.

Vertebral ligaments (Fig. 10.3)

- *Anterior longitudinal ligament:* this is attached to the anterior aspects of the vertebral bodies, and runs from C2 to the sacrum.
- *Posterior longitudinal ligament:* this is attached to the posterior aspects of the vertebral bodies, and runs from C2 to the sacrum.
- *Ligamentum flavum (yellow ligament):* this is attached to the laminae of adjacent vertebrae, forming a 'V'-shaped structure with the point posteriorly. It is more developed in the lumbar than thoracic regions.
- *Interspinous ligament:* this passes between the spinous processes of adjacent vertebrae.
- *Supraspinous ligament:* this is attached to the tips of the spinous processes from C7 to the sacrum.

In addition, there are posterior, anterior and lateral sacrococcygeal ligaments. Other ligaments are involved in the attachments of C1 and C2 to the skull.

The ligaments may become softer during pregnancy because of the hormonal changes that occur.

Epidural space

- *Boundaries:* the space extends from the foramen magnum to the sacrococcygeal membrane. It is triangular in cross-section in the lumbar region, its base anterior; it is very thin anteriorly and up to 5 mm wide posteriorly. It lies external to the dura mater of the spinal cord and internal to the ligamenta flava and vertebral

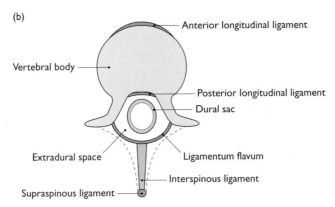

Fig. 10.3 Vertebral ligaments: (a) longitudinal section and (b) transverse section through A–B. Reproduced with permission from Yentis, Hirsch & Smith: Anaesthesia and intensive care A-Z, 2nd edn, Butterworth Heinemann, 2000.

laminae posteriorly; the posterior longitudinal ligament anteriorly and the intervertebral foramina and vertebral pedicles laterally. Magnetic resonance imaging suggests the space is divided into segments by the laminae. The space may extend through the intervertebral foramina into the paravertebral spaces.

- *Contents:* these include extradural fat, extradural veins (Batson's plexus), lymphatics and spinal nerve roots. The veins become engorged in pregnancy as a result of the hormonal changes and any aortocaval compression. Connective tissue layers have been demonstrated by radiology and endoscopy within the extradural space, in some cases dividing it into right and left portions.
- *Pressure:* a negative pressure is usually found in the epidural space upon entering it; the reason is unclear but may involve anterior dimpling of the dura by the epidural needle, sudden posterior recoil of the ligamentum flavum when it is punctured, stretching of the dural sac during extreme flexion of the back, transmitted negative intrapleural pressure via thoracic paravertebral spaces and

relative overgrowth of the vertebral canal compared with the dural sac. Occasionally a positive pressure is found.

Meninges

- *Pia mater:* this delicate and vascular layer adheres closely to the brain and spinal cord. Between it and the arachnoid mater is the cerebrospinal fluid (CSF) within the subarachnoid space containing blood vessels, the denticulate ligament laterally along its length and the subarachnoid septum posteriorly. The pia terminates as the filum terminale, which passes through the caudal end of the dural sac and attaches to the coccyx.
- *Arachnoid mater:* this membrane is also delicate and contains CSF internally. It lies within the dura externally, the potential subdural space containing vessels, between them. It fuses with the dura at S2.
- *Dura mater:* this fibrous layer has an outer component, which is adherent to the inner periosteum of the vertebrae and an inner one that lies against the outer surface of the arachnoid. The dura projects into the extradural space, especially in the midline. It ends at about S2.

Spinal cord

The spinal cord ends inferiorly level with L3 at birth, rising to the adult level of L1–2 (sometimes T12 or L3) by 20 years. Below this level (the conus medullaris) the lumbar and sacral nerve roots (comprising the cauda equina) and filum terminale occupy the vertebral canal. The main ascending and descending tracts are shown in Fig. 10.4.

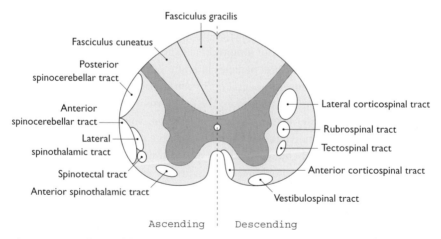

Fig. 10.4 Ascending and descending tracts, spinal cord. Reproduced with permission from Yentis, Hirsch & Smith: Anaesthesia and intensive care A-Z, 2nd edn, Butterworth Heinemann, 2000.

The blood supply of the spinal cord is of relevance to obstetric anaesthetists, since cord ischaemia may result in neurological damage:

- *Anterior spinal artery:* this descends in the anterior median fissure and supplies the anterior two-thirds of the cord. The anterior spinal artery syndrome (e.g. arising from profound hypotension) thus results in lower motor neurone paralysis at the level of the lesion, and spastic paraplegia, reduced pain and temperature sensation below the level and normal joint position sense and vibration sensation.
- *Posterior spinal arteries:* these descend along each side of the cord, one anterior and one posterior to the dorsal nerve roots.
- *Radicular branches:* these arise from local arteries (from the aorta) and feed the spinal arteries. Those at T1 and the lower thoracic/upper lumbar level (artery of Adamkiewicz – usually unilateral) are the most important. The cord at T3–5 and T12–L1 is thought to be most at risk from ischaemia. The conus medullaris and cauda equina are supplied by a vascular plexus arising from the artery of Adamkiewicz above and pelvic vessels below. In 15% of the population,

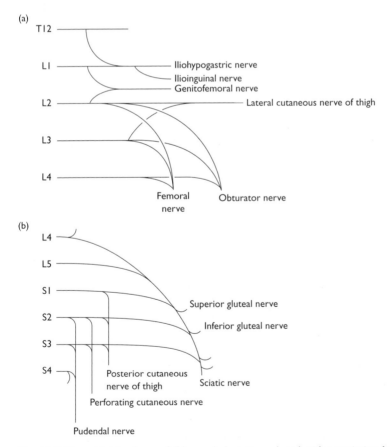

Fig. 10.5 Plan of (a) lumbar and (b) sacral plexi. Reproduced with permission from Yentis, Hirsch & Smith: Anaesthesia and intensive care A-Z, 2nd edn, Butterworth Heinemann, 2000.

the latter are the main source of arterial blood to the conus medularis and cauda equina; compression during delivery may result in permanent paraplegia.

Venous drainage is via the internal iliac, intercostal, azygos and vertebral veins.

Peripheral nerves of the lower body

The lumbar and sacral plexi are shown schematically in Fig. 10.5. They form at the posterior of the pelvis, and their branches pass round the interior of the pelvis where they may be exposed to pressure during labour and delivery (Fig. 10.6; see also Chapter 50, Peripheral nerve lesions following regional anaesthesia, p. 128).

Peripheral cutaneous innervation may be characterised according to the dermatomal distribution or peripheral nerves (Fig. 10.7 and 10.8). Both representations may vary considerably between individuals. Peripheral motor innervation may also be considered according to myotomal innervation or peripheral nerves (Table 10.1).

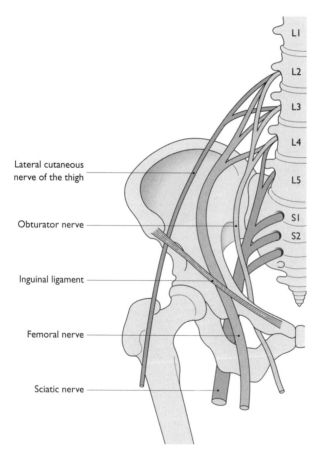

Fig. 10.6 Major nerves of the pelvis. Adapted with permission from Holdcroft & Thomas: Principles and practice of obstetric anaesthesia and analgesia, Blackwell Publishing, 2000.

Table 10.1. Motor innervation of lower limbs by myotomes and peripheral nerves

Joint	Movement	Myotomes	Nerve supply
Hip	Flexion	L1–3	Lumbar plexus
		L2–4	Femoral nerve
	Extension	L5–S2	Sacral plexus
		L5–S2	Sciatic nerve
	Abduction	L5–S2	Sacral plexus
	Adduction	L2–4	Obturator nerve
Knee	Extension	L2–4	Femoral nerve
	Flexion	L5–S2	Sciatic nerve.
		S1–2	Tibial nerve*
Ankle/foot	Dorsiflexion	L4–5	Deep peroneal nerve[†]
	Eversion	L5–S1	Superficial peroneal nerve[†]
	Plantar flexion	S1–2	Tibial nerve*
	Inversion	L4–5	Tibial nerve*

*Branch of sciatic nerve
[†]Branch of common peroneal nerve, itself a branch of the sciatic nerve

Fig. 10.7 Cutaneous innervation of lower body by dermatome. Reproduced with permission from Yentis, Hirsch & Smith: Anaesthesia and intensive care A-Z, 2nd edn, Butterworth Heinemann, 2000.

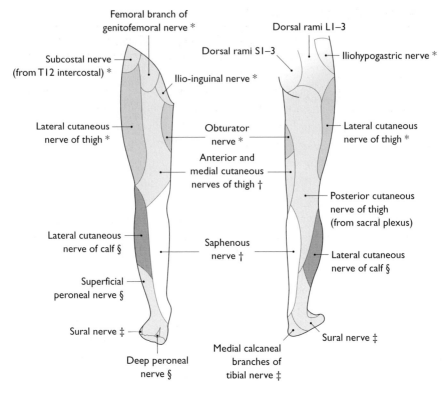

Femoral branch of
genitofemoral nerve *

Dorsal rami L1–3

Dorsal rami S1–3

Subcostal nerve
(from T12 intercostal) *

Iliohypogastric nerve *

Ilio-inguinal nerve *

Lateral cutaneous
nerve of thigh *

Obturator
nerve *

Lateral cutaneous
nerve of thigh *

Anterior and
medial cutaneous
nerves of thigh †

Posterior cutaneous
nerve of thigh
(from sacral plexus)

Lateral cutaneous
nerve of calf §

Saphenous
nerve †

Lateral cutaneous
nerve of calf §

Superficial
peroneal nerve §

Sural nerve ‡

Sural nerve ‡

Deep peroneal
nerve §

Medial calcaneal
branches of
tibial nerve ‡

* From lumbar plexus
† From femoral nerve
‡ From tibial nerve (branch of sciatic nerve)
§ From common peroneal nerve (branch of sciatic nerve)

Fig. 10.8 Cutaneous innervation of leg by peripheral nerve. Reproduced with permission from Yentis, Hirsch & Smith: Anaesthesia and intensive care A-Z, 2nd edn, Butterworth Heinemann, 2000.

Dermatomal innervation of the upper body is also important when determining the upper extent of regional blockade.

FURTHER READING

Broadbent CR, Maxwell WB, Ferrie R, *et al*. Ability of anaesthetists to identify a marked lumbar interspace. *Anaesthesia* 2000; **55**: 1122–6.

Capogna G, Celleno D, Simonetti C, Lupoi D. Anatomy of the lumbar epidural region using magnetic resonance imaging: a study of dimensions and a comparison of two postures. *Int J Obstet Anesth* 1997; **6**: 97–100.

Harrison GR. Topographical anatomy of the lumbar epidural region: an in vivo study using computerized axial tomography. *Br J Anaesth* 1999; **83**: 229–34.

Render CA. The reproducibility of the iliac crest as a marker of lumbar spine level. *Anaesthesia* 1996; **51**: 1070–1.

11   PHYSIOLOGY OF PREGNANCY

Pregnancy is associated with major physiological changes throughout the body. These are caused by both hormonal factors (influential from conception onwards) and the mechanical changes caused by the enlarging uterus (of increasing significance as pregnancy progresses). It is important to understand the normal physiological changes occurring during pregnancy in order to predict the risks and effects of analgesic and anaesthetic intervention, and also to anticipate the impact of pregnancy on any coexisting medical condition.

Hormonal changes

Following fertilisation, the corpus luteum in the ovary secretes progesterone, oestrogens and relaxin, and these hormones are secreted by the placenta when it takes over the function of the corpus luteum from 6–8 weeks' gestation onwards. The placenta also secretes human chorionic somatomammotrophin (hCS; previously known as human placental lactogen and chorionic growth hormone-prolactin).

Human chorionic gonadotrophin (hCG) can be measured by radioimmunoassay and detected in the blood 6 days after conception and in the urine 2–3 weeks after conception. It is therefore a useful early diagnostic test of pregnancy. It is produced by the syncytiotrophoblast, and levels rise rapidly during the first 8 weeks of pregnancy, falling to a plateau thereafter.

Progesterone is responsible for most of the hormonally mediated changes occurring during pregnancy. It causes:
- Smooth muscle relaxation
- Generalised vasodilatation
- Bronchodilatation
- Dilatation within the renal tract
- Sluggish gastrointestinal tract motility and constipation.

It is thermogenic, causing an increase in basal temperature during pregnancy. It may be responsible for the nausea and vomiting that are common in early pregnancy. Progesterone is a neurotransmitter and, together with increased endogenous endorphins, is implicated in the elevated pain threshold experienced by pregnant women. It also decreases the minimum alveolar concentration of inhalational anaesthetic agents. Progesterone has also been demonstrated to enhance conduction blockade in isolated nerve preparations, and it is therefore thought likely to play a role in the decreased requirement for local anaesthetic agents for spinal and epidural anaesthesia.

Progesterone levels return to pre-pregnancy values over a period of 3–4 weeks after delivery, and thus hormonally mediated changes do not reverse immediately in the puerperium.

Mechanical changes

The uterus enlarges as pregnancy progresses. The fundus is palpable:
- Abdominally by the beginning of the second trimester
- At the umbilicus by 20 weeks' gestation
- At the xiphisternum by 36 weeks.

If the fetal head engages in the maternal pelvis at the end of pregnancy, the fundal height decreases and this may alleviate some symptoms attributable to mechanical factors. In multiple pregnancies, the uterus expands to a greater extent and more rapidly, and therefore the mechanical effects are usually greater.

Following delivery the uterus involutes rapidly, and should not be palpable above the maternal umbilicus. It has usually returned to within the pelvis by 72 hours after delivery.

Cardiovascular and haemodynamic changes

Pregnancy
- Blood volume increases throughout pregnancy, to approximately 45–50% more than pre-pregnant values by term. This represents an increase in both red cell volume and plasma volume with the latter being relatively greater, thus causing the so-called 'physiological anaemia' of pregnancy. The magnitude of the increase is greater in women with multiple pregnancy and greatly reduced in women with pre-eclampsia.
- Cardiac output, heart rate and stroke volume all increase as pregnancy progresses. Cardiac output increases by approximately 40–50% by term, with most of the increase occurring by 20 weeks' gestation. The increased blood flow is distributed primarily to the uterus, where blood flow increases from approximately 50 ml/minute at 10 weeks' gestation to 850 ml/minute at term.
- Renal blood flow increases by 80% over non-pregnant levels, and this level is achieved by the middle of the second trimester. Glomerular filtration rate and creatinine clearance increase by 50% during pregnancy.
- Systemic vascular resistance falls (peripheral vasodilatation mediated by progesterone, prostacyclin and oestrogens), and there is a decrease in both systolic and diastolic blood pressures, which reach a nadir during the second trimester and then increase gradually towards term, although remaining lower than pre-pregnancy values.
- Aortocaval compression can occur from the middle of pregnancy onwards if the supine position is adopted. This is due to mechanical compression of the aorta and inferior vena cava. Venous return is dependent on the competence of collateral circulation via the azygos and ovarian veins. Recent studies have demonstrated that uterine blood flow decreases primarily as a result of aortic rather than venous compression.
- Central venous and pulmonary arterial pressures are unchanged during normal pregnancy.

Labour and delivery

- Cardiac output increases by 25–50% in labour, with an additional 15–30% increase during contractions. This increase in cardiac output is mediated through increased sympathetic nervous system activity, and is therefore significantly attenuated by epidural analgesia.
- Central venous pressure increases during contractions, partly due to sympathetic activity and partly from the transfer of up to 500 ml of blood from the intervillous space. The latter is unaffected by epidural analgesia, as is the increase in central venous pressure which occurs when the Valsalva manoeuvre is performed during pushing.
- Autotransfusion of blood (from the placenta) occurs during the third stage. The effect of this may be significant in women with cardiac disease.
- After delivery there is a sustained increase in cardiac output and central venous pressure for several hours, which is associated with hypervolaemia. The implications of these changes for women with cardiac disease are significant (see relevant sections).

Respiratory changes

Pregnancy

- Progesterone increases the sensitivity of the respiratory centre to carbon dioxide and also acts as a primary respiratory stimulant. These effects are enhanced by oestrogens, and the combined hormonal effect causes an increase in minute ventilation of 45–50%.
- The partial pressure of carbon dioxide in arterial blood (P_aCO_2) is reset to approximately 4 kPa during the first trimester and remains at that level throughout pregnancy. A partially corrected respiratory alkalosis is found in normal pregnant women.
- Functional residual capacity decreases to 80% of pre-pregnancy values as pregnancy progresses, caused by increased intra-abdominal pressure and upward displacement of the diaphragm by the enlarging uterus. Total lung capacity remains unchanged. Functional residual capacity remains greater than closing capacity throughout pregnancy whilst the woman remains in an upright position, but falls when a recumbent position is adopted. It has been estimated that airway closure may occur within normal tidal ventilation in as many as 50% of all supine pregnant women during the second half of pregnancy.
- Oxygen consumption increases progressively during pregnancy to 35% above pre-pregnancy levels.

Labour and delivery

- Massive hyperventilation occurs during labour (unless there is effective analgesia), with minute ventilation increasing by up to 350% compared with pre-labour values.

- P_aCO_2 falls to below 2 kPa in some women. This respiratory alkalosis is associated with a metabolic acidosis, since maternal aerobic requirement for oxygen (increased by hyperventilation, hyperdynamic circulation and uterine activity) cannot be met, resulting in a progressive lactic acidosis.
- Effective epidural analgesia abolishes these effects during the first stage of labour but not during the second, when the additional uterine activity and work of pushing produce a further oxygen demand that cannot be met.

Gastrointestinal changes

Pregnancy

- Lower oesophageal sphincter pressure is reduced because of the smooth muscle relaxant effect of progesterone.
- Intragastric pressure rises as a mechanical consequence of the enlarging uterus.
- The overall effect of these changes is a decrease in gastro-oesophageal barrier pressure, with a concomitant increase in risk of regurgitation and aspiration of gastric contents.
- Some 75–85% of pregnant women complain of heartburn during the third trimester, and a significant number will have a demonstrable hiatus hernia.
- Gastric emptying is not delayed during pregnancy.
- There is some evidence that gastric volume is increased, and the pH of the intra-gastric volume may be lower than in the non-pregnant individual.

Labour and delivery

- Gastric emptying is now thought to be normal in labour in most cases, unless opioids have been given.
- Opioid analgesia (regardless of route of administration) delays gastric emptying.
- Recent work suggests that gastric volume (but not acidity) may remain elevated for 48 hours after delivery.

Management options

Positioning

- It is the anaesthetist's responsibility to exercise vigilance, with special attention being paid to the hips and back. The pregnant woman has increased ligamentous laxity, and may be particularly at risk of musculoskeletal trauma if she has received epidural analgesia. This risk is considerably increased if she has received either regional or general anaesthesia, when she is unable to safeguard her position.
- No pregnant woman should lie in the unmodified supine position at term (it is rare to find a mother who will voluntarily adopt this position). The wedged supine position and the use of lateral tilt are compromises and do not reliably

relieve aortocaval compression. Women should be encouraged to remain sitting upright or in the full lateral position whenever possible. Walking and standing in labour should also be encouraged.
- Obstetricians and midwives should be asked to perform fetal scalp blood sampling and vaginal examinations with the woman in the left lateral, or at least tilted, position.
- Closing volume may occur within tidal volume when the semi-recumbent position is adopted, and consideration should be given to continuous administration of oxygen to women particularly at risk (e.g. those who are obese, and those with respiratory disease).

General anaesthesia
- Pregnant women have increased oxygen consumption and decreased oxygen reserves. They are therefore at greatly increased risk of hypoxia during periods of apnoea.
- The risk of pulmonary aspiration of gastric contents means that rapid sequence induction of general anaesthesia, preceded by measures to reduce the acidity of the gastric contents, may be required, depending on the gestation and severity of symptoms (see Chapter 56, Aspiration of gastric contents; p. 138).

12   AORTOCAVAL COMPRESSION

Aortocaval compression (supine hypotensive syndrome) was first reported in 1931. The inferior vena cava and aorta become compressed by the pregnant uterus (the vena cava may be totally occluded), causing reduction in venous return and cardiac output and thus compromising the mother, fetus or both. Vasovagal syncope may follow aortocaval compression. Maternal symptoms and signs vary from asymptomatic mild hypotension to total cardiovascular collapse, partly dependent on the efficacy of the collateral circulation bypassing the inferior vena cava. Onset of symptoms and signs is associated with lying in the supine or semi-supine position, and is relieved by turning to the full lateral position in most cases.

Problems/special considerations
- Aortocaval compression is not confined to the woman at term. The condition has been reported in the fifth month of pregnancy. Women with multiple pregnancy or polyhydramnios are at increased risk because of the increased uterine size.

- It is important to appreciate that normotension and lack of maternal symptoms do not exclude a significant fall in cardiac output and placental perfusion.
- Onset of symptoms may occur within 30 seconds, but may be delayed by 30 minutes. Severity of symptoms is not a reliable guide to severity of hypotension.
- Slight changes in maternal position may cause significant change in symptoms. A 15° lateral tilt does not reliably relieve aortocaval compression, and even a 45° tilt does not guarantee abolition of hypotension.
- Catastrophic hypotension, and even cardiac arrest, may occur if general anaesthesia is induced in a woman who is experiencing severe aortocaval compression (e.g. in the supine position). Even mild degrees of aortocaval compression can lead to severe hypotension after spinal or epidural anaesthesia.
- It is impossible to perform effective cardiopulmonary resuscitation on the undelivered woman in the supine position; use of a purpose-made resuscitation wedge is recommended. If this is not available, the uterus must be displaced off the vena cava and aorta by other means.

Management options

Women will not voluntarily adopt positions in which aortocaval compression occurs, and therefore the condition is largely iatrogenic, occurring after a woman has been placed in the supine position by her midwifery or medical attendants. A history suggestive of aortocaval compression in late pregnancy may indicate an increased risk of developing the condition during labour and delivery. All those caring for pregnant women must be aware of aortocaval compression and of the need to avoid the supine position. This is particularly important if the woman is unable to change her own position because of administration of analgesia or anaesthesia.

Uterine displacement (usually to the left, although occasionally improved symptomatic relief will be obtained by displacement to the right) must be used during all vaginal examinations and during both vaginal and operative delivery, and is especially important if regional analgesia or anaesthesia is used. This can be achieved manually or by use of table tilt or a wedge under the hip. Use of uterine displacement rather than the full lateral position is a compromise between maternal safety and obstetricians' convenience. Use of the full lateral position for Caesarean section has been reported.

Extreme vigilance is necessary when maternal symptoms are abolished by induction of general anaesthesia. During regional anaesthesia for operative delivery, complaints of faintness, dizziness, restlessness and nausea should alert the anaesthetist to the onset of hypotension. Pallor, particularly of the lips, yawning and non-specific feelings of anxiety are also warning signs of aortocaval compression. Continuous fetal monitoring may indicate signs of fetal distress when the mother adopts the supine or semi-supine position, and occasionally this may be the only indicator of the condition. Turning the mother into the full left lateral position should be the first step in the treatment of hypotension or cardiotoco-graphic abnormalities.

Key points

- No pregnant woman should lie flat on her back beyond 16–18 weeks.
- The uterus must be displaced off the aorta and vena cava during vaginal examinations and during Caesarean section. This can be done manually, with a wedge under the hip, or by using lateral tilt of the operating table.
- Cardiopulmonary resuscitation will be ineffective if the mother is supine.

FURTHER READING

Kinsella SM, Lohmann G. Supine hypotensive syndrome – a review. *Obstet Gynecol* 1994; **83**: 774–88.

13 NORMAL LABOUR

A large number of pregnant women are assessed as being 'low risk' and are predicted to have normal labours, but the diagnosis of normal labour is retrospective.

The parameters for normal labour are:
- Contractions once in every 3 minutes, lasting 45 seconds
- Progressive dilatation of the cervix
- Progressive descent of the presenting part
- Vertex presenting with the head flexed and the occiput anterior
- Labour not lasting less than 4 hours (precipitate) or longer than 18 hours (prolonged)
- Delivery of a live healthy baby
- Delivery of a complete placenta and membranes
- No complications.

First stage of labour

During the latent phase, the cervix effaces then cervical dilatation begins. The rate of cervical dilatation should be around 1 cm/h for a primiparous woman and 2 cm/h for a multigravid woman.

It is standard practice to perform a vaginal examination every 4 hours to assess the dilatation of the cervix, or more frequently if there is cause for concern.

The following routine observations are charted on the partogram:
- Fetal heart rate quarter-hourly

- Maternal pulse rate half-hourly
- Blood pressure half-hourly
- Temperature 4-hourly
- Urinalysis at each emptying of the bladder.

The fetal heart may be monitored intermittently by auscultation using Pinard's stethoscope or by cardiotocographic monitoring. The cardiotocogram (CTG) is recorded either intermittently or continuously depending on the condition of the fetus. Continuous recording of fetal heart rate may be done using either an abdominal transducer or a clip applied to the fetal head. Radiotelemetry is available in some units and this allows the woman to be mobile while her baby is monitored. Uterine contractions may be monitored externally by an abdominal transducer or internally by an intrauterine catheter. The fetal heart rate and the uterine contractions are recorded together.

Second stage of labour

The second stage of labour commences at full dilatation of the cervix and terminates at the delivery of the baby.

At full dilatation of the cervix, the character of the contractions changes and they are usually, but not invariably, accompanied by a strong urge to push. In normal labour there is an increase in circulating oxytocin secondary to Ferguson's reflex, with consequent increased strength of uterine contractions at full dilatation. Higher-dose epidural analgesia is thought to diminish the effect of this reflex.

The second stage of labour can be divided into passive and active stages and this is particularly relevant when epidural analgesia is used. With epidural analgesia, especially using older, higher-dose techniques, the labouring woman may not have the normal sensation at the start of the second stage of labour; therefore the active stage of pushing should only commence when the vertex is visible or the woman has a strong urge to push. In normal labour, the active stage usually commences at full dilatation. Traditionally, the second stage is limited to 2 hours because of the risk of fetal acidosis; up to 3 hours is often allowed in the presence of epidural analgesia in recognition of the slower descent of the fetal head. It is difficult for a woman to push efficiently for more than one hour, and after this time fetal acidosis is felt to be more likely. If there is not good progress, the advice of the obstetrician should be sought. At the delivery of the anterior shoulder, intramuscular oxytocics (e.g. Syntometrine) are given to hasten the delivery of the placenta and to stimulate uterine contraction.

Third stage of labour

The third stage of labour is the complete delivery of the placenta and membranes and the contraction of the uterus. It is usually managed actively by administering an oxytocic as above, but it may also be managed physiologically without oxytocics. This may prolong the third stage and increase the risk of postpartum haemorrhage.

During the third stage of labour there is a major redistribution of (and increase in) maternal circulating blood volume. This is potentially dangerous to those women who have cardiac disease and who may be precipitated into heart failure immediately postpartum.

Key points

- Normal labour can be anticipated but can only be diagnosed after delivery.
- The first stage comprises cervical effacement and dilatation.
- During the second stage, the baby passes through the birth canal.
- The placenta and membranes are delivered during the third stage.

FURTHER READING

Ferguson E, Owen P. The second stage of labour. *Hosp Med* 2003; **64**: 210–13.
Steer P, Flint C. Physiology and management of normal labour. *BMJ* 1999; **318**: 793–6.

14   GASTRIC FUNCTION AND FEEDING IN LABOUR

Physiological changes in pregnancy affect the volume, acidity and emptying of gastric secretions as well as sphincter mechanisms in the lower oesophagus. Interventions in labour such as analgesia may also affect these changes adversely. General anaesthesia is occasionally necessary in emergency situations, and the presence of a full stomach (and thus the risk of aspiration of gastric contents) should always be assumed in such patients (see Chapter 56, Aspiration of gastric contents, p. 138).

Problems/special considerations

Increased circulating progesterone associated with pregnancy relaxes smooth muscle and causes relaxation of the lower oesophageal sphincter, whereas placental gastrin increases the volume and decreases the pH of gastric contents. The enlarging uterus increases intragastric pressure and there is an increase in small and large bowel transit time. However, evidence suggests that gastric emptying per se is not affected by pregnancy though it may be decreased in labour if opioids are given.

Extradural analgesia with local anaesthetic solutions in labour is associated with normal gastric emptying, whereas subarachnoid or extradural opioids (fentanyl or diamorphine) in large doses cause a modest decrease in gastric emptying. Systemic opioid analgesia causes a much greater and prolonged decrease in gastric emptying. However, recent randomised studies have demonstrated large gastric volumes and a high incidence of vomiting in women allowed to eat solid food, even when pain was adequately controlled with a low-dose fentanyl/bupivacaine epidural.

Plasma progesterone concentrations return to non-pregnant values within 24 hours of delivery, and gastroesophageal reflux is considerably reduced within 48 hours of delivery. The period of risk of aspiration thus extends to an ill-defined time after delivery, and appropriate general anaesthetic management in the early postpartum period is thus somewhat controversial.

Routine withholding of food and fluids in labour has been challenged by a number of authors, particularly those who are not anaesthetists. They point out that absolute starvation is not popular with mothers, that aspiration associated with emergency general anaesthesia nowadays is uncommon and that there may be risks associated with prolonged starvation. On the other hand, there is little evidence that a period of starvation during labour is harmful, although it may be unpleasant. Starvation is associated with ketosis, but this has not been found to affect the duration or outcome of labour.

Management options

There are three approaches to the treatment of feeding in labour. The traditional approach is to assume that all women in labour are at risk of an event in labour that will require emergency general anaesthesia and that they are therefore at risk of aspiration of large volumes of acid gastric contents. As a consequence of this assumption, many women in labour are starved, allowed only sips of water to drink and given regular H_2 antagonists (e.g. ranitidine 150 mg orally 6-hourly, or 50 mg intramuscularly 8-hourly) and regular sodium citrate (30 ml of 0.3 M orally).

Another approach is to assume that women in labour require food and fluid and to give these liberally. Often no H_2-blockers are given.

A more rational approach is to stratify management on the basis of risk. Women at high risk of requiring general anaesthesia are advised to have only clear fluids and receive regular H_2-blockers. In addition, for those who do eat and drink during labour, substances that are associated with slower gastric emptying (those with high fat or sugar content) should be discouraged in favour of protein-based snacks and isotonic drinks.

If intravenous water is required in labour, the most sensible fluid to provide might be 5% or 10% dextrose. Unfortunately this has been associated with fluid overload in the mother and hyponatraemia in the neonate. However, modest volumes (<1 litre) do not significantly affect neonatal plasma sodium concentrations. Many units give relatively low volumes of intravenous saline, dextrose saline or Hartmann's solution when intravenous fluid is considered necessary.

Key points

- Women are being encouraged to eat in labour, especially by other professionals.
- Solid food ingested during labour is not predictably absorbed.
- Women treated with epidural analgesia may have normal gastric emptying unless large boluses of opioid are given.
- Opioids given parenterally markedly decrease gastric emptying.
- Acid aspiration prophylaxis should be given to all women at risk of intervention in labour.

FURTHER READING

Porter JS, Bonello E, Reynolds F. The influence of epidural administration of fentanyl infusion on gastric emptying in labour. *Anaesthesia* 1997; **52**: 1151–6.

Scrutton NJL, Metcalfe GA, Lowy C, Seed PT, O'Sullivan G. Eating in labour. A randomised controlled trial assessing the risks and benefits. *Anaesthesia* 1999; **54**: 329–34.

15   DRUGS AND PREGNANCY

Pregnancy may interact with drugs in a number of different ways. Firstly, the pregnant state confers alterations in both pharmacokinetics and pharmacodynamics; secondly, the fetus may be affected by drugs administered to the mother, and in many cases this may restrict the use of certain drugs; and thirdly, there may be further passage of certain drugs to the neonate in breast milk (see Chapter 149, Drugs and breastfeeding, p. 337). Because of these considerations, special licensing requirements exist for drugs to be used in pregnancy, which have not been met by many drugs in current use.

Pharmacokinetics

Each of the traditional components of pharmacokinetics may be altered in the pregnant, as opposed to the non-pregnant, state.

- *Absorption of drug:* this depends on the route of administration and, in general, is little affected by pregnancy. However, absorption of enterally administered drugs may be affected by pregnancy-associated gastrointestinal upsets, including vomiting. Because of the increased minute ventilation and cardiac output, absorption of inhalational agents is more rapid.
- *Distribution of drug:* this is affected by the increased blood volume and body fluid and altered plasma protein profile. The former two result in a greater volume of distribution. In addition, the fetus represents an additional compartment to which drugs will distribute, depending on their lipid solubility, pKa and protein binding. The increased cardiac output will tend to redistribute

drugs more quickly unless they are extensively bound to the tissues. During labour, acute changes in plasma pH (e.g. acidosis associated with maternal exhaustion or alkalosis associated with pain-induced hyperventilation) may affect both protein binding and degree of dissociation of drugs.

- *Metabolism of drugs:* drugs broken down in the major organs (usually the liver) should be handled normally in pregnancy, unless there is hepatic impairment, e.g. in HELLP (haemolysis, elevated liver enzymes and low platelet count) syndrome. Some drugs are metabolised by plasma cholinesterases and may thus have longer duration of action if the protein concentration is reduced, e.g. suxamethonium.
- *Elimination:* since glomerular filtration rate is increased in pregnancy, clearance of many drugs is increased unless renal function is impaired, e.g. in pre-eclampsia. An extra route of elimination is in breast milk, although this represents a relatively small amount of total drug elimination. Inhalational agents are excreted via the lungs more rapidly in the pregnant than non-pregnant state.

Pharmacodynamics

The effects of most drugs are unchanged in pregnancy. However, notable and important exceptions are anaesthetic agents. Thus the minimum alveolar concentration of inhalational agents is reduced, as is the minimal blocking concentration of local anaesthetics. The cause of this decrease in anaesthetic requirement is thought to be progesterone and/or a metabolite thereof. In addition, a given amount of epidural local anaesthetic solution produces a more extensive block than in non-pregnant subjects, possibly related to the reduction in epidural space caused by epidural venous engorgement, although progesterone has also been suggested as being involved.

Fetal effects of drugs

Drugs may affect the fetus at any stage of pregnancy. During the first trimester the developing organ systems and overall body structure are especially at risk, particularly between the third and tenth weeks; administration of certain drugs during this period may result in congenital malformations. During the second and third trimesters, the growth and development of fetal tissues may be affected. Finally, drugs given before delivery may affect fetal oxygenation indirectly (e.g. by causing maternal hypotension or respiratory depression), may affect labour (e.g. β-agonists), or may have neonatal effects after birth (e.g. opioids). Many drugs are known to be harmful when given during pregnancy, but for many others, precise information is not always available. Thus, in general, drugs are not prescribed unless the benefits are felt to outweigh any possible risk, especially during the first trimester. Where possible, older drugs of which clinicians have greater experience are preferred over newer ones, and this is also true of anaesthetic agents.

Licensing of drugs in pregnancy

Many drugs, including anaesthetic agents, are not licensed for use in pregnancy, mainly because of the prohibitive costs to the manufacturer of performing the appropriate studies required and the relatively limited addition such licensing would make to the market. For example, the data sheets of etomidate, alfentanil and fentanyl contain the sentence 'safety in human pregnancy has not been established' or words to that effect, whilst those of propofol and fentanyl specifically warn against their use in obstetrics. Even in the case of thiopental, the data sheet merely states that there is 'epidemiological and clinical evidence' of its safety in pregnancy, whereas that of atracurium, vecuronium and suxamethonium state that they should only be used in pregnancy 'if the potential benefits outweigh any potential risks'.

Key points

- Pharmacokinetics and pharmacodynamics in pregnancy may be altered from those in the non-pregnant state.
- Most drugs administered to the mother will pass to the fetus to a degree.
- Many drugs pass into breast milk.
- Most anaesthetic drugs are not licensed for use in pregnancy.

FURTHER READING

Howell PR, Madej T. Administration of drugs outside of product licence: awareness and current practice. *Int J Obstet Anesth* 1999; **8**: 30–6.

Rubin P. Drug treatment during pregnancy. *BMJ* 1998; **317**: 1503–6.

16   PLACENTAL TRANSFER OF DRUGS

The placenta is a complex structure composed of both maternal and fetal tissues. Nevertheless, it is basically a semi-permeable biological membrane and as such obeys the laws that govern transport across such membranes. Virtually all transfer of drugs across the placenta occurs by simple diffusion, and all drugs administered to the mother will reach the fetus, albeit to a variable extent depending upon the factors discussed below.

Factors determining placental transfer

Molecular weight and lipid solubility

The molecular weight of the drug, its degree of ionisation, its lipid solubility and the degree to which it is protein bound will all affect the readiness with which it will cross the placenta. The majority of anaesthetic drugs are small (molecular weights of less than 500) and lipid soluble; thus they cross the placenta readily. The main exceptions are the neuromuscular blocking drugs, which are less lipid soluble, more highly ionised quaternary ammonium compounds, and in the doses used in normal clinical anaesthesia do not cross the placenta to any significant extent. However, if used in large doses or over a prolonged period of time (e.g. to facilitate artificial ventilation in the intensive care unit) they do reach the fetal circulation in doses that may have a clinical effect necessitating ventilatory support.

Changes in maternal or fetal pH may alter the degree of ionisation and protein binding of a drug, and thus alter its availability for transfer. This is most likely to occur if the pKa of a drug is close to physiological pH, and becomes clinically relevant in the acidotic fetus. Once drug transfer to the fetus has occurred, acidosis results in increased ionisation of the drug, which is then unable to equilibrate with the maternal circulation by diffusion back across the placenta. This results in drug accumulation in the fetus (so-called ion trapping), and is particularly relevant for local anaesthetics, which all have a pKa > 7.4.

Maternal drug concentration

Drug transfer occurs down a concentration gradient (which is usually from mother to fetus but can also occur from fetus to mother). The drug concentration on the maternal side depends on the route of administration, total maternal dose, volume of distribution and drug clearance and metabolism. The highest maternal blood concentration of a drug will be achieved following intravenous administration; epidural and intramuscular administration result in similar maternal blood concentrations. Systemic drug absorption will be greater from more vascular tissues, such as the paracervical region.

The increase in blood volume and cardiac output that accompanies normal pregnancy has an effect on maternal drug concentration; the volume of distribution and plasma clearance of drugs such as thiopental is increased.

Placental factors

The area of placenta available for transfer is important. Physiological shunting occurs in the placenta, and in maternal disease such as pre-eclampsia the placenta itself may present an increased barrier to transfer. Although there is evidence that some drug metabolism occurs within the placenta itself, this is not clinically significant.

Fetal drug concentration

Once a drug has reached the fetus it is subject to redistribution, metabolism and excretion. The fetus has less plasma protein binding capacity and less mature enzyme systems than the mother, and will therefore eliminate drugs less effectively. Some transfer of drugs occurs back across the placenta to the mother if the maternal concentration falls below that in the fetus (unless ion trapping occurs – see above).

Uteroplacental blood flow

This is the other major factor influencing placental transfer. Any reduction in blood flow to the placenta will inevitably reduce transfer of drugs (and nutrients) to the fetus. Reduction in uteroplacental flow may occur as a result of generally reduced maternal blood flow (hypotension, reduced cardiac output states, aortocaval compression, generalised vasoconstriction) or direct obstruction of flow (aortocaval compression, uterine contraction, umbilical cord compression).

Problems/special considerations

All general anaesthetic agents cross the placenta readily; and in normal clinical practice their effects on the fetus are only of significance immediately after delivery. The compromised fetus, or one in whom the uterine incision to delivery interval has been prolonged, may be depressed at birth, but rarely requires more than simple resuscitative measures.

Pethidine (and all other opioids) crosses the placenta readily. It has maximal effect in the fetus 3–4 hours after maternal administration and minimal effect if given to the mother within an hour of delivery. (This is contrary to traditional midwifery teaching, which recommends that pethidine is not given if delivery is expected within 2–3 hours.) Both pethidine and its active metabolite norpethidine have prolonged half-lives in the fetus and cause respiratory depression and reduced sucking ability. Opioid side effects are reversed by naloxone.

Local anaesthetics cross the placenta by simple diffusion, but the extent of placental transfer is also dependent on maternal plasma protein binding (bupivacaine and ropivacaine are highly protein bound, and therefore cross less readily than lidocaine, which is less protein bound.)

Key points

- The major determinants of transfer by simple diffusion are the maternal–fetal drug concentration gradient, molecular weight of the drug, lipid solubility, degree of drug ionisation and extent of protein binding.
- Uteroplacental blood flow is also important.
- Opioids given to the mother for labour analgesia cross the placenta freely and may cause fetal respiratory and neurobehavioural depression, which are reversible with naloxone.

FURTHER READING

Littleford J. Effects on the fetus and newborn of maternal analgesia and anesthesia: a review. *Can J Anaesth* 2004; **51**: 586–609.

17 PRESCRIPTION AND ADMINISTRATION OF DRUGS BY MIDWIVES

In the UK, regulations for prescription and administration of drugs by midwives fall under the responsibility of the Nursing and Midwifery Council (NMC; previously the UK Central Council for Nursing, Midwifery and Health Visiting (UKCC)), which issues codes and standards relating to the practical application of acts such as the Medicines Act 1968, Misuse of Drugs Act 1971, and Medicinal Products: Prescription by Nurses Act 1992, and their subsequent amendments. Many of the the NMC's publications on the matter are not legally binding but would be taken into account if there were to be medicolegal or regulatory action concerning administration of drugs. Against this background of central control, the setting up of, and adherence to, local policies is strongly encouraged, in recognition of the differing requirements from unit to unit.

Problems/special considerations

A compromise must exist between (i) supporting the midwife's role as an independent practitioner; (ii) reducing the workload on, and requirement for, medical staff to treat common and relatively minor conditions; (iii) permitting the rapid administration of drugs that may have real benefits to mothers and reduce morbidity or mortality; and (iv) restricting the use of potentially harmful drugs or reducing the incidence of adverse effects. Whether a particular drug should be allowed to be given thus depends on the incidence, importance and potential severity of the condition for which it is indicated and the efficacy, method of administration and safety profile of the drug concerned.

Drugs that midwives can administer without medical prescription

There is regional variation according to local policies, and individual trusts bear ultimate responsibility for approving drug policies within their maternity services. However, the drugs that midwives are allowed to prescribe and administer generally fall into a number of categories (Table 17.1). Local regulations are usually decided by a panel including representatives of midwives, pharmacists and obstetricians; anaesthetic staff may also be involved, e.g. in helping with analgesic or local anaesthetic drug policies.

Midwives in different units may interpret the NMC's guidelines differently, especially with regard to epidural top-ups; thus, for example, midwives in certain units may be prepared to administer epidural drugs prescribed by a doctor (i.e. anaesthetist) whereas those in other units may not. This is not usually a problem with local anaesthetic drugs alone but has been problematic with mixtures of local anaesthetics and opioids, e.g. fentanyl, which are, first, controlled drugs, and second, unlicensed for epidural use. Recently, in the UK, there has been stricter attention to the proper handling of all preparations containing controlled drugs, even the dilute mixtures used for epidural analgesia. Interpretation of current

Table 17.1. Sample standing orders for drugs that may be prescribed and adminstered by midwives without medical prescription

Analgesics	Opioids (usually pethidine, up to two intramuscular doses)
	Paracetamol/codydramol/cocodamol
	Entonox
	Diclofenac
Local anaesthetics	Lidocaine for infiltration/local application
Gastrointestinal	Liquid antacids
	Ranitidine/cimetidine
	Laxatives
	Antiemetics
Oxytocics	Oxytocin/ergometrine
Sedatives	Temazepam
Haematological	Iron/folate preparations
	Subcutaneous heparin
	Anti-D
	Vitamin K (neonatal)
Other	Naloxone (neonatal)
	Topical clotrimazole

N.B. midwives can also administer TENS.

UK law has led to suggestions that each single top-up with such mixtures constitutes a separate administration and thus requires the syringe to be kept in a locked cupboard between top-ups, with double-checking and double-signing before each top-up. This has led some units to change from midwife-administered boluses to infusions or patient-controlled epidural analgesia. In all cases, midwives' willingness to give epidural drugs is only on the understanding that ultimate responsibility for administering the drug lies with the anaesthetist.

The regulations are regularly reviewed, with recent attention being paid to administration of intravenous fluids to reflect (i) the widespread competence of midwives in venous cannulation and (ii) the number of women choosing to deliver at home and therefore the potential for severe haemorrhage away from hospitals.

Key points

- The Nursing and Midwifery Council (NMC) issues professional guidelines and codes for administration of drugs by midwives.
- Midwives are able to administer several drugs without a doctor's prescription, according to the NMC's recommendations and local policies.
- Midwives may administer certain drugs unlicensed for use in labour, e.g. epidural fentanyl, if covered by local policies and on the written prescription of a doctor.

FURTHER READING

Nursing and Midwifery Council. *Guidelines for the administration of medicines.* London: NMC 2002.

18   LOCAL ANAESTHETICS

Bupivacaine is the most commonly used local anaesthetic in British obstetric epidural analgesic practice. Bupivacaine, lidocaine, ropivacaine and levobupivacine (the S-enantiomer of bupivacaine) are all licensed for obstetric epidural use, although heavy (hyperbaric) bupivacaine is the only local anaesthetic licensed for obstetric spinal use (levobupivacaine is licensed for non-obstetric spinal anaesthesia). These local anaesthetics are all amides. There are no local anaesthetics in the ester group in use in British obstetric anaesthesia.

Pharmacology

Local anaesthetics act by reducing permeability of the nerve cell membrane to sodium, and thus preventing development of a propagated action potential. The local anaesthetic binds to receptor sites within the sodium channels of the nerve membrane.

Increasing lipid solubility allows the local anaesthetic drug to penetrate the nerve membrane more readily, and is associated with increased potency (bupivacaine and levobupivacaine have greater lipid solubility than lidocaine and ropivacaine).

Increased capacity for protein binding increases duration of action of the local anaesthetic. Bupivacaine and levobupivacaine are 95% protein bound and ropivacaine is 94% protein bound, and these drugs therefore have a longer duration of action than lidocaine, which is only 64% protein bound.

The speed of onset of local anaesthetic activity is related to the degree of ionisation of the drug. The non-ionised form of the drug diffuses across the nerve sheath to reach the nerve membrane. The degree of ionisation is dependent on the pKa of the drug. Bupivacaine, ropivacaine and levobupivacaine each have a pKa of 8.2 and are therefore more ionised (and thus have a slower onset of anaesthetic action) at body pH than lidocaine, which has a pKa of 7.7. Addition of bicarbonate to local anaesthetic solutions speeds onset time and may improve the quality of the block.

The development of the minimum local analgesic concentration/dose (MLAC/D) technique, using an up–down sequential allocation model, has enabled relative analgesic potency ratios to be determined for epidural analgesia (and to a lesser extent, spinal analgesia/anaesthesia). In this technique, the first patient in a study group is given a set volume of a certain concentration (MLAC) or a set volume containing a certain dose (MLAD). If the target response is achieved (e.g. pain scores <1 cm on a scale of 0–10 cm), the next patient receives a 20% decrease in concentration/dose; if the target response is not achieved the next patient receives a 20% increase. The process is repeated and the ED_{50} may be derived from the resultant graph of responses. This technique has allowed the potencies of different local anaesthetics, and the effect of additives (e.g. opioids), to be compared.

The amide local anaesthetics are metabolised in the liver and excreted via the kidney.

Toxicity

Systemic toxicity of local anaesthetics is manifest as central nervous system excitability (caused by inhibition of inhibitory fibres) resulting in convulsions. This progresses to central nervous system depression if the local anaesthetic dose is increased further. Local anaesthetics also affect the cardiovascular system. Toxic doses cause depolarisation of cardiac cell membranes, systemic vasodilatation and cardiovascular collapse, and resuscitation in pregnancy is notoriously difficult.

The safety margin (i.e. the difference between systemic concentration of local anaesthetic causing central nervous system symptoms and signs and that causing cardiovascular signs) is lower for bupivacaine than for the other local anaesthetic agents in clinical use, and it is this problem that has stimulated the development of newer local anaesthetics. Bupivacaine appears to be particularly cardiotoxic in pregnancy, causing ventricular arrhythmias and asystolic cardiac arrest.

Recently, Intralipid 1–2 mg/kg over 1 minute, repeated upto twice then 0.25 mg/kg/min, has been suggested as a treatment for toxicity. It is thought to bind free drug and/or replenish myocardial energy substrates.

The addition of adrenaline to lidocaine reduces its systemic absorption and therefore permits administration of larger doses (up to 7 mg/kg body weight compared with 4 mg/kg if adrenaline is not used). This is not the case with bupivacaine, the maximum dose of which is 2 mg/kg.

Amide local anaesthetics have a minimal chance of causing allergic reactions, unlike the ester group.

Differential block

The ideal local anaesthetic for obstetric analgesia would provide complete sensory analgesia of rapid onset and long duration without any motor blockade. Although bupivacaine provides long-lasting sensory block, this is accompanied (especially at increasing dosage) by motor blockade. Ropivacaine has similar action at higher concentrations, but at lower concentrations is claimed to produce differential sensory block by preferential action on C fibres. The extent to which this is clinically significant is still unproven, and the increasing use of very low concentrations of local anaesthetic combined with opioids for labour analgesia may make any difference clinically irrelevant.

Key points

- All the local anaesthetics used in British obstetric anaesthetic practice are amides.
- Anaesthetic potency is proportional to lipid solubility.
- Duration of action is proportional to extent of protein binding.
- Speed of onset of action is proportional to the amount of non-ionised drug present.
- Systemic toxicity is manifest by central nervous system excitability followed by cardiovascular depression. The margin of safety between central nervous system and cardiovascular toxicity is lowest for bupivacaine.

19   ANTENATAL FETAL MONITORING

Recent developments have made it possible to make detailed assessments of fetal wellbeing in the antenatal period. A decision to deliver the baby early may be made on the outcome of these assessments, and the obstetric anaesthetist may be involved in this decision making.

The most commonly used tests are: serial ultrasonography, serial Doppler flow studies and cardiotocography.

Serial ultrasonography

Serial ultrasonography is a useful way of assessing fetal abnormality and continued fetal growth. The head circumference is measured in association with the abdominal circumference. If the fetus is starving, glycogen stores in the liver will be depleted and there will be an increase in the ratio of head circumference to abdominal wall circumference (asymmetrical growth retardation). There may also be a generalised growth retardation (symmetrical growth retardation).

The liquor volume is also used as an indicator of fetal wellbeing and placental function, poor placental function being reflected in a reduced liquor volume. As a measure of this volume, the anterior–posterior distance across the liquor is measured using a transducer. This measurement is called the liquor column; a column of less than 3 cm is indicative of oligohydramnios and one less than 2 cm represents very severe oligohydramnios. Amniotic fluid index may also be used to measure the liquor volume; this is the sum of the liquor column in each of the four liquor quadrants and is normally 8–20 cm.

Serial Doppler flow studies

Both maternal uterine blood flow and fetal umbilical artery blood flow may be measured using Doppler techniques. The pattern of flow reflects placental function as follows:
- Normal flow continues through systole and diastole, as there is little resistance to flow through the placenta. The systolic:diastolic flow velocity ratio (SD ratio)

is widely used to indicate resistance to arterial flow; several other derived indices (e.g. pulsatility index) have also been used to indicate fetal perfusion and oxygenation. The use of these techniques for screening for high-risk fetuses is controversial and they may be reserved for monitoring known high-risk cases.

- Just absent end-diastolic flow may indicate the need for delivery of the baby. Wide absence of end-diastolic flow suggests the need to deliver the baby urgently.
- Reversal of end-diastolic flow suggests the need for immediate delivery of the baby.

Plans for timing and mode of delivery of the baby may be based on the evidence of the Doppler studies. The anaesthetist should understand that the anaesthetic management should optimise the placental flow and that meticulous care should be taken to avoid sudden cardiovascular changes and, in particular, supine hypotension. Where there is poor, absent or reversed end-diastolic flow, it is advisable to monitor the fetal heart rate continuously during the establishment of a regional block, whether this is for labour analgesia or anaesthesia for Caesarean section.

In specialised fetal medicine units, blood flow may also be measured by using Doppler techniques in the fetal abdominal aorta, renal or middle cerebral arteries. The results of the flow measurements are difficult to interpret.

Cardiotocography

Cardiotocography is used in conjunction with other clinical evidence in a baby that is deemed to be at risk. The cardiotocograph will only record the fetal heart during the time of the trace and cannot provide historical or predictive information. The pattern of the trace may be indicative of fetal compromise and may be used to plan the mode of delivery, e.g. either induction of labour or Caesarean section.

It is important that the anaesthetist communicates with the obstetrician and understands how compromised the fetus is when asked to give analgesia or anaesthesia to these mothers. The degree of urgency for the delivery will depend on the condition of the fetus. It should be remembered that women in these circumstances may be very anxious and upset and will need extra support during delivery.

Key points

- Antenatal assessments may identify fetuses at special risk.
- Meticulous care should be taken to maintain optimal placental perfusion if investigations indicate fetal hypoxaemia.
- Communication between medical and midwifery staff is crucial.

20   CHARTING OF LABOUR

A labour record is kept to measure and record the vital signs of the mother and fetus, together with the progress of labour. It also serves as a record of events should an adverse outcome occur, especially if there is subsequent medicolegal involvement (see Chapter 157, Medicolegal aspects, p. 355; Chapter 158, Record keeping, p. 357). A list of items recorded would normally include:

- Fetal heart rate every 15 minutes
- Cervical dilatation at least every 4 hours
- Descent of the presenting part
- Colour of the liquor
- Fetal pH if relevant
- Amount of oxytocics given
- Strength and frequency of uterine contractions
- All drugs administered, including those for the epidural
- Maternal blood pressure and pulse rate
- Urine volume and analysis for ketones, protein or glucose
- Fluid input.

The most commonly used means of charting the progress of labour is the partogram, which presents the data in a graphical form. 'Normal' curves, obtained from large numbers of healthy primigravidae and multigravidae, are printed on the partogram, against which it is easier to assess the progress of labour. An example of a partogram is shown in Fig. 20.1.

Key points

- Routine recording of labour is a standard of care in maternity units.
- The partogram is used to chart labour and for reference should a bad outcome or legal proceedings occur.
- Partograms should include details of regional analgesia.

Fig. 20.1 Example of a partogram for assessing and recording progress of labour.

Concentrations per 10 mins.

5
4
3
2
1

Weak ☐
Moderate ☒
Strong ■

Duration secs.

Drugs (incl. Epidural)

Remarks:

Effects of Drug
Patients general condition

Blood pressure and pulse

200
190
180
170
160
150
140
130
120
110
100
90
80
70
60
50

Temp °C
Protein/Ketones
Volume Intake
        Output

Fig. 20.1 (*cont.*)

21   INTRAPARTUM FETAL MONITORING

Fetal monitoring is an important part of intrapartum care since labour is a stressful event for the fetus, and the ability of the fetus to maintain oxygenation is tested with each uterine contraction. Fetal wellbeing can be monitored routinely using the following methods:

- Assessment of liquor colour
- Fetal heart auscultation
- Fetal heart cardiotocography (CTG)
- Fetal blood sampling and oximetry.

Special considerations

The pregnancy and labour can be assessed as either low or high-risk. A low-risk pregnancy uncomplicated by any obstetric or medical problems will need a low level of fetal monitoring during labour, whereas a high-risk pregnancy (e.g. one complicated by hypertensive disease of pregnancy or poor intrauterine growth) will need careful intrapartum monitoring. The labour itself can be assessed as either low or high risk; it is generally recognised that a spontaneous labour is usually low risk whereas an augmented labour or an induced labour is usually high risk.

Liquor colour

When the membranes are ruptured, the liquor may be observed for the presence of meconium. The appearance of new meconium may indicate fetal hypoxia, which can cause the anal sphincter to relax, allowing the fetus to pass meconium. The appearance of thick new meconium is an indication for urgent delivery. If meconium is aspirated into the lungs of the neonate, severe lung damage may ensue; therefore it should be aspirated from the neonate's mouth before intermittent positive pressure ventilation is started. A paediatrician should be present at the delivery if meconium is present. Meconium is more commonly seen in post-term labour.

Fetal heart rate and CTG

Fetal heart monitoring is recommended as follows:

1. *Low risk (low-risk pregnancy and normal labour):* intermittent monitoring with a Pinard's stethoscope is said to be as effective as CTG monitoring. Structured intermittent monitoring involves listening immediately after a contraction for a minimum of 60 seconds and repeating this every 15 minutes in the first stage of labour (every 5 minutes in the second stage). It has been suggested that CTG monitoring in the low-risk group may lead to unnecessary intervention and increased anxiety.

2. *High risk (high-risk pregnancy and induced or augmented labours):* continuous monitoring of the fetal heart rate is recommended using a CTG, which records the fetal heart rate and the uterine contractions (and thus the effect

of the latter on heart rate). The monitor uses either an external transducer or a 'clip' applied to the fetal head. It is generally recommended that women with epidural analgesia have continuous fetal monitoring, although there is some evidence to suggest that women who have a mobile (low-dose) epidural may not need this. The need for continuous fetal monitoring during epidural analgesia is related to the cardiovascular instability that may follow administration of large doses of local anaesthetic solutions into the epidural space. There is also evidence that epidural or spinal opioids may cause transient fetal bradycardia.

There are four features of the fetal heart rate that are especially important:

- *Baseline rate:* normally 110–160 beats/min.
- *Variability:* normally 5–25 beats/min.
- *Accelerations from baseline (> 15 beats/min for 15 s):* two in 20 minutes are normally present. The significance of absent accelerations on an otherwise normal CTG is uncertain.
- *Decelerations from baseline:* normally absent. Decelerations are classified as early, variable and late. Early decelerations are synchronous with the contraction; they are benign and may be associated with compression of the fetal head in the pelvis. They mirror the uterine contractions and should be associated with good beat-to-beat variability. Variable decelerations vary in their shape, size and occurrence. They may or may not indicate fetal hypoxia. Late decelerations continue after the contraction has finished and are more ominous, especially if associated with other abnormalities, e.g. reduced variability.

Opioids or other sedative drugs may cause a flat trace with a loss of beat-to-beat variability, which makes interpretation difficult.

Thus there are three categories of pattern of CTG monitoring:

- *Normal:* all four of the above features are normal ('reassuring').
- *Suspicious:* one of the following is present (termed 'non-reassuring'):
  - Baseline: 100–109 or 161–180 beats/min.
  - Variability: <5 beats/min for 40–90 minutes.
  - Variable or early decelerations, or a single deceleration lasting 1–3 minutes.
- *Pathological:* two or more of the above features are 'non-reassuring' (see above) or one or more of the following is present (termed 'abnormal'):
  - Baseline: <100 or >180 beats/min.
  - Variability: <5 beats/min for ≥90 minutes.
  - Severe variable or late or decelerations, or a single deceleration lasting >3 minutes.

Fetal heart rate monitoring has low specificity and sensitivity. Any trace that causes concern, especially in a high-risk pregnancy, is an indication for a fetal blood sample to be taken, unless there is evidence of acute fetal compromise, in which case urgent delivery is indicated. The CTG trace should be kept for at least 25 years in case of a later medicolegal claim.

Recently, the combination of CTG and fetal electrocardiography (ST wave-form analysis) has been used to improve the sensitivity of fetal heart rate monitoring.

Fetal blood sampling

When the fetus becomes hypoxic, there is a build-up of lactic acid and a reduction in the fetal pH. Fetal blood sampling allows a more accurate assessment of fetal wellbeing than the CTG and is likely to be performed whenever there is anxiety about the CTG or when there is meconium in the liquor. The fetal blood sample may be taken with the mother in the lithotomy position or in the left lateral position. Whichever position is used, care must be taken to avoid aortocaval compression during the procedure. Recommended actions for values of fetal pH are as follows:

- >7.25 – normal; should be repeated if the fetal heart rate abnormality continues.
- 7.21–7.24 – borderline; should be repeated within 30 minutes or delivery considered if there has been a rapid fall since the last sample.
- <7.20 – indicative of significant acidosis and a need for urgent delivery of the baby.

Fetal gas tension measurement and oximetry

Non-invasive continuous transcutaneous measurement of oxygen and carbon dioxide tensions has been developed. This method requires the application of a suction ring to the baby's head; therefore the cervix needs to be dilated. The technique may not give accurate results if there is significant caput on the baby's head.

Fetal oxygen saturation may also be measured using special pulse oximeters; however, the technique is not yet reliable enough for routine use. Preliminary results suggest that fetuses normally have saturations of 30–60%.

Key points

- Good communication between the anaesthetist and obstetrician is important.
- Fetal monitoring includes assessment of liquor colour, auscultation, cardiotocography and fetal scalp blood pH measurement.
- Fetal heart rate monitoring has poor specificity and sensitivity but this may be improved by ST analysis.

FURTHER READING

Berkus MD, Langer O, Samueloff A, Xenakis EM, Field NT. Electronic fetal monitoring: what's reassuring? *Acta Obstet Gynaecol Scand* 1999; **78**: 15–21.

National Institute of Clinical Excellence. The use of electronic fetal monitoring: the use and interpretation of cardiotocography in intrapartum fetal surveillance. London: *NICE*: 2001.

Noren H, Amer-Wahlin I, Hagberg H, *et al.* Fetal electrocardiography in labor and neonatal outcome: data from the Swedish randomized controlled trial on intrapartum fetal monitoring. *Am J Obstet Gynecol* 2003; **188**: 183–92.

Steer P. ABC of labour care: assessment of mother and fetus in labour. *BMJ* 1999; **318**: 858–61.

22   PAIN OF LABOUR

The pain of primiparous labour is said to be one of the most severe pains experienced, reported to be exceeded only by the pains of traumatic amputation and causalgia. Approximately 50% of women report severe or very severe pain during labour. Painless childbirth is a reality for only a small minority of women, although labour pain can be modified by a number of non-pharmacological manoeuvres.

The pain pathways involved in labour and delivery are extensive, involving afferent fibres from T10 down to S4.

Pain pathways

The uterus, lower uterine segment and cervix are all supplied by afferent Aδ and C fibres, which accompany the thoracolumbar and sacral sympathetic outflows. The pain of the first stage of labour is therefore referred to the dermatomes supplied by the same spinal cord segments that receive input from the uterus and cervix: T10–L1 during the first half of the first stage and then the lower lumbar and sacral dermatomes as labour progresses.

The second stage of labour may also involve somatic pain caused by distension and tearing of pelvic structures and by abnormal pressure on perineal skeletal musculature.

Modification of labour pain

Psychological factors

There is considerable evidence that preparation for childbirth can significantly modify the degree of pain experienced. This was the basis of the 'childbirth without fear' movement, which was popular in the 1960s. Although there can be little doubt that fear, fatigue and anxiety enhance pain perception, for the majority of mothers it is misleading to suggest that good antenatal education will lead to painless child-birth. Such expectations may in fact have the reverse effect, since the mother may develop complete loss of self-confidence when she begins to experience significant labour pain.

Women whose pregnancy is unplanned or unwanted are likely to experience more pain, as are those who have no birth partner to support them during labour.

Conversely, the continuous presence of a midwife or female birth partner (doula) has been shown to reduce the amount of pain reported.

Cultural factors and ethnic group also have an influence on pain behaviour during labour, although it is likely that women from different cultures and of different racial groups actually experience similar levels of pain.

Promise of a finite duration of labour (as with active management of labour) may improve the ability to tolerate labour pain, although not necessarily reduce the level of pain experienced.

Physical factors

First labours are acknowledged to be more painful than subsequent labours, and older primiparae experience more painful labours than do younger women. Malpresentations, especially occipito-posterior positions, increase the pain of labour. Augmentation of labour by oxytocic drugs is reported to increase labour pain, and obstructed labour is more painful than normal labour. Tiredness is well known to reduce pain tolerance and is likely to occur if either the latent or the active phase of labour is prolonged.

There is a positive correlation between menstrual pain and labour pain, which has been postulated to be caused by excessive prostaglandin production.

Physiological factors

Progesterone may increase pain thresholds, and there is some evidence that in rats there is activation of endogenous opioid systems during late pregnancy. Experimental work in humans appears to confirm this.

Untreated pain causes an increase in circulating maternal catecholamines and other stress hormones. This may be detrimental to the mother with coexisting medical disease, and is also detrimental to the fetus. Maternal pain and acidosis are associated with reduced uteroplacental blood flow and fetal acidosis.

Key points

- Pain of childbirth is one of the most severe pains experienced.
- Pain from afferent Aδ and C fibres is referred to the dermatomes of T10 to S4 and is augmented during the second stage of labour by somatic pain from stretching and tearing of pelvic structures.
- Labour pain may be modified by antenatal education, and by the presence of a supportive partner.

FURTHER READING

Am J Obstet Gynecol 2002; 5 (Suppl): S1–S180.

23   EPIDURAL ANALGESIA FOR LABOUR

Since the introduction of epidural analgesia for labour in the 1940s, there has been continuous development of the technique. Single doses of local anaesthetic given into the caudal epidural space are now of historical interest only (although the single-shot caudal injection remains a useful adjunct to epidural analgesia), and a variety of techniques are used to provide lumbar epidural analgesia.

The use of epidural analgesia varies widely among different units in the UK, some small units having no provision and others having an epidural rate of over 50%.

Equipment

Provision of epidural analgesia for labour in the UK virtually always involves the insertion of an epidural catheter, usually with one of a variety of disposable epidural packs available. These usually include a 16 G or 17 G Tuohy epidural needle, a multi-hole catheter and a filter. Single, end-hole epidural catheters are popular in North America but are rarely used in the UK. Most epidural packs include a loss-of-resistance (LOR) device for identifying the epidural space.

If analgesia is to be provided by continuous infusion, a suitable infusion syringe or pump will be required. Dilute solutions of local anaesthetic and opioid for either intermittent top-up or infusion may be prepared 'in-house' by the hospital pharmacy or can be purchased from an outside manufacturer.

Technique

Either a midline or a paramedian technique can be used to approach the epidural space – both techniques are equally possible and acceptable in the lumbar spine, and the final choice of approach is usually determined by personal preference.

The epidural space is identified by LOR to the injection of either air or saline (Table 23.1), using either an intermittent or continuous injection technique.

With the intermittent technique (usually with air), the plunger is tested after each incremental advance of the needle. When the needle tip lies in the ligament or the ligamentum flavum, there will be resistance to injection, and this is lost when the epidural space is entered. Some anaesthetists consider that the intermittent technique is more hazardous because the needle is advanced between testing, thus increasing the risk of accidental dural puncture.

With the continuous technique, the operator's hand exerts continuous pressure on the plunger as the needle is advanced, and again detects a sudden LOR to injection as the epidural space is entered.

Once the epidural space has been identified the epidural catheter is inserted through the needle, leaving 2–4 cm within the epidural space, and is secured to the mother's back.

Table 23.1. Comparison of saline and air for loss-of-resistance (LOR) technique

	Saline	Air
Advantages	Allows the continuous technique of LOR Non-compressible. Thus no 'bounce' of the plunger when pressure is applied against resistance Retrospective surveys suggest a decreased incidence of accidental dural puncutre	Compressible, giving the plunger a characteristic 'bounce' Clear fluid dripping from the hub of the needle can only be cerebrospinal fluid
Disadvantages	Saline dripping from the hub of the needle may be confused with cerebrospinal fluid if dural tap is suspected (although testing for glucose etc. will distinguish it)	The intermittent technique must be used Has been associated with a wide range of complications, including subcutaneous emphysema, neck discomfort, air embolism, pneumocephalus, patchy block (thought to be caused by bubbles around the nerve roots) and neurological impairment The injected air is not sterile If pneumocephalus occurs,subsequent general anaesthesia with nitrous oxide may result in expansion of air bubbles

Epidural drugs

In the 1970s and early 1980s, the only drug used widely in the UK to provide epidural analgesia was bupivacaine, used in concentrations of 0.25–0.5%. During the past 20 years a variety of drug mixtures has been assessed. The most commonly used combination in the UK is now bupivacaine and fentanyl (0.1–0.125% bupivacaine with 2–2.5 μg/ml fentanyl). The reason for adding opioids to local anaesthetic is to enhance the quality of analgesia and to reduce the mass of local anaesthetic given. Initially it was hoped that this would lead to reduction in motor block and improved rates of spontaneous vaginal delivery.

Although there is a reduction in motor block, this has unfortunately not been accompanied by a dramatic reduction in instrumental delivery rate. In North America, combinations of up to four drugs (bupivacaine, sufentanil, adrenaline and clonidine) have been recommended, but the clinical benefit and wisdom of using such mixtures, given the potential for drug errors, have been questioned. More recently, ropivacaine (0.2%) has been used alone or in combination with opioids.

These 'low-dose' mixtures are given as intermittent top-ups of 10–15 ml, infusions of 10–12 ml/h, or patient-controlled epidural analgesia (PCEA). For the latter, two general types of regimen are used: boluses of 10–15 ml with no background infusion; or boluses of 4–6 ml with a background infusion of 3–8 ml/h. Suitable lockout periods are 5–20 minutes.

Infusions produce a greater consistency of analgesia and reduced workload for staff, compared with intermittent doses of stronger local anaesthetic solutions; however, this may not be the case if modern low-dose solutions are used for top-ups. Infusions are arguably safer than intermittent top-ups, since the reduction in frequency of epidural catheter dosing reduces the scope for erroneous drug administration. The use of infusions rather than top-ups appears to offer no advantage in reducing the total amount of drug administered during labour, although in hospitals where midwives are restricted to giving local anaesthetic alone, they provide a means of administering low-dose mixtures containing opioids without requiring anaesthetists to give each dose.

PCEA has been assessed over a wide range of dose variables and is a safe and effective alternative to continuous infusion techniques but with possibly less motor block.

Side effects of epidural analgesia

Epidural local anaesthetics cause sympathetic blockade and hypotension. Administration of intravenous fluids, vasopressor agents, or a combination of both, can prevent and/or treat this. Currently used low-dose combinations of local anaesthetic and opioid cause minimal haemodynamic disturbance, but it is mandatory to establish venous access before initiating epidural analgesia, although the need for routine preloading with intravenous fluids has been questioned.

Local anaesthetics also cause motor blockade, commonly graded by using various versions of the Bromage score (Table 23.2). Motor blockade can be minimised by using the lowest concentration of local anaesthetic compatible with adequate analgesia. Addition of opioid facilitates reduction of local anaesthetic dose but does not invariably lead to reduction in motor blockade.

Epidural opioids may cause nausea, vomiting, urinary retention, itching and respiratory depression. Each of these side effects occurs less commonly with fentanyl than with other opioids.

Table 23.2. Bromage score for assessing motor power following epidural analgesia

The scoring system has been modified several times from the original one, described in 1965, to account for the less intense motor block that occurs with modern, low-dose techniques.

Score	Original Bromage scoring system	Examples of modified Bromage scoring systems	
1	Unable to move feet or knees	Unable to flex ankles	Unable to move legs at all
2	Able to move feet only	Able to flex ankles but not knees	Able to move legs but unable to raise against gravity
3	Just able to move knees	Able to flex ankles and knees but unable to straight leg raise	Able to raise legs against gravity but not against resistance
4	Able to flex knees and feet fully	Able to sustain straight leg raise	Able to raise legs against gravity and resistance

The effect of epidural opioids on gastric emptying is uncertain. Boluses of fentanyl (50–100 µg) have been shown to delay gastric emptying by up to 45 minutes, but the use of low-dose continuous infusions do not appear to have this effect.

Complications

Epidural analgesia is highly effective but is an invasive technique with the potential for life-threatening complications. It must not, therefore, be used unless there is adequate care from a suitably trained birth attendant and the ability to access advanced resuscitation facilities rapidly if required.

Complications of epidural administration include:

- Failure to identify the epidural space
- Bloody tap/inadvertent intravascular injection
- Dural puncture
- Extensive conduction blockade
- Poor quality block
- Neurological complications
- Infectious complications.

These are discussed under the relevant headings elsewhere.

Outcome of labour

There is considerable debate about the effect of epidural analgesia on the outcome of labour, although there is now general (but not unanimous) agreement that epidural analgesia, especially with strong solutions of local anaesthetic, may prolong the first and second stages of labour. However, most of the relevant studies have suffered from inadequate controls, poor randomisation and a lack of blinding, factors that are well known to exaggerate treatment effects. Furthermore, the suggestion that epidural analgesia is associated with increased Caesarean section rates is not supported by the evidence. There does seem to be an association between epidural analgesia and increased rates of instrumental delivery – although allowing longer periods for the second stage has resulted in high rates of spontaneous vaginal delivery.

It is clear that the newer low-dose techniques of epidural analgesia have not been associated with dramatically increased rates of spontaneous vaginal delivery in primiparous women. Maternal satisfaction does, however, appear to be considerably greater with the newer techniques.

FURTHER READING

Evron S, Sessler D, Sadan O, *et al.* Identification of the epidural space: loss of resistance with air, lidocaine, or the combination of air and lidocaine. *Anesth Analg* 2004; **99**: 245–50.

Howell CJ, Kidd C, Roberts W, *et al.* A randomised controlled trial of epidural compared with non-epidural analgesia in labour. *Br J Obstet Gynaecol* 2001; **108**: 27–33.

Jenkins JG. Some immediate serious complications of obstetric epidural analgesia and anaesthesia: a prospective study of 145,550 epidurals. *Int J Obstet Anesth* 2005; **14**: 37–42.

Pan PH, Bogard TD, Owen MD. Incidence and characteristics of failures in obstetric neuraxial analgesia and anesthesia: a retrospective analysis of 19,259 deliveries. *Int J Obstet Anesth* 2004; **13**: 227–33.

24   EPIDURAL TEST DOSES

The purpose of the epidural test dose is to detect intravenous or subarachnoid placement of the catheter. As such, it must be formulated to produce an easily detected result when in one of these two situations, without compromising the safety of the mother or the fetus.

Problems/special considerations

- As with all screening procedures, the sensitivity and specificity of the test dose are all-important when assessing its ability to protect the mother from the unwanted effects of intravenous or subarachnoid administration. Sensitivity is the ability of the test dose to detect accurately a misplaced catheter; failure to do so represents a false-negative result. Specificity is the ability of the test dose not to produce a false-positive result, i.e. incorrectly alerting the anaesthetist when the catheter is actually in the right place.

- Accidental catheterisation of the epidural veins is common in obstetric practice, since these vessels act as collateral conduits of venous blood from the lower limbs to the heart and are therefore dilated when the inferior vena cava is compressed by the gravid uterus. Venous cannulation occurs about 1 in 20 times and is usually detected before the test dose is given, by the ability to aspirate blood.
- Subarachnoid puncture occurs about 1 in 100 times, with the incidence decreasing as the practitioner becomes more experienced. Again, the vast majority of dural punctures are detected by the free flow of cerebrospinal fluid through the needle or catheter.
- It follows that it is very rare for a test dose to be used in a situation where the catheter is actually intravenous or subarachnoid. This means that, in addition to the sensitivity and specificity of the test, it is also important to know what proportion of positive test results will actually indicate misplacement of the catheter; this is known as the positive predictive value of the test and is often lower than might be expected from the sensitivity and specificity.
- A test dose, designed to improve safety, should not in itself compromise the safety of the mother or fetus. This is a particular problem when trying to detect intravenous placement, as many tests rely on the use of adrenaline to produce tachycardia in these circumstances. Intravenous adrenaline may stress the maternal cardiovascular system and temporarily reduce placental perfusion, so doses must be carefully chosen.
- Although initial confirmation of the correct placement of the epidural catheter is particularly important, the possibility of later catheter migration should not be forgotten. Every top-up given down an epidural catheter that might be dangerous if accidentally injected intravenously or intrathecally should really be regarded as a test dose and should be fractionated if time permits, so as not to produce systemic toxicity or a dangerously high block.
- It is difficult – if not impossible – to design a test dose that will detect subdural, extra-arachnoid placement with any reliability. The possibility of subdural catheterisation must always be borne in mind and suspected when an unusual block pattern emerges.

Management options

Subarachnoid placement

This is relatively easy to detect, and it is only necessary to choose a dose of local anaesthetic that will produce a recognisable but safe block. Lidocaine 45–60 mg or bupivacaine 7.5–12.5 mg is suitable; lidocaine has the advantage of a slightly faster onset of block, but many practitioners prefer bupivacaine on the grounds that this will be the drug used for the main dose. Signs of sensory block in the lower lumbar segments and motor block of the legs should be sought after 3 minutes with lidocaine or 5 minutes with bupivacaine. This test is regarded as close to 100% specific and sensitive.

Intravenous placement

Most tests rely on the use of sympathomimetic drugs to produce changes in maternal heart rate and/or blood pressure when administered intravenously. Adrenaline 15 µg or isoprenaline 5 µg has been recommended for this purpose. Intravenous injection of 3 ml of 1:200 000 adrenaline has been shown to produce a reliable rise in heart rate of 30 beats per minute within 20–40 seconds. However, this type of test is bedevilled by the wide variability of heart rate and blood pressure brought on by the intermittent pain of contractions in labour. Even when an adrenaline-free bupivacaine test dose is used, 12% of patients will demonstrate a rise in heart rate that would count as a positive response. The specificity of this test is low, with a positive predictive value of only 55–73%, and reliance on adrenaline to detect intravenous placement will result in 5–9% of all epidural catheters being removed unnecessarily.

Sensitivity is also low but can be improved by ensuring that the heart rate is measured between contractions and by using the change in peak heart rate (as measured over a 2-minute period before and after the test injection) rather than a simple change from a random baseline rate as the basis of the test.

Subjective symptoms have also been used to detect intravenous placement, and some test dose regimens rely on this. Fentanyl 100 µg produces obvious sensations of drowsiness within 1 minute when given intravenously, and lidocaine 45–60 mg may cause tingling in the perioral region. These methods are far from reliable, however, and the increased sensitivity of pregnant women to local anaesthetic toxicity should always be borne in mind when using the systemic effects of lidocaine as a test.

Finally, 1–2 ml of air has been used as a test for intravenous placement, with a Doppler probe (readily available in the labour suite in the form of a fetal heart monitor) placed over the mother's right ventricle to detect the characteristic sounds of air entering the heart. This is rarely advocated now.

Best practice

Nowhere is the old maxim 'eternal vigilance is the price of safety' more apposite than in the prevention and detection of misplacement of the epidural catheter. Careful aspiration via the catheter before administering a dose of local anaesthetic and a continuous high index of suspicion are vital adjuncts to an effective test dose policy.

No single regimen has been proven to be superior, but a test dose of 3 ml of bupivacaine 0.25% with 1:200 000 adrenaline is often considered the best compromise. This may be too small a dose of bupivacaine to produce obvious spinal anaesthesia if there is accidental subarachnoid injection and may also be unreliable in detecting intravenous injection (see above). Many obstetric anaesthetists therefore recommend abandoning a formal test dose, and instead, fractionating all epidural doses. The current practice of using low concentrations of local anaesthetic (usually 0.1–0.125% bupivacaine) means that accidental intravenous or subarachnoid administration is unlikely to produce any serious adverse maternal or fetal effects.

Midwives should be trained to recognise the early signs of local anaesthetic toxicity and to fractionate all doses to ensure safety if the catheter migrates through a dural tear.

Key points

- A test dose must be safe, with a high sensitivity and specificity; high specificity is difficult to achieve when the condition being sought is uncommon.
- Accidental subarachnoid placement is relatively easy to detect with a test dose.
- Intravenous placement is more difficult to detect and requires the use of a sympathomimetic drug and careful attention to detail when measuring changes in maternal heart rate.
- Subdural placement cannot be reliably detected with a test dose.
- Catheter migration can occur, and every epidural top-up should be regarded as a test dose.
- No test dose regimen is infallible.

FURTHER READING

Birnbach DJ, Chestnut DH. The epidural test dose in obstetric patients: has it outlived its usefulness? *Anesth Analg* 1999; **88**: 971–2.

25   COMBINED SPINAL–EPIDURAL ANALGESIA AND ANAESTHESIA

The combined spinal–epidural (CSE) technique was first described over 60 years ago. Although it is commonly assumed that CSE means a needle-through-needle technique, there are theoretically several ways of instituting CSE:

1. Insertion of an epidural needle into the epidural space, insertion of a long spinal needle through the epidural needle into the subarachnoid space and finally insertion of an epidural catheter through the epidural needle after the spinal needle has been removed. This is the most commonly used technique in the UK.
2. Insertion of an epidural needle (and usually an epidural catheter) into the epidural space followed by separate insertion of a spinal needle into the subarachnoid space, either at the same or at a different lumbar interspace. This is favoured by a minority of UK anaesthetists.
3. Insertion of a spinal needle into the subarachnoid space followed by insertion of an epidural needle and catheter. This is rarely practised.
4. Specialised needles (e.g. the Eldor needle), which consist of an epidural needle with a side channel welded onto it, through which the spinal needle is passed. This has theoretical advantages, but is not in widespread use.

5. The use of a single needle to identify and inject drugs into the epidural space, then advancing it through the dura to make a subarachnoid injection. This is rarely practised today.

CSE offers the certainty and speed of onset of spinal analgesia or anaesthesia and the flexibility and continuity of an epidural catheter. For the needle-through-needle technique, successful aspiration of cerebrospinal fluid (CSF) upon insertion of the spinal needle confirms correct placement of the epidural needle, which may be reassuring in difficult cases.

Problems/special considerations

- Anaesthetists should be entirely familiar with the management of both spinal and epidural analgesic and anaesthetic techniques before considering CSE. Either a needle-through-needle or separate space technique can be used according to the equipment available and the anaesthetist's preference. The separate space technique has the advantage of not requiring special needles but the disadvantage of inflicting two sets of injections upon the woman. The needle-through-needle technique involves only a single injection but requires long (approximately 120 mm) and more expensive spinal needles either singly or as part of specialised CSE kits.
- Any standard Tuohy needle can be used, although most of the leading needle manufacturers produce kits containing specially matched spinal and epidural needles for needle-through-needle CSE. Some of these include locking devices for fixing the two needles together so that once CSF is obtained, the spinal needle cannot move in or out during subarachnoid injection, which might increase the chance of inadequate block; however, these devices may reduce the 'feel' as the spinal needle is advanced through the dura. Typically, an 18 G or 16 G Tuohy needle and a 25 G or 27 G spinal needle are used, as for separate epidural and spinal techniques. It is essential to check that the spinal needle will project beyond the end of the epidural needle by an adequate amount to achieve dural puncture (usually 12–15 mm).

Management options

Analgesia

The use of CSE for labour analgesia varies. Some maternity units employ the technique routinely, others never. The benefits include rapid onset of pain relief (usually within 5 minutes) and absence of significant motor block in most cases. The major disadvantage is the additional potential for complications introduced by deliberate dural puncture. The use of a spinal needle in addition to an epidural needle also adds to the cost of labour analgesia.

The original regimen for the spinal component recommended in the UK was 25 µg of fentanyl and 2.5 mg of bupivacaine (1 ml of 0.25% solution), made up to a volume of 2 ml with saline; further experience has suggested that smaller doses of fentanyl (5–10 µg) may be adequate and that 3–5 ml of the standard 'low-dose' epidural mixture (bupivacaine 0.1% with fentanyl 2 µg/ml) may also be suitable and not require a separate ampoule of fentanyl to be obtained from the locked controlled drug cupboard. These combinations will provide approximately 60–90 minutes' analgesia, in most cases with little motor blockade. (Spinal opioids alone are very rarely used in the UK, although they may be considered in some high-risk women with coexisting medical disease. In the USA sufentanil is widely used.) When further analgesia is needed, a low concentration of bupivacaine with fentanyl is given via the epidural catheter, either by bolus top-ups or an infusion.

Those who do not routinely use CSE analgesia point to the above disadvantages and to the fact that epidural analgesia is usually effective within a few contractions. Many anaesthetists, however, would consider CSE for women who request regional analgesia late in the first stage of labour, or for those needing regional analgesia for instrumental delivery.

Anaesthesia

The use of CSE for Caesarean section combines the speed of onset and reliability of spinal anaesthesia with the ability to extend the block and provide postoperative analgesia through an epidural catheter. There are three different techniques of CSE for Caesarean section:

1. The spinal injection is performed using a 'full' spinal dose of local anaesthetic, and the epidural catheter is used as a back-up in the event of inadequate anaesthesia and also to provide postoperative analgesia.
2. A smaller volume of local anaesthetic (e.g. 1 ml heavy bupivacaine 0.5%) is used intrathecally, with the intention of producing a limited spinal block (usually to about T8–10). Anaesthesia is then extended gradually with local anaesthetic via the epidural catheter. This results in greater haemodynamic stability, which may be advantageous in women with cardiac disease, and a more controllable extent of blockade, which may be beneficial in women with neurological or respiratory disease.
3. A small dose of local anaesthetic (e.g. 1 ml heavy bupivacaine 0.5%) is given intrathecally using a needle-through-needle technique; when the spinal needle is withdrawn approximately 10 ml saline is injected through the epidural needle to extend the height of block suitable for surgery, by compressing the dural sac. The epidural catheter is then placed as usual. Proponents of the 'EVE' (epidural volume extension) technique claim greater cardiovascular stability and less motor block, while those who do not use it claim a greater incidence of perioperative discomfort.

Complications

If specific 'locking' CSE kits are not used, it may be awkward for the inexperienced practitioner to grip the spinal and epidural needles in such a way as to stop the former moving during subarachnoid injection. Possibly as a result of this, or because of the greater time taken to complete the procedure after spinal injection if insertion of the epidural catheter is difficult, it has been claimed that there is a higher failure rate of the subarachnoid component of CSE than with single-shot spinal anaesthesia, but this does not appear to be a problem as experience with the technique is gained.

CSE carries similar risks to both spinal and epidural injection alone. A number of early reports of meningitis following CSE suggested that there might be an increased risk of this complication with CSE compared with a single-shot spinal; however, since CSE is widely used this could equally be an artefact of reporting. There have also been reports of neuropraxia and neurological damage with CSE, presumed to be related to needle length and design. A particular concern relates to the difficulty in identifying the correct lumbar interspace that even experienced anaesthetists may have, and the risk that the chosen level may be above the termination of the spinal cord. In such a case, there should be no extra risk from epidural analgesia in labour, for example, so long as an accidental dural tap does not occur, but if CSE is used, there is a risk of neurological damage from the spinal needle.

It must be remembered that the epidural catheter is untested at the time of insertion, and there is always the risk of an 'epidural' dose passing into the subarachnoid space, as for any epidural catheter – increased perhaps by the presence of a dural hole (though this complication remains a rarity despite widespread usage of CSE). In addition, the physical compressing effect of epidural solutions on the spread of spinal anaesthesia (as in the EVE technique above) means that should the subarachnoid block be inadequate, small boluses ($<5\,\text{ml}$) of local anaesthetic should be used to top up the epidural catheter.

Key points

- Needle-through-needle combined spinal–epidural (CSE) requires only a single injection but is more expensive than separate space techniques.
- CSE analgesia provides pain relief usually within one or two contractions but is a more invasive and complex technique than epidural alone.
- CSE anaesthesia combines the advantages of spinal anaesthesia (speed of onset and quality of anaesthesia) with the ability to extend the level and duration of anaesthesia via the epidural route.

FURTHER READING

Cook TM. Combined spinal-epidural techniques. *Anaesthesia* 2000; **55**: 42–64.

Eisenach JC. Combined spinal-epidural analgesia in obstetrics. *Anesthesiology* 1999; **91**: 299–302.

Rawal N, Van Zundert A, Holmstrom B, Crowhurst JA. Combined spinal epidural technique. *Reg Anesth* 1997; **22**: 406–23.

26 SPINAL ANALGESIA

Single-shot spinal analgesia is rarely used alone for labour since its duration is usually much shorter than that of labour itself. However, it may be useful in the later stages of labour when delivery is felt to be imminent, or to provide rapid onset of analgesia in a mother who is desperate and losing control, thus enabling her to cooperate whilst an epidural catheter is inserted.

Use of an intrathecal catheter to allow repeated boluses (or infusion) of local anaesthetic or other mixtures is an attractive concept, since the advantages of spinal block (rapid onset, profound block) are potentially combined with those of epidural block (flexibility, titrated effect). In practice, however, continuous spinal block is uncommon in the UK although it has its enthusiasts, especially in the case of high-risk mothers in whom sudden drops in systemic vascular resistance are particularly unwelcome.

Problems/special considerations

The main considerations for single-shot spinal analgesia are the risk of postdural puncture headache and the choice of solution, given the requirement for maximal analgesia and minimal motor block and other side effects (see Chapter 26, Combined spinal–epidural analgesia and anaesthesia, p. 63).

Modern intrathecal catheters are very fine (e.g. 28–32 G) and thus may be difficult to handle and insert. They are usually supplied in a kit with a spinal needle; originally these needles had cutting tips, but they are now available with pencil-point tips in an attempt to reduce the incidence of postdural puncture headache. However, even with fine catheters, 22–26 G spinal needles are required. Some catheters include a removable wire to make them stiffer for insertion. A catheter-over-needle kit also exists, in which a 27–29 G needle protrudes from the distal end of a 22–24 G catheter; the catheter is slid over the needle into the subarachnoid space whilst advancement of the needle is prevented by a wire attached to its end.

A continuous catheter technique may also be used with a standard epidural kit (e.g. 16 G or 18 G catheter), either because specialist kits are unavailable or when an accidental dural puncture has occurred during attempted epidural block. A reduced incidence of headache after placement of an intrathecal catheter has been claimed when this is done, possibly related to inflammation around the dural puncture site, which leads to faster healing; however, this is uncertain since evidence is mostly anecdotal.

The main factor that has led to the withdrawal of microspinal catheters in the USA and that has contributed to the technique's unpopularity in the UK is the association between their use and the development of subsequent cauda equina syndrome. This is thought to be caused by a combination of factors, including the use of lidocaine (more common in the USA), the known neurotoxic effect of high concentrations of lidocaine on neural tissue experimentally (more so than bupivacaine), the pooling of drug around the sensitive nerves of the cauda equina associated with very fine catheters placed caudally, and the use of excessive doses of drug in an attempt to extend an inadequately extensive block (resulting in more pooling around the nerves).

Management options

Management after single-shot spinal anaesthesia is discussed elsewhere (see Chapter 35, Spinal anasthesia for caesarean section, p. 90).

For continuous techniques, once the catheter has been inserted, it should be clearly labelled, since accidental injection of an epidural–style dose may be disastrous. For labour analgesia, a standard spinal dose can be given as for a combined spinal–epidural. Subsequent analgesia may be provided with repeated boluses of 0.5–1.5 ml bupivacaine 0.1–0.25% ± fentanyl 10–20 µg as required. Infusions (e.g. 0.1–0.25% bupivacaine ± fentanyl at 1–5 ml/h) have also been used. Unless the technique is commonly used in a particular unit, it is prudent for all top-ups to be given by an anaesthetist, since midwifery and other staff are likely to be unfamiliar with it.

For Caesarean section, incremental doses of bupivacaine ± opioid may be given to achieve the required level of block, as slowly as is felt appropriate for the clinical circumstances.

Whatever the indication, directing the catheter caudally should be avoided, as should repeated injections of concentrated solutions of local anaesthetic if the block is inadequate. Greater than normal doses of local anaesthetic should not be given.

Key points

- Continuous spinal techniques are acceptable (if unpopular) for both labour and operative delivery.
- Advantages include good quality of block, ability to titrate the dose and avoiding the risk of inadvertent total spinal block.
- Disadvantages include difficulty handling the catheters, risk of postdural puncture headache, risk of cauda equina syndrome, cost, and mistaking the catheter for an epidural one.
- Care should be taken to avoid pooling of local anaesthetic around sacral nerve roots.

FURTHER READING

Denny NM, Selander DE. Continuous spinal anaesthesia. *Br J Anaesth* 1998; **81**: 590–7.

Horlocker TT, McGregor DG, Matsushige DK, *et al.* Neurologic complications of 603 consecutive continuous spinal anesthetics using macrocatheter and microcatheter techniques. *Anesth Analg* 1997; **84**: 1063–70.

27 CAUDAL ANALGESIA

The caudal route was the first approach used for epidural analgesia and anaesthesia in childbirth and was described in 1901. It has now been largely superseded by the lumbar route but still has a place, especially to supplement a lumbar block that is deficient sacrally. It is also popular with some anaesthetists for outlet instrumental deliveries, although spinal block is more commonly performed. Finally, it may be a useful route in women who have abnormal lumbar spines, e.g. after back surgery.

Problems/special considerations

The basic technique is no different from that used in non-obstetric patients, although there may be increased fat and fluid deposition over the sacral area associated with pregnancy, which may make the procedure technically more difficult. Insertion of the needle into the head of the fetus has been reported. The caudal route is often avoided in labour because of a perceived increase in the risk of infection, although there is no evidence to support this.

Effects and complications of caudals are similar to those of lumbar blockade, although larger volumes of local anaesthetic are required (e.g. 25–35 ml for boluses). In addition, caudal blocks are less reliable because of the variable anatomy of the sacral canal and the difficulty of extending the block cranially.

Key points

- Caudal analgesia is occasionally used to supplement lumbar epidural block or for outlet instrumental deliveries.
- Techniques similar to those in the non-pregnant population are used.

28 SPINAL AND EPIDURAL OPIOIDS

Epidural opioids have been increasingly widely used in combination with local anaesthetics to provide both labour and post-Caesarean section analgesia. Spinal opioids have also been used to enhance surgical anaesthesia and to provide postoperative analgesia, and more recently to provide analgesia for labour (in combined spinal–epidural techniques). Spinal and epidural opioids alone do not provide adequate pain relief for the late first stage and second stage of labour.

All opioids have significant maternal side effects, ranging from mild nausea to life-threatening respiratory depression. These side effects may occur following administration of opioids by any route, although the published literature has tended to focus on adverse effects associated with neuraxial administration. In the UK, fentanyl is the opioid most commonly used to provide labour analgesia, with diamorphine or fentanyl being used for intra- and postoperative analgesia.

Epidural morphine is less commonly used because of the greater perceived risk of late respiratory depression, although spinal morphine appears to be very safe.

Sufentanil is used widely in the rest of Europe and in North America, but is not available in the UK.

Site of action

Opioids act at the opioid receptors in the substantia gelatinosa of the spinal cord. Drugs injected into the epidural space have to penetrate the dura to reach the site of action. Ease of dural penetration will depend on lipid solubility and molecular weight, with highly lipid-soluble molecules (such as fentanyl) entering the subarachnoid space most readily. Once the opioid has reached the cerebrospinal fluid (CSF), the more lipid-soluble drugs will fix readily in the spinal cord, whereas less lipid-soluble drugs (such as morphine) remain in the CSF and are carried in a cranial direction with CSF flow, reaching the lateral ventricles in about 6 hours. This accounts for the slow onset of action, higher incidence of nausea, vomiting and pruritus, and late respiratory depression seen with morphine.

The epidural space is highly vascular in the pregnant woman, and there is significant systemic uptake of epidurally administered opioids (with similar blood concentration curves to those seen after parenteral administration). In addition, some opioid is bound to fat in the epidural space and does not reach the spinal cord. The ratio of epidural to spinal dose of opioid is thus in the order of 5–10:1.

Commonly used epidural and spinal bolus doses are:
- Fentanyl: epidural 50–100 µg, spinal 15–25 µg
- Diamorphine: epidural 2–3 mg, spinal 0.2–0.5 mg
- Morphine: epidural 3–4 mg, spinal 0.075–0.1 mg.

Benefits

Several studies have confirmed that epidural administration of opioids alone provides analgesia for early labour but is inadequate for the later stages of labour. However, the combination of local anaesthetic and opioid is synergistic. This is clearly advantageous, allowing improved quality of analgesia, reduced consumption of local anaesthetic, reduced motor block and reduction in opioid side effects.

Typical combinations used are:
- 0.1% Bupivacaine with fentanyl 2 µg/ml
- 0.0625% Bupivacaine with fentanyl 2.5 µg/ml.

Improved maternal mobility may increase maternal satisfaction with labour analgesia, although studies have so far failed to demonstrate significant improvement in rates of spontaneous vaginal delivery. The mechanism of local anaesthetic/opioid synergy is unclear.

Epidural and intrathecal opioids are claimed to provide superior postoperative analgesia, although there are so many variables involved and different measures of analgesic outcome that it is difficult to assess this reliably.

Side effects

Side effects of both epidural and intrathecal opioids are dose dependent and are more severe for less lipophilic drugs such as morphine. With the exception of urinary retention (which is not dose related), all the side effects seen after neuraxial administration of opioids may occur following parenteral administration (although itching is common only when opioids are given epidurally or intrathecally). A unique side effect is the potential for reactivation of herpes simplex labialis 2–5 days after the epidural administration of morphine. Several theories have been proposed, but the exact mechanism is uncertain.

Use of an opioid receptor antagonist such as naloxone reliably reverses the side effects of epidural and intrathecal opioids, but reversal of analgesia may occur. This has encouraged symptomatic treatment of individual side effects, typically using antihistamines such as chlorphenamine 4 mg orally or 10 mg parenterally. Low doses of propofol (10 mg) and ondansetron have been reported to reduce opioid-induced itching but the evidence for benefit is inconclusive.

Respiratory depression

Fentanyl has the shortest duration of action following epidural or subarachnoid administration (approximately 4 hours) and the lowest potential to cause respiratory depression, although cases have been reported. Epidural morphine is well recognised as being associated with a small risk of respiratory depression for up to 12–24 hours after administration, but will also provide analgesia for a similar period of time. Diamorphine has an intermediate duration of action and there have been no reported cases of delayed respiratory depression, although early cases have occurred – usually in combination with other sedatives.

The potential for this life-threatening side effect of centrally administered opioids has led to a general prohibition on the concomitant use of opioid and sedative drugs by any other route. It has also caused considerable controversy about the intensity and duration of monitoring and nursing care required for patients who have received epidural or spinal opioids. Respiratory depression manifests itself as increasing sedation (due to carbon dioxide retention) rather than reduced respiratory rate; therefore in the absence of facilities for prolonged high-dependency nursing (which few obstetric units possess), it is sensible to nurse the mother in a postnatal bed that can be readily observed from the central nursing station, and in the company of other mothers, rather than in a side room. Many obstetric anaesthetists consider that the small but real risks of late respiratory depression associated with epidural morphine outweigh the benefits of using it in preference to diamorphine or fentanyl, although there are many studies confirming the safety of spinal morphine.

If respiratory depression occurs it is important to use either repeated doses or an infusion of naloxone to reverse it, because of the prolonged action of the opioid compared with its antagonist.

Gastric emptying

This is delayed after epidural or intrathecal boluses of opioids, although there is some evidence that low-dose infusions of fentanyl do not impair gastric emptying.

Placental transfer

Although centrally administered opioids cross the placenta, this occurs in a dose-dependent manner. Administration of an epidural bolus of fentanyl 100 µg 20 minutes before delivery results in umbilical artery concentrations well below those needed to cause neonatal respiratory depression. Similarly, although opioids can be found in breast milk after maternal epidural administration, the amounts are negligible.

Key points

- There is synergy between neuraxial opioids and local anaesthetics.
- Side effects occur following all routes of administration.
- Side effects are dose dependent, with the exception of urinary retention.
- Reactivation of herpes simplex may occur following administration of epidural morphine.
- Morphine has a slower onset, longer duration of action and increased incidence of side effects compared with fentanyl; the action of diamorphine is intermediate.

FURTHER READING

Boyle RK. A review of the anatomical and immunological links between epidural morphine and herpes simplex labialis in obstetric patients. *Anaesth Intens Care* 1995; **23**: 425–32.

Chaney MA. Side effects of intrathecal and epidural opioids. *Can J Anaesth* 1995; **42**: 891–903.

de Leon-Casasola OA, Lema MJ. Postoperative epidural opioid analgesia: what are the choices? *Anesth Analg* 1996; **83**: 867–75.

29   INHALATIONAL ANALGESIC DRUGS

The most commonly used agent for inhaled analgesia in the UK is Entonox, which is a mixture of 50% nitrous oxide and 50% oxygen. Its advantages are that it is inexpensive, is almost universally available (including for use in the community), has a long record of safety, and is acceptable to many mothers and midwives. Its low blood solubility means that blood levels rapidly reach a maximum after inhalation and fall once a contraction has passed and inhalation has ceased. It does not appear to have any detrimental effect on the fetus. The main disadvantage of Entonox is that it provides only limited pain relief. In addition, some mothers are phobic about the use of 'gas'.

Volatile anaesthetic agents such as methoxyflurane and trichloroethylene have been used for analgesia in labour, but these drugs have been withdrawn for non-obstetric reasons. They were administered using a draw-over vaporiser and breathing system and provided analgesia of slow onset because of their high blood solubility, with residual effects between contractions. Other volatile agents, more recently sevoflurane, have also been studied, but none are widely used. A premixed preparation of isoflurane and Entonox (Isoxane) has been described but this too is not widely available.

Problems/special considerations

- Nitrous oxide is a relatively weak analgesic, helping 30–50% of mothers who use it. Use of more than 50% nitrous oxide improves analgesic efficacy, but at the cost of increased maternal sedation and decreased inspired concentration of maternal oxygen. The use of the 50:50 mixture of nitrous oxide and oxygen represents a compromise between analgesic efficacy and maternal and fetal safety.
- Entonox is presented as a premixed agent, available in cylinders for community use and piped from central tanks in hospital maternity units. The mixture is stable under most conditions, but at very low temperatures the constituent gases separate out. This is relevant for community midwives practising in parts of the UK in winter, who must be aware that they need to invert Entonox cylinders several times before use to ensure adequate mixing. The mother administers the gas to herself from a demand valve via either facemask or mouthpiece. Maternal sedation may occur even with 50% nitrous oxide, and it is therefore important that, in order to avoid the risk of aspiration, Entonox is self-administered, not administered by the midwife or by the woman's partner.
- Some mothers find inhalation of dry gases unpleasant, and in asthmatics this may provoke bronchospasm. Entonox also causes unacceptable nausea in a small number of women.
- The efficacy of Entonox can be improved by instructing the mother to start inhaling as soon as she becomes aware of a contraction, and to continue inhalation until the contraction subsides. It is also important to ensure that if a facemask is used it is applied snugly to the face to avoid entraining air.
- Although Entonox crosses the placenta readily, it is excreted by the neonatal lungs after delivery. Entonox does not have adverse effects on the fetus, but the maternal hyperventilation associated with its use may cause placental vasoconstriction and impair fetal oxygenation in an already compromised fetus. Similarly, the combination of pethidine and Entonox has been associated with a high incidence of maternal arterial oxygen desaturation and should be avoided if there is evidence of fetal compromise.
- There has been recent concern about the pollutant effects of Entonox. Many labour wards do not have any means of scavenging exhaled Entonox, and this is increasingly considered unacceptable. Scavenging equipment is available but obviously has resource implications.

- Volatile anaesthetic agents cause dose-dependent uterine relaxation, although this can be overcome at low concentrations by oxytoxic drugs. They also have cardiorespiratory side effects, although these are usually minimal at low concentrations.

Key points

- Entonox provides acceptable (but incomplete) analgesia to up to half of the mothers who use it. It is appropriate for low-risk mothers in uncomplicated labour and for mothers awaiting regional analgesia.
- Entonox should not be recommended for either high-risk mothers or as a supplement to inadequate systemic analgesia.

FURTHER READING

Yentis SM, Clyburn P. The use of Entonox™ for labour pain should be abandoned. *Int J Obstet Anesth* 2001; **10**: 25–9.

30   SYSTEMIC ANALGESIC DRUGS

A variety of opioid analgesics have been used in the UK to reduce the pain of labour, and none have been found adequate for the majority of mothers. Pethidine is the most commonly used systemic analgesic in England and Wales, whereas in Scotland diamorphine is also common. Shorter acting opioids such as fentanyl, alfentanil and remifentanil have also been used. All opioid analgesics, given in equianalgesic doses, have similar advantages and disadvantages, and the widespread use of pethidine is largely historical.

The major advantages of systemic opioid analgesia for labour are ease of administration, low cost, midwife autonomy of use and acceptability by many mothers. The major disadvantages of systemic opioid analgesia for labour are failure to provide adequate analgesia for many women, general opioid side effects for the mother and rapid placental transfer to the fetus.

Problems/special considerations

Dosage and administration

- Midwives in the UK are authorised to give a total of 200 mg pethidine to a labouring mother, provided that the dose is divided, without a doctor's prescription. It is common practice to give 100 mg intramuscularly as the first dose. Blood levels of pethidine following intramuscular injection are unpredictable, and it is not possible reliably to achieve therapeutic levels with this standardised approach to administration. There is also little correlation between the weight of the mother, the amount of pethidine given and subsequent plasma concentration of pethidine.

Intravenous administration of pethidine, either by medical staff or as patient-controlled analgesia (PCA; e.g. 10–20 mg with a lockout of 10 min), is more likely to achieve therapeutic plasma concentrations of the drug, but the intramuscular route remains the most commonly used.

- Diamorphine is also used in some units, in doses of 5.0–7.5 mg intramuscularly. Diamorphine is claimed to be more effective than pethidine, but direct comparisons are few.
- Fentanyl has been used intravenously to provide labour analgesia. Use of bolus doses of 20–50 μg at least 5–6 minutes apart has been reported to cause less neonatal depression than intravenous boluses of pethidine (25–50 mg). The general risks and benefits of opioid analgesics in labour apply, although severe neonatal depression is uncommon.
- Use of intravenous alfentanil via PCA has been described but is rare.
- Remifentanil offers theoretical advantages for PCA in labour (very rapid onset of action and ultra-short half-life); furthermore, studies suggest that fetal/neonatal effects are few since the drug is rapidly metabolised after crossing the placenta. However, maternal side effects may still occur, necessitating close monitoring, and the efficacy of remifentanil is still questionable, as for all opioids. Doses of 30–50 μg have been used with a lockout of 2 minutes.

Side effects

These are common to all opioid drugs. Maternal side effects include:

- Altered respiratory pattern – hypoventilation occurs between contractions, but inadequate analgesia is accompanied by hyperventilation during contractions
- Reduced gastric motility
- Nausea and vomiting
- Sedation, dysphoria and euphoria
- Muscle rigidity may occur after remifentanil.

Drugs such as promethazine and promazine are still frequently administered with pethidine in an attempt to reduce the incidence of nausea and vomiting, and these drugs considerably enhance the sedative effects of pethidine, sometimes to the extent that the mother has no clear recall of the events surrounding delivery.

All opioids cross the placenta freely; fetal effects include:

- Loss of heart rate variability – the typical 'flat' cardiotocographic trace that results may make interpretation of any other changes difficult
- Neonatal respiratory depression, especially if given within 2–4 hours of delivery for pethidine or diamorphine (reversible with naloxone, although it is important to remember that naloxone is a short-acting drug and may need to be given either as an infusion or in repeated boluses)

- Depression of neonatal neurobehavioural scores for up to 3 days – the significance of this is not clear
- Lower likelihood of successful breastfeeding in babies whose mothers have received pethidine in labour, although there may be other psychosocial factors relevant to these findings.

Pethidine has a long-acting metabolite, norpethidine, which accumulates in both the mother and fetus and has significant opioid activity. Its half-life is 21 hours in the mother and 63 hours in the fetus, compared with 3–7 hours and 13–23 hours respectively for pethidine. Norpethidine also has proconvulsant activity, and therefore on theoretical grounds pethidine is not an ideal analgesic for women with epilepsy or pre-eclampsia.

Management options

The advantages of intramuscular opioid analgesia (simplicity of administration, low cost and acceptability to many midwives and mothers) have to be balanced against the disadvantages for both mother and baby, and the fact that the quality of analgesia is generally poor, although it may be useful in very early labour or pre-labour. For mothers with significant medical disease and those at increased risk of operative delivery, regional analgesia is usually preferable. However, women unable to have regional analgesia (e.g. those with coagulation disorders) may benefit from PCA as an alternative.

Women receiving systemic opioid analgesia should be considered at risk of gastric stasis and advised accordingly regarding oral intake. Concurrent administration of H_2-antagonists should also be considered. In some units, metoclopramide is given concurrently to women receiving opioids as a non-sedating antiemetic.

Key points

- Pethidine is the most commonly used opioid analgesic for labour in the UK.
- Other opioids have similar risks and benefits.
- Patient-controlled analgesia may improve efficacy and reduce side effects.
- Systemic opioid analgesia is not advisable for women at increased risk of operative delivery.
- Routine administration of antacid prophylaxis to women receiving systemic opioid analgesia is advisable.
- Neonatal respiratory depression and impaired neurobehavioural scores may follow maternal administration of opioids.

FURTHER READING

Bricker L, Lavender T. Parenteral opioids for labor pain relief: a systematic review. *Am J Obstet Gynecol* 2002; **186**: S94–109.

Littleford J. Effects on the fetus and newborn of maternal analgesia and anesthesia: a review. *Can J Anaesth* 2004; **51**: 586–609.

Volmanen P, Alahuhta S. Will remifentanil be a labour analgesic? *Int J Obstet Anesth* 2004; **13**: 1–4.

31 NON-PHARMACOLOGICAL ANALGESIA

Many women wish to avoid intervention in labour, including use of pharmacological methods of analgesia. The use of psychoprophylaxis ('childbirth without fear') dates from the 1950s, and since that time a variety of relaxation techniques have been introduced. More recently, relaxation techniques, self-hypnosis, acupuncture, aromatherapy, reflexology and water labour and birth have become more common. The availability of transcutaneous electrical nerve stimulation (TENS) for labour analgesia is now widespread.

Problems/special considerations

Fear of the unknown is a major factor in the experience of pain. Provision of antenatal education about the process of labour and the common complications that occur is an essential first step in provision of analgesia for labour. Translations of information leaflets and availability of interpreters must be considered, especially in units delivering a significant number of women for whom English is not their first language. It is desirable to have an independent translator rather than a family member whenever possible. Videos about pain relief in labour are readily available and provide information in a format that is familiar and accessible to the majority of the population. Attendance at parentcraft classes should be encouraged.

Relaxation techniques

These range from simple breathing exercises to formal yoga techniques. There is a vast range of literature in the lay press about such techniques. The association between tension, anxiety and pain is well recognised, and the use of relaxation techniques should be encouraged for all pregnant women.

Self-hypnosis

Practitioners of hypnosis differentiate between a hypnotic state and deep relaxation. Hypnosis has been successfully used not only for pain relief in labour but also to provide anaesthesia for Caesarean section. There seems little doubt about the efficacy of the technique in well-motivated women, but hypnosis is time consuming, requires considerable antenatal preparation and is not freely available to the majority of women.

Acupuncture, aromatherapy and reflexology

Acupuncture has much evidence to support its use in certain areas of medicine, but properly conducted studies in obstetric practice are rare. What evidence there is mostly concerns manual acupuncture and suggests a beneficial effect on pain and analgesic requirements in labour.

Practitioners of aromatherapy and reflexology are becoming more numerous, and include an increasing number of midwives. The usefulness of such analgesic techniques is dependent on the availability of a practitioner. Many women gain considerable emotional support and satisfaction as well as analgesia from these forms of pain relief, and there is no reason to discourage their use in women who are in normal labour.

Water

The use of the birthing pool has become increasingly popular since the 1980s. Enthusiasts for the pool claim reduced rates of virtually all forms of medical intervention in labour, whereas some obstetricians view the pool as an unnecessary additional hazard for the labouring mother. The evidence regarding the first stage of labour suggests a reduction in labour pain and analgesic requirements with no effect on outcome of labour or neonatal status.

For decades mothers have been advised to have warm baths to help them relax in early labour, and use of the pool for labour analgesia is an extension of this advice. Women who have had a lot of back pain during pregnancy often find the birthing pool particularly helpful. Continuous fetal monitoring is not possible in a birthing pool, and therefore the mother with an at-risk fetus should be advised against using the pool. Similarly, the use of the pool is inadvisable in mothers needing intravenous infusions or any form of continuous maternal monitoring. Mothers requesting pharmacological analgesia should be asked to leave the birthing pool.

TENS

Transcutaneous electrical nerve stimulators have been used for chronic pain for many years and their use in labour is now also common. Particular benefit is claimed for women with 'backache labour' associated with a posterior position and for women with a prolonged latent phase of labour.

The advantage of TENS is the absence of any effect on the fetus and the lack of any significant side effects for the mother. Meta-analysis of randomised controlled trials of TENS in labour does not confirm its efficacy, but it has a high degree of acceptance by mothers and midwives and at least may delay requests for systemic or regional analgesia.

Doulas

It is recognised that the constant presence of a supportive and encouraging second person reduces the pain scores of women in labour. Some cultures ban the father from the labour room and provide a female partner for the labouring woman. There has been a resurgence of interest in use of birth partners, or doulas, in both the USA and the UK. The constant presence of the midwife during labour is also thought to reduce demand for analgesia and other interventions.

Management options

Anaesthetists should be aware of the benefits and limitations of non-pharmacological analgesia and be able to advise mothers when use of these methods of pain relief is or is not appropriate. It is important that anaesthetists realise that maternal satisfaction with pain relief in labour is not necessarily related to the degree of analgesia obtained.

Non-pharmacological methods of pain relief have the major advantage of minimal or absent fetal and maternal adverse effects, and as such their use by mothers in normal, uncomplicated labour should be encouraged. Prolonged use of these methods of pain relief by mothers with pregnancy or labour complications may increase the risk of ultimate recourse to general anaesthesia for delivery. For this group of women a change from non-pharmacological to regional analgesia is advisable.

Key points

- Although evidence for the efficacy of non-pharmacological methods of analgesia is not strong, many women request them.
- Antenatal education should include all methods of analgesia available in a particular unit.

FURTHER READING

Carroll D, Tramer M, McQuay H, Nye B, Moore A. TENS in labour pain: a systematic review. *Br J Obstet Gynaecol* 1997; **104**: 169–75.

Cluett ER, Nikodem VC, McCandlish RE, Burns EE. Immersion in water in pregnancy, labour and birth. *Cochrane Database Syst Rev* 2004; (**2**): CD000111.

Cyna AM, McAuliffe GL, Andrew MI. Hypnosis for pain relief in labour and childbirth: a systematic review. *Br J Anaesth* 2004; **93**: 505–11.

Lee H, Ernst E. Acupuncture for labor pain management: A systematic review. *Am J Obstet Gynecol* 2004; **191**: 1573–9.

III   Operative delivery and third stage

32   INSTRUMENTAL DELIVERY

Vaginal delivery may be facilitated by the use of forceps or a suction cup (ventouse). Forceps deliveries can be divided into outlet, low, mid-cavity or high (rotational), although high forceps deliveries are in decline in many centres in favour of Caesarean section.

In the UK, approximately 10% of deliveries are performed with forceps or ventouse, but the figure is very variable in different units and is greatly affected by individual policies with respect to the maximum allowable duration of the second stage, the use of Syntocinon to augment contractions and criteria for Caesarean section.

In general, instrumental delivery can be indicated by maternal factors (exhaustion, failure to descend, illness precluding Valsalva manoeuvre) or fetal factors (fetal distress, prematurity). The commonest indication is prolongation of the second stage, often defined as longer than 2 hours for a primigravida (3 hours with an effective epidural), or one hour for a multigravida (2 hours with an epidural).

Problems/special considerations

Analgesia

Analgesia produced by low-dose epidural solutions may be adequate for low-outlet ('lift-out') forceps or ventouse delivery, but mid- or high-cavity forceps delivery requires dense surgical anaesthesia. A good pelvic block is essential, and the perineum should be tested before inserting the instrument. For anything other than an outlet forceps or ventouse, the sensory block should extend up to T10. Although it is common practice in many centres for the anaesthetist to anticipate the need for forceps delivery by writing up a single dose of 0.25–0.5% bupivacaine to be given by the midwife if needed, it is better for the anaesthetist to be present when anything other than the most straightforward instrumental delivery is being performed. Mothers now anticipate that instrumental delivery should be as pain free as Caesarean section under regional analgesia, and are proving increasingly litigious if this is not the case.

Analgesia, Anaesthesia and Pregnancy: A Practical Guide Second Edition, ed. Steve Yentis, Anne May and Surbhi Malhotra. Published by Cambridge University Press. © Cambridge University Press 2007.

Trial of forceps

When it is anticipated that instrumental delivery may be difficult, provision should be made for immediate conversion to Caesarean section. The procedure should be carried out in the operating theatre and regional anaesthesia should be adequate for rapid operative delivery.

Aftercare

It should be remembered that the extensive episiotomy that usually accompanies instrumental delivery, coupled with the inevitable tissue trauma, often results in significant pain in the immediate postpartum period. Non-steroidal anti-inflammatory drugs should be used prophylactically if there are no contraindications, and epidural opioids may be required. Postpartum haemorrhage can result from cervical or vaginal tears.

Instrumental delivery and regional analgesia

There is no doubt that, in most centres, there is a higher rate of instrumental delivery in mothers who opt for regional analgesia. Although it is very difficult to exclude potential confounders (e.g. it is likely that women who need epidural analgesia are those with other factors that predispose to instrumental delivery, such as slow progress, malpresentation, multiple gestation, relative cephalopelvic disproportion etc.) a causal link cannot be excluded. This must be weighed against the improved quality of analgesia compared with alternatives, the beneficial effect of epidural analgesia on fetal acid–base balance, and the ability to avoid general anaesthesia in many cases should Caesarean section be required.

Management options

For deliveries other than outlet forceps and ventouse, with a functioning epidural *in situ*, it is an easy matter to intensify the block by administering a solution such as 10 ml of 0.25–0.5% bupivacaine. Pelvic spread may be encouraged by sitting the mother up, and it is therefore important to establish the block before putting the legs into stirrups. A small dose of fentanyl may help to provide perineal analgesia if spread is recalcitrant.

Where no epidural is in place, spinal anaesthesia is most appropriate, using a dose in the region of 1.5 ml of hyperbaric 0.5% bupivacaine in the sitting position, $\pm$ 10–15 µg fentanyl. Other than in exceptional circumstances, general anaesthesia should not be used, since it does not allow the mother to cooperate by pushing at the right time and is an excessively invasive approach for a relatively minor procedure.

Pudendal block may be performed by the obstetrician if there is no anaesthetist available or if the mother is already prepared in the lithotomy position. The technique has considerable drawbacks, however, having a high failure rate and needing at least 10–20 minutes to become effective. Pudendal block may also be used to supplement an existing epidural with sacral sparing, and infiltration of the perineum with local anaesthetic is a useful adjunctive technique before performing an episiotomy.

In all cases, care must be taken to ensure that aortocaval compression is avoided, e.g. by tilting the mother's pelvis with a wedge.

Key points

- A good pelvic block is essential and should be confirmed by testing.
- Conversion to Caesarean section may be required.
- Anaesthesia should be established before elevating the legs.

FURTHER READING

Liu EH, Sia AT. Rates of caesarean section and instrumental vaginal delivery in nulliparous women after low concentration epidural infusions or opioid analgesia: systematic review. *BMJ* 2004; **328**: 1410–12.

33   CAESAREAN SECTION

The Caesarean section (CS) rate in the UK in 2004–5 was ~23% (about one-third 'elective' – see below), though with wide regional variation. There has been general concern over the increasing CS rates in most developed countries and the associated complications, notwithstanding the benefits that CS might also have in individual cases. Since CS is such an important procedure in obstetrics, and anaesthetic-related maternal deaths commonly involve emergency CS, it is important that obstetric anaesthetists have an understanding of the practical aspects relating to obstetric indications and techniques.

Classification and delivery time

Traditionally, CS has been classified as elective (i.e. a date is given beforehand) or emergency (the rest). The latter group is thought by many obstetricians and obstetric anaesthetists to be too broad, since it includes cases in which immediate delivery is required (e.g. severe fetal compromise or cord prolapse) as well as cases in which there is little urgency (e.g. early spontaneous labour in a mother with a breech scheduled for elective CS the next day). This has led to reclassification of CS into four grades (Table 33.1); this classification has been adopted by all the major UK bodies involved in this field. Although intended as an audit tool (e.g. to monitor outcomes and allocation of staff), the classification has been used to guide management (e.g. second operating theatre opened for grade-1 cases). However, attempts to link the grades to acceptable maximum times to delivery (e.g. 15 min for grade 1) are hampered by the unwillingness of obstetricians to commit themselves to 'acceptable' delays for grades 2 and 3 in

Table 33.1. Classification of Caesarean section

1   Immediate threat to life of woman or fetus
2   Maternal or fetal compromise which is not immediately life-threatening
3   Needing early delivery but no maternal or fetal compromise
4   At a time to suit the woman and maternity team

N.B. applies to the time of decision to operate; e.g. an episode of fetal compromise caused by aortocaval compression responding to therapy, followed some hours later by Caesarean section for failure to progress, would be graded as 3, not 2. Similarly, a case booked as an elective procedure for malpresentation could eventually be classified as grade 3 if the mother goes into labour before the chosen date of surgery. Also applies whether or not the woman is in labour.

case of a bad outcome. In addition, maximum times to delivery are controversial and not based on good science: the often quoted maximum of 15–30 minutes for fetal compromise is derived largely from work in the 1960s in which animal fetuses were exposed to varying durations of intrauterine hypoxia and the degree of subsequent fetal damage assessed. Most cases of cerebral palsy are now known to be related to factors arising before labour. A number of audits within maternity units have found that meeting the particular standard set is extremely difficult to achieve in practice because of delays at each stage of the process (e.g. calling the anaesthetist/anaesthetic assistant, moving the mother to the operating theatre, preparing the surgical equipment, etc.). Finally, the defined time period itself varies: the time from decision to skin incision; from decision to delivery; and from informing the anaesthetist to skin incision or delivery have all been quoted in various recommendations or guidelines.

More recently, analysis of data from the Royal College of Obstetricians and Gynaecologists' Sentinel audit of CS in the UK suggests that poorer maternal and neonatal outcomes are associated with decision-to-delivery intervals exceeding 75 minutes, but not intervals of 31–75 minutes. Nevertheless, 30 minutes has repeatedly been recommended as an 'audit standard'.

Indications

CS may be performed for the benefit of the mother, the fetus or both (Table 33.2), although in practice maternal indications will ultimately affect the fetus adversely if not relieved, and vice versa. For elective CS, 39 weeks is commonly chosen as the optimum gestation, reflecting a balance between the benefit to the neonate of a longer gestation and the greater risk of spontaneous labour and emergency surgery.

Procedure

For lower segment CS, skin incision is usually low transverse (i.e. in the L1 dermatome) but may be midline. Once exposed, the rectus sheath is split longitudinally

Table 33.2. Indications for Caesarean section

Previous Caesarean section
Elective
Following trial of labour
Other
Maternal disease
Worsening pre-existing disease, e.g. cardiac
Associated with pregnancy, e.g. pre-eclampsia
Placenta praevia or abruption
Maternal exhaustion/choice
Obstructed labour/failure to progress
Malpositions
Multiple pregnancy
Fetal compromise
Cord prolapse

and stretched laterally and the peritoneum incised. The uterus is incised transversely in its thin lower segment. A 'classical' CS involves a midline incision, and the uterus is incised longitudinally in its upper segment. Classical CS is associated with a greater risk of haemorrhage, infection and ileus but is quicker to perform and easier than lower segment CS. It may be indicated if the lower segment is poorly formed (e.g. in premature delivery), or in placenta praevia, transverse/unstable lie or uterine fibroids.

Uterine incision is accompanied by removal by suction of amniotic fluid if the membranes have not ruptured (mothers and partners may find the noise alarming if unexpected). Delivery of the baby may be difficult if the head has descended well into the pelvis, and may require forceps. If the placenta has already started to separate, the uterus may contract around the baby's head; increased inspired concentration of volatile agent has been used to relax the uterus during general anaesthesia; glyceryl trinitrate 50–100 μg intravenously or sublingually, repeated as necessary, has also been used to good effect.

The time between induction of general anaesthesia and delivery (I–D interval) may affect fetal wellbeing since, if very short, the induction agent may be present in the fetus at high levels; if the interval is very long, fetal accumulation of inhalational agents may occur. The time from uterine incision to delivery (U–D interval) is thought to be more important, since placental disruption may occur once the uterus is incised; fetal acidosis is unlikely if the U–D interval is less than 3 minutes.

Following delivery of the baby, oxytocin is given (5 U slowly intravenously). Rapid injection of larger doses may cause severe tachycardia and may be no more effective than smaller doses. Uterine contraction may be aided by vigorous rubbing of the uterus; an oxytocin infusion may be required (e.g. 40 U in 500 ml saline at 100 ml/h), especially after prolonged augmented labour, multiple delivery, in the presence of polyhydramnios and with a previous history of postpartum haemorrhage or multiple deliveries.

Once the baby and placenta have been delivered, the uterus is checked for tears and sutured. Many obstetricians prefer the ease of access conferred by exteriorising the uterus, although this may be accompanied by discomfort and nausea/vomiting during regional anaesthesia, bradycardia and increased incidence of air embolism. The obstetrician should always check with the anaesthetists before performing this manoeuvre.

Problems/special considerations

- Surgical problems relating to the procedure itself include difficulty caused by adhesions (especially following previous CS or other abdominal surgery), haemorrhage, surgical trauma to the baby, difficulty delivering the baby with the risk of fetal hypoxia or physical trauma, difficulty delivering the placenta and damage to neighbouring structures. There may be large veins on the anterior wall of the uterus and wide transverse incisions may extend to the uterine angles when the baby is delivered, leading to severe bleeding. Usual blood loss is ~400–700 ml (increased with general anaesthesia) but is notoriously difficult to estimate accurately. There is an increased risk of placenta accreta in women who have had previous CS, especially if the placenta overlies the previous scar. Overall the risk of further surgery is increased from ~3 per 10 000 after CS to ~50 per 10 000 after vaginal delivery, with the risk of hysterectomy increased from 1–2 per 10 000 to up to 80 per 10 000 (though it isn't clear how much the reason for CS may also influence the need for further surgery).
- Anaesthetic problems include those of general or regional anaesthesia generally. Pain during CS under regional anaesthesia has replaced awareness under general anaesthesia as the main reason for litigation associated with CS. Chest pain and/ or electrocardiographic changes may occur; their cause is unknown (although small air emboli or coronary artery/oesophageal spasm has been suggested) and they may occur independently of each other. Elevations of maternal troponin I levels have also been reported. Shoulder-tip pain may occasionally occur, probably related to blood irritating the diaphragm. Other possible problems related to the procedure include air or amniotic fluid embolism and allergic phenomena.
- Postoperative problems are as for any surgery and include infection (prophylactic antibiotics have been shown to reduce infection and should be given) and thromboembolism (heparin is given prophylactically to women at high risk in some units and to all women in others). If the former, the Royal College of Obstetricians and Gynaecologists' guidelines should be followed. National Institute of Clinical Excellence guidelines suggest that observations (including assessment of pain and sedation) should be half-hourly for 2 hours after CS, then 1–2 hourly.

Management options

The choice of anaesthetic technique depends on the degree of urgency, whether an epidural catheter is already in place, specific obstetric (e.g. complicated surgery anticipated) or anaesthetic (e.g. known difficult intubation, previous back surgery) factors, the personal preference of the anaesthetist and the wishes of the mother (see Chapters 34–36). Absolute figures are unavailable, but it is thought that >90% of CS are performed under regional anaesthesia in the UK, reflecting the above preferences and the widely perceived greater safety of regional over general anaesthesia for CS. Particular concerns are the possibly inadequate exposure of anaesthetic trainees to general anaesthesia for CS, the greater tendency of trainees to use general anaesthesia (especially for emergency CS) than more experienced consultants, and the anxiety caused when this occurs. There is also concern that the incidence of failed intubation in obstetrics is increasing and that this may be related to the above factors.

Key points

- Caesarean section rate in the UK is ~23%.
- Indications may be maternal, fetal or both.
- Complications include shoulder-tip, abdominal or chest pain, air or amniotic fluid embolism, haemorrhage, surgical trauma and awareness.

FURTHER READING

Lucas DN, Yentis SM, Kinsella SM, et al. Urgency of Caesarean section: a new classification. J R Soc Med 2000; **93**: 346–50.

National Institute for Clinical Excellence. *Clinical guideline 13: caesarean section.* London: NICE 2004.

Shibli KU, Russell IF. A survey of anaesthetic techniques used for caesarean section in the UK in 1997. *Int J Obstet Anesth* 2000; **9**: 160–7.

Yentis SM. Whose distress is it anyway? 'Fetal distress' and the 30-minute rule. *Anaesthesia* 2003; **58**: 732–3.

34   EPIDURAL ANAESTHESIA FOR CAESAREAN SECTION

Although no longer the technique of choice for elective Caesarean section, the popularity of epidural analgesia for pain relief in labour means that many women presenting for emergency Caesarean section have an epidural *in situ*. A greater understanding of methods to enhance the speed of onset and quality of epidural block has reduced the need for general anaesthesia in this group of mothers; extension of the block is the technique of choice, unless epidural analgesia during labour has been of poor quality or there is a very urgent indication for delivery within 5–10 minutes.

Problems/special considerations

- Poor block with breakthrough pain is more common than with spinal anaesthesia, and a careful assessment of block is therefore particularly important in this group. Whereas in spinal anaesthesia it is reasonable to assume that the block is consistent between the upper and lower limits, this is not the case with an epidural. The block should be 'mapped out' to ensure that there are no missed segments or patchy areas and the extent of block carefully recorded. The mother must be warned of the risk of pain before starting the procedure, and the anaesthetist should be prepared to supplement the block with further top-ups, intravenous analgesia or even general anaesthesia. Pain during Caesarean section is the commonest failure cited in negligence suits against obstetric anaesthetists in the UK.
- Hypotension is slower in onset and normally less severe than with spinal anaesthesia, but vasoconstrictors are still frequently required, and great care should be taken to avoid aortocaval compression.
- The possibility of migration of the epidural catheter, whether into the subdural, intrathecal or intravenous compartments, must be borne in mind, especially when large, concentrated doses of local anaesthetic are being used. Doses should be fractionated or given by slow injection and the level of block regularly checked. It is unacceptable to leave a mother for any reason once the process of establishing the block has started.

Management options

Suitability of the technique

Unlike spinal anaesthesia, the operation cannot be started as fast as if general anaesthesia is used. In the true emergency, therefore, such as massive placental abruption or prolapsed cord, spinal or general anaesthesia remains the technique of choice. Having said this, the use of a bolus dose of 15–20 ml concentrated solution (e.g. bupivacaine 0.5% or lidocaine 2%) over 2–3 minutes can convert a moderate T10 block to a block suitable for surgery within about 10–15 minutes in most cases. Use of carbonated solutions and mixtures of lidocaine and bupivacaine have been shown to speed onset for elective Caesarean section, but clinical trials in emergency Caesarean section are few. It is clear that there is considerable variation in onset times between patients. Slow injection of a bolus necessitates cutting corners, with the precautions mentioned above about fractionating doses. The risks and benefits to the mother and fetus of epidural versus general anaesthesia in these circumstances must be carefully considered, and these can be among the most difficult clinical decisions taken by anaesthetists.

A 'fresh' spinal anaesthetic may be preferable to attempting to top up a poorly functioning epidural catheter, since the chance of inadequate anaesthesia during surgery is greater if analgesia has been poor during labour. Also, if extension of the epidural proves to be inadequate and a spinal anaesthetic is then chosen, the spread of the spinal dose may be more unpredictable after large volumes of solution have already been injected epidurally.

Contraindications to epidural anaesthesia are discussed in Chapter 35, Spinal anaesthesia for Caesarean section (p. 90). In practice, there are very few mothers in whom an epidural cannot be 'topped up' for operative delivery.

Preoperative preparation

This is also discussed in Chapter 35, Spinal anaesthesia for Caesarean section (p. 90). It is particularly important in these patients to mention the risk of intra-operative pain and to have a plan to deal with this should it occur. Because of the occasional need for general anaesthetic supplementation, full antacid precautions must be employed; these should include oral sodium citrate and an intravenous H_2 antagonist in the emergency situation. Assessment of the airway for possible intubation difficulty is also mandatory. Prophylactic vasopressors are rarely needed but should be available, and a large-bore intravenous cannula must be inserted to allow rapid fluid infusion.

Choice of drugs

Bupivacaine 0.5% has been the mainstay for many years for epidural Caesarean section, but large doses (often in excess of the recommended upper limits) are frequently required, and the block may not be ideal. Lidocaine 2% has a faster onset for elective cases, but the volumes required mean that adrenaline must be added to minimise systemic absorption. In both cases, volumes in the region of 20–25 ml are usually needed to establish a sufficiently extensive block. Slow bolus injection (including through the needle) has been shown to produce more rapid and reliable block (with lower final volumes) than boluses of 5 ml repeated every 5–10 minutes, but with attendant risks if the injection is misplaced. Carbonated solutions of bupivacaine and lidocaine have been shown to produce a more rapid onset of a denser block for elective and emergency Caesarean section respectively. A 'recipe' consisting of 10 ml 0.5% bupivacaine, 10 ml 2% lidocaine, 0.1 ml 1:1000 adrenaline and 2 ml 8.4% bicarbonate is often used; when given over 3 minutes to supplement an effective labour epidural, 15–20 ml of this solution will usually produce a bilateral block to T4 to cold within 8–10 minutes. However, it has been argued that this practice increases the risk of drug errors during mixing, and preparation of fresh solution itself delays injection and thus onset of block. Ropivacaine and levobupivacaine appear to have no advantage over bupivacaine other than improved toxicity. Fentanyl 50–100 µg is often added, although it is uncertain whether this is useful if regular doses have been given during labour, and intra-operative nausea and vomiting may be increased.

Administration of the epidural anaesthetic

If a catheter is being sited *de novo*, it is often best done on the labour ward or in a suitable area outside the operating theatre, since the slower onset of epidural anaesthesia would otherwise mean that the mother would have to lie on the operating table for some time while waiting for the block to take effect. In most cases the epidural catheter is already *in situ*; if this is the case, then it has been argued that the epidural may be topped up in the delivery room before transfer, thus saving what may be important time. This practice is controversial, however, since the delivery room is not an ideal place for dealing with extensive block, severe hypotension or local anaesthetic toxicity. The anaesthetist must, of course, remain with the mother from the point of topping up an epidural with concentrated solutions, wherever this is done, and ensure adequate monitoring.

Testing the block

Because of the possibility of missed segments and unilateral block, the extent of sensory loss should be mapped with great care, including sacral segments. The upper and lower levels on both sides should be determined and the intermediate dermatomes tested also. Bilateral lower limb motor block is a useful indicator of adequate sacral spread and should be confirmed before starting the operation; sacral sparing may be treated with epidural fentanyl 50 μg. A block to cold from T4 to S5, with loss of touch sensation up to T5, should be the target, and the extent of the block must be documented. The epidural catheter allows further doses to be given, and appropriate positioning of the patient, although not as effective as with spinal anaesthesia, may encourage spread into recalcitrant areas.

During the operation

Hypotension is rarer than with spinal anaesthesia, but blood pressure should be carefully monitored and treated expeditiously. Inadequate block may become apparent during peritoneal incision, and exteriorisation of the uterus, a manoeuvre much favoured by certain obstetricians, is often poorly tolerated. A delicate surgeon can make all the difference if the block is borderline, and good communication between medical staff is rarely more important. Nausea and vomiting, if associated with vagal stimuli such as exteriorisation of the uterus or peritoneal manipulation, may be treated with glycopyrronnium 200–600 μg.

After the operation

If opioids have not been given, an epidural dose of a long-acting, lipid-soluble drug such as diamorphine 2–3 mg may be given along with oral/rectal non-steroidal analgesics if not contraindicated. The same precautions regarding discharge from recovery and monitoring should be followed as for spinal anaesthesia. The epidural catheter lends itself to further low-dose local anaesthetic/opioid top-ups or infusion, but this can only be done if there are facilities and staff to care for the patient safely. These should be similar to those that are available for mothers with an epidural in labour.

Key points

- The full extent of the block must be tested.
- Pain during the operation is more common than with spinal anaesthesia, and the patient must be warned.
- Slow-bolus epidural injection may be used to produce a good quality block within 10–15 minutes but may be more hazardous than fractionated injection.

FURTHER READING

Lam DT, Ngan Kee WD, Khaw KS. Extension of epidural blockade in labour for emergency Caesarean section using 2% lidocaine with epinephrine and fentanyl, with or without alkalinisation. *Anaesthesia* 2001; **56**: 790–4.

Lucas DN, Ciccone GK, Yentis SM. Extending low dose epidural analgesia for emergency Caesarean section–a comparison of three solutions. *Anaesthesia* **1999**: 54: 1173–7.

Pan PH, Bogard TD, Owen MD. Incidence and characteristics of failures in obstetric neuraxial analgesia and anesthesia: a retrospective analysis of 19,259 deliveries. *Int J Obstet Anesth* 2004; **13**: 227–33.

Patel M, Craig R, Laishley R. A comparison between epidural anaesthesia using alkalinized solution and spinal (combined spinal/epidural) anaesthesia for elective caesarean section. *Int J Obstet Anesth* 1996; **5**: 236–9.

Sanders SD, Mallory S, Lucas DN, *et al.* Extending low-dose epidural analgesia for emergency caesarean section using ropivacaine 0.75% *Anaesthesia* 2004; **59**: 988–92.

35   SPINAL ANAESTHESIA FOR CAESAREAN SECTION

In 1996, a survey of British obstetric anaesthetists showed that 74% would use single-shot spinal anaesthesia as their first choice for elective or, if time permitted, urgent Caesarean section; this technique therefore probably accounts for the majority of all anaesthetics for Caesarean sections in the UK.

Problems/special considerations

- Rapid onset of widespread vasodilatation coupled with the effect of aortocaval compression means that hypotension is an almost inevitable accompaniment to spinal anaesthesia in the mother unless specific precautions are taken. Avoidance of the supine position, frequent blood pressure measurement and instant availability of intravenous fluid and vasopressors are prerequisites for the safe use of this technique.
- Careful assessment of the level of block is essential before starting the operation. Despite an apparently adequate block, pain may still occur, although this is less likely than if an epidural anaesthetic has been used. Mothers should be warned of this possibility in advance, and adequate treatment, even to the extent of inducing general anaesthesia, must be offered.

Pain during Caesarean section under regional anaesthesia is currently the commonest successful cause of litigation against obstetric anaesthetists in the UK.

- The incidence of postdural puncture headache (PDPH) is related to the size and type of needle used. 'Pencil-point' and conical tip needles, such as the Sprotte and Whitacre, are associated with a much lower rate of headache than Quincke needles with a cutting tip, so much so that a 24 G pencil-point needle is probably better than a 27 G Quincke needle.
- Meningitis and encephalitis are extremely rare. However, once the dura mater has been penetrated, the cerebrospinal fluid (CSF) is particularly susceptible to contamination, and it is considered good practice to use a completely aseptic technique, including the wearing of mask, gown and gloves.

Management options

Suitability of the technique

In experienced hands, spinal anaesthesia can be almost as fast as general anaesthesia, and there are few occasions when the urgency of the situation means that there is no time for this technique. If the mother already has an epidural *in situ* then, time permitting, this should be topped up in preference to establishing a new block. If time is short, a single-shot spinal has been suggested as an alternative to general anaesthesia in a mother with an epidural *in situ*. If spinal supplementation of an existing epidural block is thought appropriate, it may be necessary to use a reduced dose, as there have been case reports of very high blocks in these circumstances. Spinal anaesthesia is contraindicated in patients with hypovolaemia, coagulation disorders (whether iatrogenic or pathological) and systemic sepsis. Although regional anaesthesia has traditionally been avoided if massive blood loss is expected, such as in the case of placenta praevia, many modern anaesthetists would now use a spinal block in this situation, particularly since uterine contractility is greatly enhanced if general anaesthesia with volatile agents is eschewed.

Although traditionally favoured as being better for the baby than general anaesthesia, there is evidence that spinal anaesthesia may be associated with greater neonatal acidosis than after epidural or general anaesthesia, possibly related to the rapidity of onset and cardiovascular changes. However, the rapid onset and more profound block compared with epidural anaesthesia, and the greater maternal safety profile compared with general anaesthesia, make spinal anaesthesia the technique preferred by most obstetric anaesthetists for Caesarean section.

Preoperative preparation

Full fasting and antacid precautions should be taken, and the preoperative assessment should include bedside tests for difficult intubation, since general anaesthesia may be needed, albeit rarely, if the block is unsatisfactory. An explanation of the technique should be given, and the mother should be warned about the risks of hypotension with associated nausea and vomiting, and PDPH. The possibility of pain during the operation must be mentioned, although she should be reassured that this is unusual and will be treated if necessary with intravenous opioids or even general anaesthesia. Most mothers will want their partners present for the delivery, and it is good practice to involve them in these discussions so that they are aware of what may happen.

Preparation

Automated non-invasive blood pressure, electrocardiography and pulse oximetry are mandatory. Most anaesthetists prefer to perform spinal anaesthesia with the patient on the operating table, since this minimises the need for movement after the local anaesthetic has been administered. Sitting or lateral positions are both acceptable, although the former may be easier if the bony landmarks are difficult to palpate. In the 'Oxford position', the patient lies laterally with slight head-down tilt but with the upper spine pushed into an upward curve by pillows under the head and shoulder; this is said to encourage a good block while protecting the patient from spread above the upper thoracic dermatomes.

Intravenous access

Good intravenous access is essential, and a preload of 1000–2000 ml has been traditionally used. Colloid solutions may be more efficacious than crystalloids at preventing hypotension. A vasopressor must be to hand; many practitioners now prefer phenylephrine to ephedrine because of a more fovourable neonatal pH. The vasopressor may be added to the intravenous infusion, given as a bolus immediately after the spinal injection, or saved until the onset of hypotension. Prophylactic use is becoming increasingly common and has been shown to be more effective at preventing hypotension than fluid preloading; it has been suggested that prophylactic vasopressors obviate the need for fluid preloading.

Administration of the spinal anaesthetic

Full asepsis should be used, and an interspace below L3 should be chosen to ensure that the needle tip is well below the termination of the cord. A pencil-point or conical tip needle is best but, if there is no choice, the smallest available Quincke needle should be inserted, with the bevel orientated in the cranial–caudal plane to reduce the risk of PDPH. Once free-flowing CSF has been identified, the chosen dose of local anaesthetic should be administered over 30–60 seconds. 'Dry tap' or pain during insertion or injection should be a signal to withdraw the needle and try again.

Drugs

Hyperbaric bupivacaine 0.5% is the only drug licensed for spinal use in the UK, and a dose of 12.5–15 mg (2.5–3 ml) is usually sufficient. Recent reports of prolonged neurological deficit with hyperbaric 5% lidocaine suggest that this drug should be avoided in the intrathecal space. Fentanyl 10–20 µg (higher doses increase analgesia slightly but with marked increases in side effects) or preservative-free morphine/diamorphine 0.1–0.3 mg may be added for postoperative analgesia. The mother should be moved quickly but carefully into a left-wedged supine position, ensuring that there is no head-down tilt, and the blood pressure checked at 1–2 minute intervals. Some practitioners prefer to turn the mother into a full lateral posture, avoiding the wedged supine position until just before draping and incision.

Testing the block

To minimise the risk of pain, the block should extend up to T4 on both sides when a cold sensation or pin-prick is applied; a block to fine touch extending to T5 has been shown to be associated with a low incidence of intraoperative pain. Although a complete block below the upper level is fairly certain when spinal anaesthesia is used, it is good practice to check that the sacral segments are covered and that the mother cannot straight leg raise against gravity. A recalcitrant block can be extended by using a variety of techniques such as turning from side to side, coughing, a Valsalva manoeuvre or judicious head-down tilt. The extent of the block and the modality used for testing must always be recorded.

During the operation

The patient should be watched for premonitory signs of hypotension, such as pallor, yawning or nausea. Bradycardia often indicates a high block affecting the sympathetic cardiac accelerator fibres. The mother may complain that her chest 'feels heavy'; this sensation is common when the intercostal muscles are affected, and reassurance should be offered. Complaints of discomfort or pain should be treated with boluses of intravenous fentanyl or alfentanil at first; pain is more likely during peritoneal traction, swabbing of the paracolic gutters or exteriorisation of the uterus.

After the operation

Positional changes may cause sudden cranial spread of the block even at this late stage. A fully-staffed recovery area is mandatory, and the sitting position may be carefully adopted if the blood pressure is stable. The mother should not be moved to the ward until cardiovascular stability is certain and the block is receding. Blood pressure recordings should be continued on the ward at 30-minute intervals until leg movements have returned. Respiratory rate and conscious level should be checked hourly for 12–24 hours if spinal opioids have been used, and no other opioids should be used during this period without consultation with an anaesthetist. Anaesthetic follow-up for symptoms of PDPH or persistent block should continue for 48 hours.

> **Key points**
>
> - Hypotension is almost invariable unless actively prevented with vasopressors.
> - The extent of the block must be tested and recorded, and the patient should be warned of the risk of pain.
> - Pencil-point or conical tip needles should be used to minimise the risk of postdural puncture headache.

FURTHER READING

Belzarena SD. Clinical effects of intrathecally administered fentanyl in patients undergoing Cesarean section. *Anesth Analg* 1992; **74**: 653–7.

Reynolds F, Seed PT. Anaesthesia for Caesarean section and neonatal acid-base status: a meta-analysis. *Anaesthesia* 2005; **60**(7): 636–53.

Rocke DA, Rout CC. Volume preloading, spinal hypotension and Caesarean section. *Br J Anaesth* 1995; **75**: 257–9.

Russell IF. Levels of anaesthesia and intra-operative pain at Caesarean section under regional block. *Int J Obstet Anesth* 1995; **4**: 71–7.

36   GENERAL ANAESTHESIA FOR CAESAREAN SECTION

There has been a general trend away from general anaesthesia in both the UK and North America over the past few decades because of the associated potential morbidity and mortality, with >90% of Caesarean sections now being performed under regional anaesthesia.

General anaesthesia is usually reserved for those women who adamantly refuse a regional technique, or for those in whom such a technique is contra-indicated e.g. by medical disease or lack of time. Perceived contraindications to regional anaesthesia are becoming fewer in number as enthusiasm for it increases.

Problems/special considerations

- *Airway difficulty:* the incidence of failure to intubate the trachea is approximately 1 in 300–500 in the obstetric population, compared with a ten-fold lower incidence in the general surgical population. Reasons for this are not completely clear but are thought to include the following:
  - The pregnant woman has a tendency to fluid retention and generally increased vascularity. Attempts at laryngoscopy, intubation or passage of oro/nasogastric tubes are more likely to result in soft tissue trauma and bleeding.
  - Full dentition is the norm; dental hazards may be increased by expensive restorative dentistry. Increased breast mass and the application of cricoid pressure may make insertion of the laryngoscope difficult. Positioning of the

patient on the operating table to avoid aortocaval compression may increase the likelihood of incorrectly applied cricoid pressure.

- Psychological pressure on the anaesthetist, especially in the emergency situation, may increase the chances of failed intubation.
- Current anaesthetic teaching is that anaesthetists must declare failure early and wake the patient; thus cases in which intubation might be successful with the aid of other staff/equipment in non-obstetric settings are being counted as failed intubations in the delivery suite.

    Pressure to achieve tracheal intubation may lead to prolonged attempts during which hypoxia occurs. Fatalities typically arise from failure of oxygenation rather than failure of tracheal intubation.

- *Pulmonary aspiration of gastric contents* (see Chapter 56, Aspiration of gastric contents, p. 138; Chapter 14, Gastric function and feeding in labour, p. 35).
- *Hypovolaemia* (see Chapter 73, Major obstetric haemorrhage, p. 173): the extent of blood loss in fit young people is usually underestimated. Induction of general anaesthesia in an unresuscitated hypovolaemic mother may precipitate catastrophic cardiovascular collapse. Tachycardia should alert the anaesthetist to the possibility of hypovolaemia, although the significance of tachycardia may be difficult to assess in an extremely anxious mother.
- *Awareness:* the risks of awareness during general anaesthesia for Caesarean section are thought to be minimal if modern techniques are used (see Chapter 57, Awareness, p. 141). Suitable opioid analgesia should be administered to the mother after delivery of the baby. Meticulous anaesthetic record keeping is vital. Most cases of supposed intraoperative awareness are in fact episodes occurring during recovery from anaesthesia, but claims of intraoperative awareness are difficult to refute if the anaesthetic record is inadequate. Some authorities recommend that all mothers are warned preoperatively of an extremely small risk of intraoperative awareness, and that this warning is recorded in the preoperative assessment.
- *So-called 'minor' problems:* general anaesthesia is associated with a tendency towards longer immediate recovery, more pain, more postoperative nausea and vomiting, and more neonatal depression than regional anaesthesia. In addition, the parents do not experience the moment of birth as with spinal or epidural anaesthesia.

Management options

There are few recognised options for provision of general anaesthesia for Caesarean section in the UK.

Preoperative assessment

In every case, a preoperative anaesthetic assessment must be made, no matter how urgent the requirement for anaesthesia. This need not be lengthy but should include questioning about any relevant medical, obstetric and dental history, previous anaesthesia, history of drug allergy, recent food intake and indication (and urgency) for Caesarean section.

An assessment of the airway must be made for every woman, for example by asking her to open her mouth widely and extend her neck. Assessment of blood loss should be made when relevant and intravenous fluid resuscitation initiated if appropriate.

Therapy to raise intragastric pH and minimise intragastric volume is given. It is usual to administer ranitidine (or cimetidine) or omeprazole preoperatively, either orally or parenterally, depending on timing. Metoclopramide is also given in many units. Some obstetric units advocate the administration of antacid prophylaxis routinely to every woman in labour, but this is controversial. 0.3 M sodium citrate (30 ml) is administered immediately before preoxygenation and induction of anaesthesia to neutralise any gastric contents.

Induction of anaesthesia

- It is customary to induce anaesthesia for Caesarean section in the operating theatre. The obstetric anaesthetist should check the anaesthetic machine in the obstetric theatre at least once a day. A suitably trained anaesthetic assistant must be present before induction of general anaesthesia. There should be an intubation trolley equipped with a range of differently sized tracheal tubes, intubation aids, laryngoscopes and equipment for dealing with failed intubation. The uterus must be displaced off the aorta and vena cava either manually (uncommon in the UK) or by a wedge placed under the woman's right hip, or by laterally tilting the operating table.
- A large-bore intravenous cannula (14 G or 16 G) that is connected to a freely running infusion must be in place before induction of anaesthesia starts.
- Adequate preoxygenation (3 minutes or 4–5 vital capacity breaths) must always precede induction of anaesthesia, regardless of urgency for delivery. It is crucial to ensure a tight fit of the facepiece and if a circle system is being used, at least 12 l/min of oxygen.
- Monitoring of the mother should include blood pressure, capnography, electrocardiography, pulse oximetry and end-tidal volatile concentration.
- Rapid sequence induction of anaesthesia using thiopental in an adequate dose (350–500 mg unless there is hypovolaemia or a fixed cardiac output) and suxamethonium 1–1.5 mg/kg is standard practice in the UK. These drugs may be supplemented with hypotensive agents and/or opioid analgesics in mothers with pre-eclampsia or cardiac disease. Cricoid pressure is applied before consciousness is lost and maintained until the airway is secured and tracheal intubation confirmed (see Chapter 37, Cricoid pressure, p. 98).

  Propofol has been used but has been associated with a less favourable neonatal acid–base profile – though the clinical significance of this is disputed. In addition, it has been claimed that propofol's short duration of action might increase the risk of awareness before adequate brain levels of volatile agent are reached, especially if intubation is difficult – though this too is controversial.

Use of non-depolarising neuromuscular blocking drugs, e.g. vecuronium or rocuronium, has been advocated, on the basis that intubation conditions will be maintained for long enough to achieve intubation if the latter is unsuccessful on the first attempt. However, most authorities favour the use of suxamethonium because the intubation conditions it produces are felt to be the best, within the shortest time, and if intubation fails the return of muscle power favours earlier self-ventilation.

- Every obstetric anaesthetist should be familiar with both failed intubation and failed ventilation drills and should mentally rehearse these before every induction of general anaesthesia in the obstetric patient. Every obstetric theatre should have monitoring equipment that includes measurement of end-tidal carbon dioxide, and there should be access to specialised airway equipment, e.g. cricothyroid cannulae and a fibreoptic endoscope.

- Most obstetric anaesthetists in the UK use 50% nitrous oxide in oxygen plus a volatile anaesthetic agent of choice to ventilate the lungs, reverting to conventional mixtures of 70% nitrous oxide in 30% oxygen after delivery of the baby. The volatile agent should be continued throughout anaesthesia.

- A short-acting non-depolarising neuromuscular blocking drug should be used when the suxamethonium has worn off, and if the surgeon is fast it may not be necessary to use further neuromuscular blockers after the initial dose of suxamethonium. Deaths have occurred from inadequate reversal of neuromuscular blockade following the use of long-acting drugs. Use of a peripheral nerve stimulator is recommended.

- Oxytocin (Syntocinon) is usually given as a slow intravenous bolus of 5–10 IU at delivery of the baby, and may be followed by an intravenous infusion of 100–150 IU/h for 4–6 h at the request of the obstetrician.

- Adequate analgesia should be given following delivery of the baby; the combination of a long-acting opioid such as morphine and a non-steroidal anti-inflammatory drug (NSAID) such as diclofenac is used in many units. It is important to obtain consent to rectal administration of drugs preoperatively. Intravenous paracetamol has recently become available in the UK and may also be given intraoperatively.

- At the end of surgery, residual neuromuscular blockade is reversed and the mother is turned into the left lateral position before the trachea is extubated. It is important to remember that the risk of aspiration is present at extubation and possibly during the initial phase of recovery from anaesthesia, as well as during induction of anaesthesia. Extubation of the trachea should not be performed until there is evidence of return of protective reflexes.

- The mother must be nursed in a properly equipped recovery room by trained staff before returning to the postnatal wards. Deaths have occurred due to inadequately staffed and equipped recovery facilities.

- Postoperative analgesia must be provided; patient-controlled opioids are popular, and NSAIDs appear to be particularly effective in combating 'afterpains' of uterine involution. NSAIDs should not be used in severe pre-eclamptics and severe asthmatics. Bilateral ilioinguinal block has been suggested as a simple, safe and effective way to provide postoperative analgesia.

- Heparin should be given preoperatively if it is known that general anaesthesia will be given, as for any operation; if general anaesthesia is unexpected the first dose may be given during surgery or shortly afterwards.

Key points

- All obstetric patients requiring general anaesthesia should be considered high risk.
- Emergency general anaesthesia is associated with increased morbidity and mortality.
- Failure to intubate the trachea is ten times more common in the obstetric population compared with a general surgical population.
- There are very few absolute indications for general anaesthesia for Caesarean section.

---

37   CRICOID PRESSURE

The cricoid cartilage is the only cartilaginous part of the upper airway to be a complete ring and so pressure on its anterior aspect results in compression of the upper oesophagus/hypopharynx against the vertebral body of C6 posteriorly. First described by Sellick in 1961 (hence 'Sellick's manoeuvre'), cricoid pressure is widely used as a means of preventing passive regurgitation (and thus aspiration) of gastric contents during induction of general anaesthesia in at-risk patients. It is thus a standard technique in obstetric anaesthesia, although precisely when the period of risk begins and ends is controversial. In addition, whether cricoid pressure is actually necessary at all has also been questioned, since it is not routinely practised in many continental European countries without apparent increases in morbidity and mortality.

Method

As originally described by Sellick, the assistant's forefinger is placed over the cricoid cartilage and firm pressure exerted posteriorly, with the thumb and middle finger supporting on either side. The optimal time to start exerting pressure is somewhat controversial since cricoid pressure is uncomfortable when the patient is awake, whereas regurgitation may occur if it is applied too late. As a compromise, many advocate gentle pressure until consciousness is lost, with firmer pressure thereafter (as Sellick originally described), although there is evidence that gentle pressure itself may cause relaxation of the lower oesophageal sphincter. Estimates of the force required to prevent regurgitation range from 20 N to over 40 N. Various devices have been described that apply the correct amount of force but they are not widely used.

More recently, use of two-handed cricoid pressure has been suggested as improving efficacy whilst causing less difficulty with intubation (although controlled studies are few). Whilst applying pressure as described above, the assistant's second hand is placed behind the patient's neck, resisting any flexion of the cervical spine as cricoid pressure is applied. The two-handed technique does, however, mean that the anaesthetic assistant has both of his/her hands occupied should the anaesthetist need any more equipment.

Although the use of cricoid pressure is standard practice, it may hinder tracheal intubation; first, because the assistant's hand may obstruct insertion of the laryngoscope blade into the mouth, and second, because if incorrectly applied it can distort the laryngeal anatomy. If pressure is excessive, it may also flex the neck (or hyperextend it if two-handed cricoid pressure is used). It is therefore important that anaesthetic assistants are properly trained in its application; studies have demonstrated considerable variation in assistants' ability but also considerable improvement following training.

In cases of failed intubation, release of cricoid pressure should be considered, especially if placement of a laryngeal mask airway is considered, since this too may be hindered. Release is also advocated if there is active vomiting since oesophageal rupture has been reported; however, cricoid pressure should only be released on the anaesthetist's instruction.

Key points

- Cricoid pressure should be applied as consciousness is lost.
- A force of 20–40 N is required.
- Incorrect application may impede intubation.
- Assistants should be properly trained in its application.

FURTHER READING

Benhamou D, Vanner R. Controversies in obstetric anaesthesia: cricoid pressure is unnecessary in obstetric general anaesthesia. *Int J Obstet Anesth* 1995; **4**: 30–3.

Brimacombe JR, Berry AM. Cricoid pressure. *Can J Anaesth* 1997; **44**: 414–25.

Sellick BA. Cricoid pressure to control regurgitation of stomach contents during induction of anaestheisa. *Lancet* 1961; **ii**: 404–6.

38   FAILED AND DIFFICULT INTUBATION

Towards the end of the 20th century the number of deaths associated with failed intubation declined, though more recently there has been concern that the incidence of failed intubation is again increasing. It is important to remember that patients do not die from failed intubation; they die from hypoxia or acid aspiration if the failed intubation is unrecognised or the corrective measures are inadequate.

Problems/special considerations

Tracheal intubation is more difficult in obstetric anaesthesia and the incidence of failed or difficult intubation is usually quoted as between 1 in 250 and 1 in 500 obstetric general anaesthetics, compared with 1 in 2000 to 1 in 3000 for non-obstetric general anaesthetics. There are many reasons for difficulties with intubation and the increased risk of developing hypoxia (Table 38.1). Laryngoscopy and placement of a tracheal tube may thus be more difficult, whilst hypoxaemia develops more rapidly than in general surgical patients. This is compounded by the anaesthetist's being under considerable stress during induction of anaesthesia.

The consequences of failed intubation in obstetrics are serious for both maternal and fetal health. Obstetric anaesthetists have been encouraging regional anaesthesia to reduce the numbers of general anaesthetics administered. There is a decreased percentage of general anaesthetics administered, although the absolute numbers of general anaesthetics may not have fallen dramatically. However, there are now many obstetric units where very few general anaesthetics are given and this, although a commendable trend, has led to a reduction in training opportunities, especially given the reduced exposure of modern trainees to clinical workload generally.

Management options

If general anaesthesia is to be administered then it is important to do the following:
- Attempt to predict difficult intubation
- Use an anaesthetic technique that will minimise the risk of failing
- Have a failed intubation drill.

Table 38.1. Causes of increased incidence of problems relating to tracheal intubation in obstetric anaesthesia

Anatomical	Physiological	Iatrogenic
Difficulty inserting laryngoscope: • Large breasts • Weight gain/increased fatty tissue • Oedema (especially pre-eclampsia) • Complete dentition • Cricoid pressure	Increased risk of aspiration Increased oxygen demand Reduced lung capacity	Incorrectly applied cricoid pressure Urgency leading to haste Inexperience of staff
Poor laryngoscopic view: • Weight gain/increased fatty tissue • Laryngeal oedema • Cricoid pressure causing distortion • Swollen mucosa		

Prediction of difficult intubation

Prediction of difficult intubation is attempted using the same clinical examination as in the non-pregnant patient:

- Mallampati score
- Coexisting neck pathology
- State of dentition
- Mouth opening
- Thyromental distance.

Unfortunately, even in combination these tests have low predictive value (i.e. relatively few of the cases predicted as being difficult will actually be difficult), partly because of the poor function of the tests and partly because difficult intubation is uncommon, even in obstetric cases. Mallampati scores have been shown to change during pregnancy and even during labour.

Anaesthetic technique

The delivery suite theatre should be well equipped for a difficult intubation, and the equipment should include a variety of aids to intubation as well as equipment to aid oxygenation if a problem arises. Skilled assistance for the anaesthetist is essential.

The anaesthetist should ensure that the patient is well positioned and that adequate doses of induction agent and neuromuscular blocking drug (although alternatives such as rocuronium have been used suxamethonium is still the standard agent) are given after a full 3 minutes' preoxygenation or 4–5 vital capacity breaths. Proper fitting of the facemask is important to ensure efficient preoxygenation. The correct application of cricoid pressure by a trained assistant is important, since badly applied cricoid pressure can make laryngoscopy difficult.

In order to avoid a catastrophe there should be a plan that comes into effect as soon as failure to view the larynx or to intubate the trachea becomes evident. The time from the realisation of difficulties to the admission of a failed intubation is the most critical aspect in the safe management of the patient. It is at this point that a previously rehearsed 'failed intubation drill' should commence.

Failed intubation drill

There exist a multiplicity of failed intubation drills, some more complicated than others, but the essential requirement of all of them is to maintain oxygenation. If necessary, cricoid pressure should be altered or released, since oxygenation takes precedence over protection from aspiration. The key factors in any failed intubation drill are:

- Assessment of the airway and severity of the difficulty
- Deciding whether to try alternate approaches to intubation, at all times maintaining oxygenation
- Defining a specific time limit on efforts to persist with intubation attempts
- Calling for help.

It is important to remember that the primary duty of the anaesthetist is to the mother; thus the initial course of action is to allow the mother to wake up, irrespective of the risk to the fetus, and to proceed with a regional anaesthetic. Exceptions to this would be if the mother herself requires the surgery as a life-saving procedure (e.g. major haemorrhage) or if the person making the decision to continue is of sufficient experience and seniority. Proceeding with a Caesarean section under laryngeal mask or facemask anaesthesia risks aspiration if cricoid pressure becomes inefficient and risks airway obstruction developing during the procedure. Trainees should be reassured that they will always be supported if they wake a mother up after a failed intubation.

A simple failed intubation drill is illustrated in Fig. 38.1. Traditionally, such drills called for the patient to be turned to the left lateral position, but most anaesthetists are more familiar with managing the airway in the supine position. Therefore most drills now do not include turning the patient as part of initial management, although this still represents the safest position in which the mother should wake up. A second (quick) attempt at laryngoscopy would be indicated if the anaesthetist

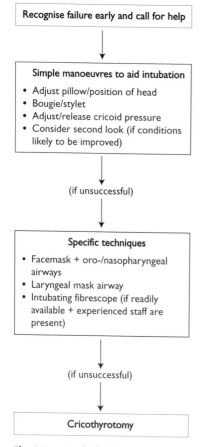

Fig. 38.1 Simple failed intubation drill.

feels that the patient's position could be improved or a special blade or intubation aid would achieve intubation. A second dose of suxamethonium should only be given in exceptional circumstances.

Key points

- The patient does not die from failure to intubate the trachea but from failure to stop trying to intubate.
- Oxygenation must be maintained at all times.
- The failed intubation drill should be regularly rehearsed.

FURTHER READING

Barnardo PD, Jenkins JG. Failed tracheal intubation in obstetrics: a 6-year review in a UK region. *Anaesthesia* 2000; **55**: 690–4.

Harmer M. Difficult and failed intubation in obstetrics. *Int J Obstet Anesth* 1997; **6**: 25–31.

Kuczkowski KM, Reisner LS, Benumof JL. Airway problems and new solutions for the obstetric patient. *J Clin Anesth* 2003; **15**: 552–63.

39   AWAKE INTUBATION

Awake tracheal intubation might be considered in obstetric practice in two situations: management of the mother with a known airway problem and acute management of the failed intubation. The need for awake intubation is considerably reduced by the greater proportion of procedures (mainly Caesarean section) performed under regional, rather than general, anaesthesia. Indeed, regional anaesthesia is often considered the immediate technique of choice following failed intubation. Conversely, some authorities would consider a known difficult airway as an indication for awake intubation, since the airway may otherwise be at risk during an inadequate or extensive regional block, and having to deal with a difficult intubation in an uncontrolled manner mid-Caesarean is especially hazardous and stressful.

Problems/special considerations

The basic techniques used are the same as for the non-pregnant patient. Nerve blocks and transtracheal injection may be difficult because of the increased subcutaneous tissue deposition of pregnancy. Because of the nasal vascular engorgement and tendency to nosebleeds that are common in pregnancy, the oral route is often preferred, but nasal intubation is an acceptable route. If the awake procedure follows a failed intubation, there may be considerable airway bleeding and oedema resulting from trauma. In the past, the risk of aspiration of gastric contents has made obstetric anaesthetists wary of obtunding the protective reflexes with local anaesthesia for awake intubation, but this is felt to be safe if excessive sedation is avoided.

Management options

If not already given, antacids/H_2-receptor antagonists should be given, and intramuscular hyoscine 20–40 µg or intramuscular/intravenous glycopyrronium 100–300 µg may be used to reduce secretions.

During the procedure, the same attention to avoidance of aortocaval compression and to fetal monitoring and wellbeing is required as for any procedure in the labour ward. Particular efforts are required to reassure the mother and her partner since the situations in which awake intubation is required are especially stressful.

Fibreoptic intubation is generally considered the technique of choice. Once the trachea has been intubated and the tube's cuff inflated, general anaesthesia can be induced. It should be remembered that there is a risk of airway obstruction following tracheal extubation, which should be performed only when the mother is awake and in the left lateral position. A bougie or similar device may be placed through the tracheal tube before extubation to facilitate reinsertion of the tube should this be required. Impaired protective reflexes may persist for an hour or more after local anaesthetic techniques have been used in the airway.

Key points

- The indications for awake intubation in obstetrics are controversial.
- The principles of awake intubation are similar to those in non-pregnant women.

40   POST-CAESAREAN SECTION ANALGESIA

Adequate pain relief following Caesarean section is particularly important because the mother needs to be sufficiently comfortable to care for her baby; she is also at increased risk of thromboembolism, and effective analgesia facilitates early mobilisation.

Problems/special considerations

- Psychological considerations are important. The mother who has been delivered by elective Caesarean section under regional anaesthesia, with preoperative preparation and discussion about postoperative analgesia, cannot be directly compared with the mother who has been delivered by emergency Caesarean section under general anaesthesia after many hours of labour and a failed trial of forceps delivery. (In the worst scenario she may also have received an episiotomy.)

- Most published studies of post-Caesarean section analgesia are, for logistical reasons, performed in women having elective section, and the results should therefore be interpreted cautiously.
- The ideal analgesic should of course be extremely effective, universally applicable, cheap to use and free from unwanted side effects. The ideal analgesic does not exist, and the demand for freedom from unwanted effects is particularly important in obstetric patients. It is important to remember that unwanted effects include need for intravenous cannulae and infusions, urinary catheters and additional monitoring equipment. Safety is vital in a patient population that is young and fit with newly born dependants. Other side effects, which may be acceptable to an elderly general surgical population (e.g. pruritus, nausea and sedation), are unacceptable to women wishing to care for babies.

The use of various opioids by the subarachnoid or epidural routes has become routine, but the level of nursing care required by women who have received this method of analgesia remains controversial. The relative risk and timing of respiratory depression associated with different opioids varies, but none can be considered completely safe in this respect. Equally, all centrally administered opioids cause nausea, vomiting and pruritus, although to differing degrees. Although there can be no doubt that high-dependency care, either in a high-dependency unit, or given in a normal postnatal ward by one-to-one or one-to-two patient supervision, is ideal, many obstetric units are unable to provide this. Protagonists of spinal opioids point out that all opioids, given by any route, have the capacity to cause respiratory depression, and that no special precautions are taken after the administration of intramuscular opioids. Various compromises are made at a local level.

Management options

A combination of opioids and non-steroidal anti-inflammatory drugs (NSAIDs) is used in the majority of women to provide analgesia following Caesarean section. Analgesics prescribed regularly are more likely to be given than those prescribed 'as required', but midwives should be educated about assessment and management of postoperative pain and encouraged to give analgesics as prescribed. Published research has failed to demonstrate clearly the superiority of any one route or of any one drug or drug combination.

Caesarean section under general anaesthesia

The most commonly used drugs in this situation are intraoperative intravenous opioids (e.g. morphine 10–20 mg or diamorphine 5–10 mg), an NSAID (e.g. diclofenac 100 mg given rectally at the end of surgery) and either intramuscular or patient-controlled intravenous opioids postoperatively. Regular paracetamol and NSAIDs act synergistically with both strong and weak opioids and may be given orally or rectally. Specific consent should be sought before administering rectal drugs, and this may preclude the immediate postoperative use of these drugs in the emergency situation.

NSAIDs are contraindicated in women with severe pre-eclampsia because of their effect on platelet function and should also be used with caution in asthmatics. The potentially adverse effect of NSAIDs on renal function should be considered in women who are hypovolaemic and in those who have compromised renal function.

Bilateral ilioinguinal blocks have been shown to improve postoperative pain control, and should be considered for all cases under general anaesthesia. Rectus sheath blocks may also be used, although this is more difficult immediately after Caesarean section than in elective gynaecological surgery.

In the emergency situation there may be an epidural catheter in place but insufficient time to extend a block for anaesthesia, but this does not preclude use of the catheter for postoperative analgesia using epidural opioids.

Caesarean section under regional analgesia

It is common anecdotal evidence that women experience less pain following Caesarean section under regional anaesthesia than under general anaesthesia, although this is difficult to substantiate. The pre-emptive action of epidural or spinal anaesthesia remains unproven. Subarachnoid fentanyl (10–20 µg) is used to improve the quality of intraoperative anaesthesia, but its action does not extend significantly into the postoperative period. This had led to many North American anaesthetists using a combination of subarachnoid fentanyl and morphine (0.1–0.2 mg), which provides very effective analgesia for up to 24 hours, but is considered by some anaesthetists to be associated with the highest risks of nausea, vomiting, pruritus and respiratory depression. In the UK, subarachnoid diamorphine (200-400 µg) is commonly used, providing analgesia both during surgery and extending 6–8 hours postoperatively.

Epidural or combined spinal–epidural anaesthesia allows greater flexibility for postoperative analgesia. Epidural local anaesthetic alone is unsuitable since women are unable to mobilise and dislike the sensation of being numb. Fentanyl (e.g. 50–100 µg) is relatively short acting (3–4 hours) but is reported to have the lowest incidence of side effects; morphine (e.g. 2–4 mg) has delayed onset of action but long duration (18–24 hours) and a higher incidence of side effects, including delayed respiratory depression. Diamorphine (e.g. 2–3 mg) is available in the UK, although in few other countries in the world, and has an intermediate duration of action and incidence of side effects. Sufentanil is widely used in North America but is not available in the UK.

Patient-controlled administration of epidural opioids (e.g. fentanyl or pethidine) has been described, but this is uncommon in the UK.

Regardless of choice of opioid, analgesia is improved by the addition of an NSAID (subject to the same precautions outlined above) and by the regular administration of simple analgesics such as paracetamol.

Key points

- The mother needs to be alert and comfortable in order to feed, care for, and bond with her baby.
- Opioids and non-steroidal anti-inflammatory drugs are the mainstay of postoperative analgesia.
- Opioids are associated with respiratory depression, nausea and vomiting with all routes of administration.
- The epidural and subarachnoid routes are also associated with pruritus and possible delayed respiratory depression.

FURTHER READING

Gadsden J, Hart S, Santos AC. Post-Cesarean delivery analgesia. *Anesth Analg* 2005; **101** (Suppl): S62–S69.

Lane S, Evans P, Arfeen Z, Misra U. A comparison of intrathecal fentanyl and diamorphine as adjuncts in spinal anaesthesia for Caesarean section. *Anaesthesia* 2005; **60**: 453–7.

Leung AY. Postoperative pain management in obstetric anesthesia – new challenges and solutions. *J Clin Anesth* 2004; **16**: 57–65.

National Institute for Clinical Excellence. Clinical guideline 13: caesarian section. London: NICE 2004.

41   REMOVAL OF RETAINED PLACENTA

Failure to deliver the placenta often follows a rapid uncomplicated delivery. It is one of the causes of postpartum haemorrhage, and unless there is a prompt response to conservative management the placenta must be removed surgically under regional or general anaesthesia.

Problems/special considerations

- The need for anaesthesia and surgery at this stage of childbirth is frequently unanticipated by the mother and her partner and may be a significant psychological blow.
- The presence of the placenta in the uterus prevents the latter from contracting effectively so there may be excessive bleeding from any areas of separation.

Occasionally, retained placenta is complicated by uterine inversion (either partial or complete). Unless the uterus is rapidly replaced manually the mother will become severely hypotensive and may become bradycardic. A similar clinical picture may be seen with so-called 'cervical shock', in which there is increased vagal tone caused by the placenta being stuck in the cervix.

Management options

Early conservative management is appropriate if bleeding is not excessive and vital signs are stable. An intravenous infusion of oxytocics may be started, and putting the baby to the breast for suckling sometimes stimulates delivery of the placenta. Turning the woman into the left lateral position is anecdotally reported to assist spontaneous placental delivery, and emptying the bladder may also be helpful.

Surgical removal of the placenta should take place in theatre, not in the delivery room. Choice of anaesthetic technique should be based on assessment of the relative risks of general and regional anaesthesia. Intravenous access via a large cannula (at least 16 G) with a freely flowing infusion is mandatory before starting any anaesthetic technique.

If epidural analgesia has been used for labour this should be extended for surgery. There is usually no reason to separate mother and baby if regional anaesthesia is used, and there should be no delay in initiating breastfeeding. Adequate fluid replacement is essential, particularly as the sympathetically induced vasodilatation accompanying regional blockade will aggravate any existing hypovolaemia. Suitable solutions for topping up the epidural catheter include 2% lidocaine with 1:200 000 adrenaline, or 0.5% bupivacaine with or without fentanyl. An upper extent of block to T8 is required since uterine manipulation may be considerable.

In the absence of epidural analgesia, spinal anaesthesia should be instituted, unless the mother is significantly hypovolaemic (see below). It is often more comfortable for the mother to have spinal anaesthesia induced in the lateral rather than sitting position. A dose of 1.5–2 ml 0.5% heavy bupivacaine is usually adequate. The mother can be turned to the supine position immediately; the risk of hypotension when the legs are placed in the lithotomy position should be anticipated, and treated promptly with intravenous ephedrine.

If there is evidence of hypovolaemia and continuing bleeding despite adequate resuscitation, general anaesthesia should be used and a consultant anaesthetist contacted. The mother is assumed to have a full stomach and the same technique as for Caesarean section should be used, including antacid prophylaxis and rapid-sequence induction of anaesthesia. Blood should be cross-matched and preferably two large (14 G) intravenous cannulae inserted, and the case managed as for any obstetric haemorrhage.

If there is uterine inversion, general anaesthesia is often required to aid replacement of the uterus, unless the mother is stable and regional analgesia is already present.

Key points

- There is a risk of massive bleeding from retained placenta.
- Resuscitation should take place before induction of anaesthesia.
- Spinal or epidural anaesthesia (to at least T8) is appropriate in haemodynamically stable patients.
- General anaesthesia (with cricoid pressure and tracheal intubation) is indicated in hypovolaemic patients.

IV   Anaesthetic complications

42   BLOODY TAP

Cannulation of an epidural vessel may occur with either the needle or the catheter during siting of an epidural. Its incidence is uncertain since widely varying figures have been quoted (e.g. 5–45%), possibly related to different methods of locating the epidural space, different needles or different definitions. It is thought to be less likely when the paramedian approach is used, when 5–10 ml fluid is injected before threading the catheter and when smaller needles are used.

Bloody tap is important because if unrecognised, injection of local anaesthetic solution intravenously instead of epidurally may result in systemic toxicity (depending on the drug and dose) as well as not producing a block; and continued bleeding from a punctured vessel (e.g. after the epidural has been resited) may theoretically lead to an epidural haematoma if coagulation is impaired.

Problems/special considerations

Diagnosis is not usually a problem, especially if the needle has punctured a vessel. Puncture of a vessel by the catheter may be marked by discomfort as the vessel wall is pierced. Blood may then be aspirated from the catheter – although this is not always the case, hence the use of a test dose. Similarly, the absence of a bloody tap does not guarantee correct placement of the catheter.

Management options

If blood flows from the needle there is no option other than to remove the needle and reinsert it at a different interspace. If blood is obtained again, it may represent a new vascular puncture or blood from the original puncture. If blood is aspirated from the catheter, withdrawing the catheter in 0.5 cm increments, and flushing it with saline after each increment until aspiration is no longer possible, may remove the catheter from the vessel whilst still leaving enough length in the epidural space for effective anaesthesia. If this is not possible, then it should be resited in another interspace.

Analgesia, Anaesthesia and Pregnancy: A Practical Guide Second Edition, ed. Steve Yentis, Anne May and Surbhi Malhotra. Published by Cambridge University Press. © Cambridge University Press 2007.

Key points

- In cases of bloody tap, flushing and incremental withdrawal of the catheter may avoid having to resite the epidural.
- Bloody tap may not always be present when the catheter is placed intravascularly.

43   DURAL PUNCTURE

Dural puncture usually refers to puncture of the dura and the underlying arachnoid mater. It may be deliberate during subarachnoid anaesthesia or accidental during epidural anaesthesia. The incidence in the latter case is traditionally said to be around 1% in teaching centres but many authorities consider this to be unacceptably high, with an incidence of 0.5–1% being more realistic and <0.5% attainable in experienced hands. Most would routinely include dural puncture in their discussion with patients of the risks associated with regional anaesthesia.

Most accidental dural punctures are caused by the epidural needle, although it is possible for an epidural catheter to migrate through the dura. In vitro studies suggest that this can only occur if there has been prior (unrecognised) dural puncture or partial tear of the dura by the needle. Rotating the Tuohy needle once its tip is within the epidural space has been implicated in this and is now generally considered undesirable. Reduced incidence of accidental dural puncture has been associated with use of saline rather than air for loss of resistance (LOR), and possibly use of the paramedian rather than midline approach.

Problems/special considerations

Dural puncture poses three main problems if it occurs:
- *Diagnosis:* dural puncture is usually heralded by a 'give' as the needle passes through the dura, and passage of cerebrospinal fluid (CSF) through the needle. For subarachnoid block, these two signs may be influenced by the design of the needle. In a combined spinal–epidural technique, it is usually easier to identify the dura by feel, especially in less experienced hands, since the starting position of the spinal needle in relation to the dura is more precisely known.

When a 16–18 G Tuohy needle is accidentally passed into the sub-arachnoid space, there is usually free flow of CSF, which poses no diagnostic difficulty. However, studies during deliberate dural puncture when placing lumbar drains prior to neurosurgery have revealed that occasionally, free flow is not obtained. Thus the appearance of slowly dripping clear fluid at the hub of the needle may represent CSF from a dural puncture or backflow of saline injected into the epidural space during a LOR technique and may cause confusion, especially during a difficult procedure. In this situation, testing for temperature, glucose and protein content and pH (the last three by using urinary testing strips) will reliably distinguish CSF from saline (even saline that has been injected into the epidural space).

Occasionally, typical postdural puncture headache (PDPH) may be the first evidence that dural puncture has occurred, although this more often reflects either inexperience on the part of the operator in not recognising accidental dural puncture or the operator not wishing to 'own up' in the hope that PDPH will not occur.

- *Management:* the aims of management of accidental dural puncture during establishment of epidural anaesthesia should include provision of adequate analgesia, safety of the patient and, if possible, reduction of risk from the adverse consequences of the dural puncture, as discussed below.
- *Adverse consequences:* adverse consequences of dural puncture are PDPH (which occurs in 50–80% of cases of accidental dural puncture in parturients) and its sequelae such as cranial nerve palsies, convulsions and subdural or intracranial haemorrhage.

Management options

Traditional management of accidental dural puncture comprises removing the needle and placing an epidural catheter at the adjacent (cranial) interspace. Once the block is no longer required, saline may be infused under gravity in an attempt to reduce the incidence and severity of subsequent PDPH (e.g. 50 ml over 5–10 minutes and/or 1000 ml over 12–24 hours), by displacing spinal CSF into the cranium and/or tamponading the CSF leak. This has been shown to reduce the incidence of PDPH by up to a half, although not consistently amongst the various studies.

Other management options include converting the initial block to subarachnoid ± inserting the catheter into the subarachnoid space for a continuous subarachnoid block, e.g. by using 1–2 ml of standard low-dose epidural solution as top-ups or 1–2 ml/h by infusion. Inserting the catheter has been associated with a reduced incidence of PDPH, and it has been suggested that a possible mechanism is via initiating an inflammatory reaction around the catheter, but this association has been largely in uncontrolled retrospective studies. If the catheter is placed intrathecally, it must be clearly labelled and the whole team informed since there is a risk that it might be mistaken for an epidural catheter. The use of epidural or spinal opioids has also been claimed to reduce the incidence of PDPH, although the evidence for this is also weak.

The place of prophylactic epidural blood patch (via the catheter after delivery) is controversial. Advocates point to the high incidence and severity of PDPH in this population, whereas opponents cite the difficulty it might cause with analgesia (e.g. postoperatively), the fact that some women will receive an intervention they may not need, the possible risk of infection if the catheter is left in place throughout a prolonged labour and the reduced efficacy of prophylactic blood patch.

Because of the sometimes unpredictable nature of the block and the departure of the management from routine labour ward protocols, the epidural catheter should be clearly labelled, e.g. with 'dural tap', and all subsequent top-ups administered by an anaesthetist. The woman, her partner and the attending midwives/obstetricians should be informed that accidental dural puncture has occurred.

Traditionally, women who have had an accidental dural puncture have been advised to accept instrumental delivery to avoid pushing, but this is now generally considered unnecessary.

After delivery, there is no benefit in restricting the mother to bed since this does not prevent PDPH. Similarly, although dehydration can exacerbate PDPH there is no evidence that overhydration has any beneficial effect. The mother should be visited regularly and given full support, and if PDPH occurs she should be offered the various management options available. She should also be informed about the possible serious sequelae of dural puncture, but reassured that they are rare. It is equally important that the anaesthetist is honest with his/her colleagues, since attempting to conceal accidental dural puncture may only serve to delay appropriate management. Each unit should have a clear protocol for managing accidental dural puncture, and there should be a system in place for recording and monitoring such cases, usually involving a senior anaesthetist. Postpartum follow-up at 6–10 weeks is recommended in order to check that symptoms have resolved and to advise about future pregnancies.

Key points

- Incidence of accidental dural puncture should be less than 1%.
- Immediate management includes resiting the epidural or inserting the catheter into the subarachnoid space.
- Saline infusion may decrease the incidence of headache if a catheter is placed epidurally.
- All top-ups should be administered by an anaesthetist.
- The mother should be allowed to mobilise freely and advised to avoid dehydration.
- Mothers should be followed regularly and any headache managed promptly.

FURTHER READING

Choi PT, Galinski SE, Takeuchi L, *et al.* PDPH is a common complication of neuraxial blockade in parturients: a meta-analysis of obstetrical studies. *Can J Anaesth* 2003; **50**: 460–9.

Jeskins GD, Moore PA, Cooper GM, Lewis M. Long-term morbidity following dural puncture in an obstetric population. *Int J Obstet Anesth* 2001; **10**: 17–24.

Paech M, Banks S, Gurrin L. An audit of accidental dural puncture during epidural insertion of a Tuohy needle in obstetric patients. *Int J Obstet Anesth* 2001; **10**: 162–7.

Turnbull DK, Shepherd DB. Post-dural puncture headache: pathogenesis, prevention and treatment. *Br J Anaesth* 2003; **91**: 718–29.

44 POSTDURAL PUNCTURE HEADACHE

Postdural puncture headache (PDPH) is typified by severe headache, usually frontal and bilateral, which is worsened by standing and relieved by lying. There may be associated neck stiffness, nausea, tinnitus, visual disturbances and photophobia. It is thought to arise from intracranial hypotension resulting from leakage of cerebrospinal fluid (CSF) through the dural hole, with stretching of the cranial nerve roots and meninges in the upright position. Thus the incidence and severity of PDPH are greatest following dural puncture with large cutting needles that leave large holes in the dura (70–90% in parturients after accidental dural puncture with a 16 G Tuohy needle), whereas small non-cutting needles are associated with a low incidence (under 1% with 25–27 G pencil-point needles). Parturients are more susceptible to PDPH than any other patient group.

There may be associated cerebral vasodilatation, leading to similarities being made between PDPH and migraine.

Symptoms usually begin within 1–2 days of dural puncture and last less than 1–2 weeks, although PDPH may occasionally persist for many months or even years.

Problems/special considerations

- Symptoms may be severe enough to prevent the mother mobilising and caring for her baby; this is particularly unwelcome in the early postpartum period. Discharge from hospital may be delayed, increasing costs and the risks of hospital-acquired infection and thromboembolism.
- Rarely, more sinister sequaelae may occur. These include cranial nerve palsies, convulsions and subdural or intracranial haemorrhage, which may lead to death.

Management options

It is important that a full history is taken and neurological examination performed, since there are many causes of postpartum headache (Table 44.1). Neurological referral may be wise in difficult cases. PDPH is suggested by a history of dural puncture and typical symptoms, especially the postural element. However, it may follow apparently unremarkable epidural anaesthesia; the incidence is unknown, although it may involve a number of factors including: lack of recognition at the time of dural puncture; lack of reporting dural puncture for fear of retribution; a possible tear of the dura but not arachnoid at the time of epidural insertion, with rupture of the arachnoid subsequently; and migration of the epidural catheter intrathecally during labour. It has been suggested that an otherwise typical PDPH that only becomes severe hours after getting up is caused by a very small dural hole with slow leak of CSF, e.g. after spinal anaesthesia with a very fine needle. A useful confirmatory sign is the lessening of headache produced by gradually compressing the upright patient's upper abdomen. This is thought to displace spinal CSF into the cranium by causing venous engorgement in the extradural space.

Table 44.1. Causes of postpartum headache

Tension, stress, fatigue, depression

Intracranial hypotension, e.g. postdural puncture headache

Intracranial hypertension, e.g. tumour, haematoma, cortical vein thrombosis, benign
  intracranial hypertension

Migraine

Infection, e.g. meningitis, sinusitis, encephalitis

Pre-eclampsia

Electrolyte imbalance, hypoglycaemia

Magnetic resonance imaging and computerised tomography scanning have been used to diagnose intracranial hypotension and to demonstrate cerebrospinal fluid leaks (in the latter case involving further diagnostic dural puncture), but are not widely used.

Initial management includes simple analgesics such as paracetamol and non-steroidal anti-inflammatory drugs. Constipation (which causes straining) should be prevented if possible by avoiding opioids such as codeine or by offering lactulose. Although dehydration can exacerbate the headache, there is no evidence that over-hydration has a beneficial effect. Other medical management includes oral caffeine 150–300 mg 6–8 hourly, which has been shown to improve the symptoms although not cure them. Caffeine may cause nausea and vomiting in overdosage and has been implicated in convulsions occurring after dural puncture. Successful use of the anti-migraine serotonin-receptor agonist sumatriptan (6 mg subcutaneously) has been described anecdotally, as has adrenocorticotrophic hormone (ACTH; 1–5 μU/kg in 1000–2000 ml saline given intravenously over one hour). However, despite anecdotal reports of ACTH's synthetic analogue Synacthen being successful, a randomised controlled trial found no benefit of Synacthen 1 mg intramuscularly.

Invasive procedures involve infusion or injection of various substances into the extradural space, firstly to shift CSF from the spine into the skull and secondly to tamponade leakage of CSF through the dural hole and even to seal the hole. Saline infusions have been used both diagnostically and therapeutically, and dextran has been used in an attempt to provide longer-lasting relief. However, epidural blood patch (EBP) is now generally accepted as the definitive treatment in persistent PDPH, with a success rate of 70–100%, although headache may recur. Many anaesthetists would now proceed to EBP early (e.g. within 24–48 hours of symptoms) if there is a good history rather than delay for several days as was common previously.

Full discussion with, and support of, the patient is of prime importance, since she may be more distressed by apparent indifference to the severity of her symptoms than by the complication itself. She should be regularly visited and the various options discussed, preferably by a senior anaesthetist. If she decides against an EBP, she should be reassured that she may come back at any time should her symptoms persist. She should also be told about the rare possibility of serious sequelae.

It is not known whether EBP prevents these, although this is generally assumed if symptoms resolve. Postpartum follow-up at 6–10 weeks is recommended in order to check that symptoms have resolved and to advise about future pregnancies.

Key points

- Postdural puncture headache occurs in 70–90% of parturients after accidental dural tap with a 16 G Tuohy needle.
- The postural element is the most important confirmatory feature.
- Initial management includes paracetamol, non-steroidal anti-inflammatory drugs, avoidance of dehydration, ± caffeine.
- Definitive treatment is with epidural blood patch.

FURTHER READING

Choi PT, Galinski SE, Takeuchi L, *et al.* PDPH is a common complication of neuraxial blockade in parturients: a meta-analysis of obstetrical studies. *Can J Anaesth* 2003; **50**: 460–9.

Rucklidge MW, Yentis SM, Paech MJ. Synacthen Depot for the treatment of postdural puncture headache. *Anaesthesia* 2004; **59**: 138–41.

Turnbull DK, Shepherd DB. Post-dural puncture headache: pathogenesis, prevention and treatment. *Br J Anaesth* 2003; **91**: 718–29.

45 EPIDURAL BLOOD PATCH

Injection of blood into the epidural space as a treatment for postdural puncture headache (PDPH) was first suggested in the 1960s, following the observation that the incidence of PDPH was lower when dural tap followed a bloody tap. In fact, this relationship was later found not to be so, but epidural blood patch (EBP) has became widely accepted as an effective treatment for PDPH (even after years), despite early fears about adverse effects.

The mechanism of action of EBP is uncertain; traditional teaching is that the blood seals the dural hole, preventing further leakage of cerebrospinal fluid. However, an alteration of cerebrospinal haemodynamics by EBP has been suggested, accounting for EBP's immediate effect and the observation that lumbar EBP is effective even following cervical dural puncture.

Problems/special considerations

- Current opinion favours early use of EBP for PDPH (e.g. within 1–2 days if headache is severe), although the place of prophylactic EBP via the epidural catheter after delivery is controversial. Although the incidence of postdural puncture headache in parturients is high (70–90%), prophylactic EBP may interfere with anaesthesia and analgesia if this is required postpartum and EBP may be less effective when performed prophylactically. In addition, the blood might represent an infection risk if the catheter remains *in situ* and prophylactic EBP represents an intervention that is unnecessary in 10–30% of mothers.

- Contraindications are those of epidural analgesia generally; in particular, the risk of epidural abscess is often quoted if the mother is pyrexial. In that situation, other methods of treating PDPH may be tried; alternatively, prophylactic use of antibiotics has been suggested. Some authorities advocate routine sending of blood for microbiological culture in case bacteraemia is present, although this practice is not universal.
- Adverse effects of EBP include those of epidural analgesia (including failure or another dural puncture), back pain, transient nerve root pain and pyrexia. Transient bradycardia has been reported but its significance is uncertain.

Management

Other causes of postpartum headache should be excluded (see Table 44.1, p. 115). Two operators are required. Whilst one locates the epidural space in the usual way, the other prepares to draw 20 ml of blood under aseptic conditions. The blood is injected slowly and the patient is asked to report any unpleasant effects. The interspace at or below the level of the original dural puncture is usually recommended, since injected blood has been shown to track mainly upwards after injection. In general, the more blood that is injected the greater the chance of success; most would attempt to inject 15–20 ml if no adverse effects allow. Flushing the epidural needle with saline as it is withdrawn has been suggested, to avoid leaving a plug of blood, which can act as a conduit for infection.

The patient is usually kept lying for 2–4 hours after EBP (reduced efficacy has been suggested if mobilisation is immediate). The success rate of EBP has been reported as 70–100%; typically, there is complete relief of headache, although some degree of headache may return in up to 30–50% of women. Repeat EBP is sometimes required, rarely more than once. The procedure is performed on an outpatient basis in some units.

The mother should be fully informed of the benefits and risks of EBP (including the fact that proper randomised trials are few, as concluded by a recent Cochrane review). A senior anaesthetist should perform the EBP for two reasons: first, the original epidural may have been difficult, and a second dural puncture occurring during EBP would be at best embarrassing; second, the mother has suffered considerable distress and deserves the reassurance of knowing that a senior anaesthetist is handling her case. Since the headache may return after EBP, she should be invited to contact the anaesthetist if this occurs.

Key points

- Epidural blood patch should be performed by a senior anaesthetist.
- Strict asepsis is required.
- 15–20 ml of blood is injected if tolerated.
- The mother is kept supine for 2–4 hours after patching.
- Epidural blood patch is thought to affect cerebrospinal haemodynamics $\pm$ plug the dural hole.
- Treatment is effective in 70–100% of cases but headache may recur in 30–50%.

FURTHER READING

Banks S, Paech M, Gurrin L. An audit of epidural blood patch after accidental dural puncture with a Tuohy needle in obstetric patients. *Int J Obstet Anesth* 2001; **10**: 172–6.

Cooper G. Epidural blood patch. *Eur J Anaesthesiol* 1999; **16**: 211–15.

Duffy PJ, Crosby ET. The epidural blood patch. Resolving the controversies. *Can J Anaesth* 1999; **46**: 878–86.

Sudlow C, Warlow C. Epidural blood patching for preventing and treating post-dural puncture headache (Cochrane Review). In: *The Cochrane Library*, Issue 1, 2004. Chichester, UK: John Wiley & Sons, Ltd.

46   EXTENSIVE REGIONAL BLOCKS

Obstetric anaesthetists, in routinely extending neuraxial analgesia up to the level of T4, are accustomed to dealing with regional anaesthetic blocks that other practitioners would regard as excessively high. It is inevitable that occasionally the block will extend beyond the anticipated area, either due to inadvertent subarachnoid or subdural administration or merely because of the unpredictability of spread in some individuals. Although many such blocks may be quite benign and not cause any cardiovascular or respiratory embarrassment, it is important that they are detected in order to pick up misplacement of the local anaesthetic, which may cause more serious problems later.

'Total spinal block' is strictly defined as a spinal block that results in unconsciousness and central depression of respiratory and myocardial activity, accompanied by massive vasodilatation. Since the same may also result from epidural and subdural blocks, and one should not wait until unconsciousness before acting, the terms 'high regional block' or 'extensive regional block' are preferred. A practical definition of these terms would be a regional block that results in the need for tracheal intubation or other airway intervention. The reported incidence of such blocks is between 1 in $\sim$2000 and 1 in $\sim$13 000, probably reflecting differences in definitions used in the studies from which these figures arise.

Problems/special considerations

- The effect and spread of local anaesthetic drugs is enhanced in pregnancy and this should be borne in mind when planning doses for a spinal or epidural block.
- An apparently fixed spinal block may extend further if the patient is moved, even 30 minutes or more after the local anaesthetic has been administered. This particularly applies to rotation through the fully supine position from one side to the other and may be due to dural compression resulting from dilatation of the epidural veins, which act as a collateral circulation during aortocaval compression.
- Early features of extensive block include weakness/tingling of the upper arms and shoulders, breathing difficulties, slurred speech and sedation. Symptoms and signs may develop late and insidiously.
- Hypotension may be severe and may be associated with reduced placental perfusion and fetal hypoxia/ischaemia. Urgent delivery may be necessary both to relieve maternal hypotension and to protect the fetus.
- Airway management following total spinal block is made more difficult in pregnancy because of the increased risk of aspiration and the difficulty in maintaining a clear airway without tracheal intubation.

Epidural analgesia/anaesthesia

Relatively large doses of local anaesthetic drugs are used which, if they find their way into the wrong compartment, can cause a dangerously extensive block.

Prevention is the key, and this is achieved by maintaining a high index of suspicion and regarding every dose of local anaesthetic as subarachnoid until proven otherwise. The potential problems are best discussed under the following headings:

- *Epidural analgesia:* a test dose suitable for distinguishing subarachnoid placement should be used after the epidural catheter is inserted, and the effect should be assessed before further local anaesthetic is given. Each epidural dose should be given sufficiently slowly to allow detection of a spinal block before it spreads to a dangerously high level; doses should be administered at intervals of 5 minutes or longer, with the mother moving between increments. These precautions should be used with every dose in labour, since catheter migration has been known to occur between doses. The use of low-dose local anaesthetic/opioid mixtures reduces the risk to the mother if inadvertently given intrathecally; the local anaesthetic concentration should be the lowest for the effect required.
- *Epidural top-up for instrumental or Caesarean delivery:* volumes of up to 20 ml concentrated solution may be injected over 3 minutes, the risk of extensive block being weighed against the need for rapid extension for surgery. It has been suggested that the top-up can safely be given in the labour room and the patient

transferred to theatre while the block is extending, although this is controversial, since the ability to monitor and/or resuscitate may not be ideal before/during transit. It is essential that the anaesthetist is by the patient at all times and ensures adequate monitoring and lateral tilt. Regular testing of the block is mandatory.

- *Epidural after dural puncture with the Tuohy needle:* if an epidural catheter has been resited following inadvertent dural puncture, the risk of high block is increased, both because the local anaesthetic can leak through the puncture and because the catheter can migrate. Epidural doses/infusions should be reduced and given by an anaesthetist.

- *Subdural block:* this is thought to occur in up to 1% of 'epidurals'. It may occur when the epidural catheter is passed into the potential space between the dura mater and the arachnoid, probably after the needle has torn the dura. The block is characteristically slow (20–30 minutes) in onset and spreads cranially much higher than expected, often involving the lower cervical dermatomes. Extensive motor block is, however, uncommon, and hypotension is usually mild. The block tends to spare the lumbar and sacral segments and may be patchy; consequently, pain relief is often poor. If analgesia is acceptable, it is tempting to leave the catheter *in situ* and to continue to use smaller doses. This technique should be avoided, however, because of the risk of a top-up rupturing the arachnoid, with subsequent development of an extensive subarachnoid block.

- *Inadvertent subarachnoid block:* this is rarer than subdural block, largely because the anaesthetist is usually alerted by the free flow of cerebrospinal fluid from the hub of the catheter. The consequences are far more hazardous, however, since the resulting block is very rapid in onset, has a considerable motor component and is normally associated with severe hypotension.

Spinal anaesthesia

High blocks associated with spinal anaesthesia are related to greater spread rather than deposition of local anaesthetic into the wrong space. This may result from use of hypobaric solutions, or compression of the dural sac from the outside as a result either of recent epidural top-up or of aortocaval compression, or it may represent an extreme of normal variation as anaesthetists have sought higher and higher blocks in order to avoid pain during surgery. The continuous presence of the anaesthetist and the immediate availability in the operating theatre of the necessary equipment and assistance ensure that further supportive measures are readily available if needed.

Prevention of excessive block is achieved by using the minimum necessary dose of local anaesthetic, which should be hyperbaric to allow control of spread. Excessive barbotage should also be avoided. Maintenance of the natural kyphosis of the thoracic spine if in lateral tilt, or the use of pillows under the shoulders and head if in the full lateral position, will help prevent the local anaesthetic spreading higher than the T4 dermatomes. Head-down tilt is very occasionally needed to encourage a recalcitrant block to spread high enough for surgery, but this should be used with great care and reversed as soon as the desired effect has been achieved. The same precautions apply if the mother is rolled through the full supine position as part of the positioning or if she is coughing or otherwise performing a Valsalva manoeuvre; these can result in sudden cranial spread of the block, and this can even happen at the end of a procedure when the block has been established for some time.

The ideal dose of spinal solution to use after a recent (failed) epidural top-up is uncertain. There have been reports of extensive blocks if normal spinal doses are used, presumably as a result of dural compression, but there have also been reports of normal responses or even inadequate anaesthesia if smaller doses are used.

Management options

- The basics (ABC) of resuscitation should be remembered. Aortocaval compression should be prevented and the full lateral position is best if cardiopulmonary resuscitation is not needed.
- Oxygen should be given by facemask and tracheal intubation performed early if a raising block progresses; waiting until the patient is unconscious may risk airway obstruction and/or aspiration of gastric contents.
- Cardiovascular support includes copious intravenous fluids, vasopressors such as ephedrine or phenylephrine (adrenaline may be needed if hypotension is resistant) and cardiopulmonary resuscitation if cardiac arrest or severe myocardial depression is compromising cerebral oxygenation.
- Delivering the fetus should be considered to protect it from hypotension and to relieve aortocaval compression.

Key points

- All epidural doses should be divided into safe aliquots if time permits.
- Subdural catheter placement is common and may progress to subarachnoid block.
- Spinal blocks can spread cranially even 30 minutes after administration.
- Careful and regular monitoring of the height of block is required after institution of spinal or epidural anaesthesia.
- Delivery of the fetus may protect it from ischaemia and may also benefit the mother.

FURTHER READING

Jenkins JG. Some immediate serious complications of obstetric epidural analgesia and anaesthesia: a prospective study of 145,550 epidurals. *Int J Obstet Anesth* 2005; **14**: 37–42.

Yentis SM, Dob DP. High regional blockade – the failed intubation of the new millennium? *Int J Obstet Anesth* 2001; **10**: 159–61.

47   INADEQUATE REGIONAL ANALGESIA IN LABOUR

Although epidural analgesia has an excellent track record for relieving the pain of labour, a proportion of epidurals fail to deliver adequate pain relief. Approximately 10% of women will have initially unsatisfactory blocks, and around 2% of these will be persistently inadequate. Poor blocks can be conveniently grouped into three categories, which may also represent different aetiologies, namely, limited unilateral spread, unilateral block and inadequate spread.

Problems/special considerations

- *Limited unilateral spread:* only one or two dermatomes, usually lumbar, are successfully blocked, and this is typically unilateral. Limited unilateral spread is responsible for the poorest quality blocks, and the effect is often so limited that a cursory test might suggest that there is no block at all. The block is usually confined to the lumbar dermatomes closest to the insertion site of the catheter and is due to the tip of the catheter 'escaping' from the epidural space via the intervertebral foramen. The incidence of this complication is related to the length of catheter inserted into the epidural space.
- *Unilateral block:* cranial and caudal spread is satisfactory, but the block is limited to one side of the body only. Contrast studies of this type of block have shown that it is associated with distribution of fluid to one side of the epidural space only. The most likely explanation is the existence of a dorsal midline septum arising from the posterior aspect of the dura mater, which acts as a barrier to the free spread of local anaesthetic. Unilateral block has also been shown to be more common in cases of scoliosis and this is also presumed to be due to anatomical barriers to spread of local anaesthetic in the epidural space. Missed segment, whereby one or more segments remains unblocked despite normal analgesia above and below, is much rarer than unilateral block but may also be related to the isolation of some nerve roots from the local anaesthetic by longitudinal septae.
- *Inadequate spread:* the cranial or caudal extent of spread is insufficient and cannot be extended with further doses. Contrast studies have suggested that there may be a horizontal septum preventing flow in these cases. Limited cranial or caudal spread is also often seen in patients who have undergone spinal surgery and is presumed to be due to scarring in the epidural space.

Catheters with single terminal eyes are commonly used in the USA, whereas most UK practitioners prefer multi-holed, blind-ending catheters. Studies have demonstrated a higher incidence of unsatisfactory blocks with the former, mostly due to unilateral blocks and missed segments. This is probably due to a 'streaming' effect, whereby all the solution is directed along a single track, encouraging longitudinal spread at the expense of lateral flow.

Management options

The key to managing poor blocks is early detection. All mothers who have had an epidural block in labour should be checked by the anaesthetist within 30 minutes of the first dose and the level of analgesia tested with a suitable stimulus. Any complaint of persistent pain at any time during the labour should prompt further testing.

A limited unilateral block is usually due to an excessive amount of catheter having been inserted into the epidural space. Anything greater than 5 cm is generally regarded as likely to lead to transforaminal escape of the catheter tip. Even multi-holed catheters can be freely pulled back to leave 2–5 cm in the space in an attempt to overcome this problem. Unfortunately, once a 'track' has been established for the local anaesthetic solution, it may persist despite the catheter being pulled back, and the only solution may be to remove the catheter and resite it in a different space. Even if the catheter was originally inserted to the optimum distance, the possibility of it being drawn further into the epidural space should not be discounted; this has been shown to happen as a result of traction imposed by movements of the vertebrae and activity of the spinal muscles.

Unilateral block can occasionally be overcome by lying the patient on the affected side and administering large volumes of local anaesthetic, with or without opioid. It is presumed that this encourages spread of the solution up and down the epidural space and thus beyond the boundaries of any midline septum or allows any breaches in the septum to be exploited. These manoeuvres will be effective in only about 50% of cases and, even in these, there will always be a marked tendency for the block to affect one side more than the other. In the more recalcitrant unilateral block, the catheter may need to be resited in another space. To prevent the same problem from arising again, a paramedian approach from the unblocked side is recommended. The original catheter may be left in place to prevent the same problem arising on the other side.

Inadequate caudal spread can often be helped by using epidural opioids. In more difficult cases, a caudal catheter can be sited via the sacral hiatus, and doses of local anaesthetic can be divided between the two routes. A similar approach using a low thoracic epidural can also be employed for inadequate cranial spread.

In general, when the above manipulations have been unsuccessful, a paramedian approach may help, since the catheter has been shown to travel a straighter course in the epidural space when inserted via this route. A combined spinal–epidural technique may be used to overcome poor spread or missed segments, and a continuous spinal catheter may be used as the last resort when all else fails.

Other causes for poor block should not be overlooked. Continuous infusion techniques may fail if the syringe pump is not functioning properly, has been incorrectly set up or has become occluded. The commonest reason for a previously satisfactory block failing is the epidural catheter falling out – another good reason for checking the catheter first.

Finally, it should be remembered that an inadequate epidural for labour may be inadequate for Caesarean section should one be required in an emergency; in such situations it might be appropriate to consider spinal anaesthesia instead. Furthermore, in women with a high risk of Caesarean section the anaesthetist should have a low threshhold for resiting an epidural if the latter is less than perfect during labour.

> **Key points**
>
> - Blocks should be checked regularly to allow early detection of failure.
> - In the event of a poor block, especially when previously satisfactory, the catheter should be checked.
> - Poor spread is often due to an excessive length of catheter in the epidural space. A length of 2–5 cm is optimum.
> - Resiting the catheter early is often a better option than repeated 'fiddling'.

FURTHER READING

Pan PH, Bogard TD, Owen MD. Incidence and characteristics of failures in obstetric neuraxial analgesia and anesthesia: a retrospective analysis of 19,259 deliveries. *Int J Obstet Anesth* 2004; **13**: 227–33.

Riley ET, Papasin J. Epidural catheter function during labor predicts anesthetic efficacy for subsequent cesarean delivery. *Int J Obstet Anesth* 2002; **11**: 81–4.

48   BACKACHE

Backache is not a trivial symptom. It is the commonest cause of time off work in the UK, and can be particularly debilitating for the nursing mother.

Backache is very common, and a high proportion of women have significant backache before pregnancy, with surveys putting this figure at around 15%. During pregnancy, the prevalence of backache rises to 51%.

Long-term backache after childbirth (defined as backache lasting longer than 3 months) occurs in about a third of women and this increases to half if there is a history of backache before or during the pregnancy. The incidence of new, long-term backache in women with no symptoms of backache before or during pregnancy is much lower, at around 5–10%.

Problems/special considerations

Prospective studies have found no significant increase in the risk of backache when epidural analgesia is used in labour, nor an association with motor block.

Despite this, there is a popular belief among parturients, midwives and even obstetricians that there is a causative link between epidural analgesia in labour and subsequent backache, largely arising from retrospective surveys of mothers in the late 1980s. Many women who develop intractable backache shortly after an anaesthetist has inserted a needle into their back will, not surprisingly, believe that the two are connected, and commonly refer to their backache as starting 'after the epidural' instead of 'after the baby'.

This is not to say, of course, that a poorly administered epidural cannot cause trauma that might lead to backache or that backache should be ignored after an epidural. In particular, acute tenderness over the epidural site should always raise the suspicion of an epidural abscess or haematoma, especially when accompanied by pyrexia and signs of nerve root irritation or cauda equina syndrome. Finally, rare incidental causes such as a tumour should not be overlooked.

Management options

Women with backache often present to the anaesthetist in the antenatal period. Referral to the obstetric physiotherapist, lumbar support, simple analgesia and transcutaneous electrical nerve stimulation (TENS) may all be of help.

With the evidence as it currently stands, there is no need to warn women of the risk of backache when preparing to perform epidural or spinal anaesthesia. However, many women ask about this complication, especially at antenatal classes, and the best approach is to inform them of the high risk of long-term backache associated with pregnancy and childbirth and to reassure them that epidurals do not appear to increase this risk.

The woman who presents with severe backache or a long history of back trouble in the antenatal clinic should be warned that it is very likely that this will continue after childbirth. Epidural analgesia should not be contraindicated in these cases but it may sometimes be more painful having an epidural sited in a sensitive back. A 'mobile' technique should be preferred, to allow the patient to move freely in labour, and care should be taken to avoid unnatural postures that will unduly stress the ligaments. Support of lumbar lordosis and prevention of hyperextension at the hips is helpful.

Midwives should be alerted to refer acute, localised backache after epidural to the anaesthetist. Management should include a full neurological examination, early referral to a neurologist and an early magnetic resonance imaging scan to exclude haematoma or abscess.

Localised tenderness and limitation of movement may be due to a small haematoma in the interspinous ligament or paraspinous muscles and these will often respond to physiotherapy.

> **Key points**
>
> - Backache is very common after childbirth.
> - There is no apparent link between epidural/spinal analgesia and long-term postpartum backache.
> - Tenderness associated with pyrexia should raise the suspicion of abscess.

FURTHER READING

Howell CJ, Dean T, Lucking L, *et al.* Randomised study of long term outcome after epidural versus non-epidural analgesia during labour. *BMJ* 2002; **325**: 357

Loughnan BA, Carli F, Romney M, Dore CJ, Gordon H. Epidural analgesia and backache: a randomized controlled comparison with intramuscular meperidine for analgesia during labour. *Br J Anaesth* 2002; **89**: 466–72.

MacEvilly M, Buggy D. Back pain and pregnancy: a review. *Pain* 1996; **64**: 405–14.

49   HORNER'S SYNDROME AND CRANIAL NERVE PALSY

Horner's syndrome is the combination of partial ptosis, myosis (small pupil), enophthalmos and hypohydrosis, and represents interruption of the ipsilateral sympathetic supply to the head anywhere along its length. There may also be associated nasal stuffiness and reduced taste sensation on the ipsilateral side (Gustav's sign). Horner's syndrome may occasionally occur during an otherwise unremarkable epidural block.

Palsies of cranial nerves V and VI have been reported following uncomplicated obstetric epidural anaesthesia, although much less commonly than Horner's syndrome. In addition, cranial nerve palsies are well known to occur (albeit uncommonly) following dural puncture, and cases (including cranial nerve VII palsy) have been reported after accidental dural tap during childbirth. An idiopathic lower motor neurone lesion of cranial nerve VII (Bell's palsy) may occur rarely in pregnancy but there is no evidence that it is related to regional anaesthesia.

Problems/special considerations

The mechanism for Horner's syndrome occurring during apparently normal and non-extensive epidural anaesthesia is uncertain; partial subdural cranial extension of local anaesthetic solution has been suggested, although there may be no other features of atypical block. The sympathetic innervation of the iris is variable and may arise from C8 to T5; in addition, sympathetic fibres are thought to be more sensitive to local anaesthetics than somatic fibres. Increased incidence in pregnancy has been suggested and may be related to the greater susceptibility of pregnant women to local anaesthetics generally or to more extensive central neural blocks in particular. Cranial nerve palsy is also thought to be related to excessively high blockade; palsy of cranial nerve V is commonly associated with Horner's syndrome. Cranial nerve palsy following dural puncture is thought to be related to stretching of the nerve caused by traction of intracranial contents and is usually associated with postdural puncture headache.

Lesions may go unnoticed or may cause alarm to the patient, her partner or labour ward staff. In addition, if another possibly unrelated complication or event were to occur or if general anaesthesia were administered subsequently, the pupillary signs especially may cause confusion.

Management options

For cases occurring during uncomplicated epidural anaesthesia, no specific treatment is required other than reassurance, since the signs themselves are harmless and disappear when the epidural block wears off. Although there are other more sinister causes of Horner's syndrome and cranial nerve palsies, they are rare and would not be expected to cause signs to appear so acutely in the absence of other symptoms or signs, and last such a short time. Palsies associated with dural puncture should be managed as for the headache; it has been suggested that resolution of the palsy is less likely if epidural blood patch is delayed.

There is no evidence that the occurrence of Horner's syndrome or cranial nerve palsy during one labour epidural predisposes the patient to the same thing during subsequent epidurals.

It must not be forgotten that some individuals naturally have unequal pupils or an asymmetrical face; it is therefore worth asking the patient and her partner whether the signs are new. Once diagnosed, simple observation is all that is required, bearing in mind that the intense interest of medical and midwifery staff may cause more anxiety than the syndrome itself.

Key points

- Horner's syndrome:
  - Comprises partial ptosis, myosis, enophthalmos and hypohydrosis
  - May occur during an otherwise unremarkable epidural
  - Is harmless and requires no treatment if related to epidural anaesthesia.
- Cranial nerve palsy:
  - Most commonly involves nerves V or VI although the incidence is less than that of Horner's syndrome
  - Requires no treatment if of short duration and associated only with regional anaesthesia.

FURTHER READING

Day CJE, Shutt LE. Auditory, ocular, and facial complications of central neural block. *Reg Anesth* 1996; **21**: 197–201.

Dunbar SA, Katz NP. Failure of delayed epidural blood patching to correct persistent cranial nerve palsies. *Anesth Analg* 1994; **79**: 806–7.

Loo CC, Dahlgren G, Irestedt L. Neurological complications in obstetric regional anaesthesia. *Int J Obstet Anesth* 2000; **9**: 99–124.

50 PERIPHERAL NERVE LESIONS FOLLOWING REGIONAL ANAESTHESIA

Although spinal and epidural needles and catheters must, by virtue of their mode of action, pass close to nerve roots, the incidence of neurological damage appears to be very low. Surveys have suggested that around 1 in 2000 obstetric epidurals/ spinals is complicated by numbness, paraesthesia or weakness in the distribution of a single nerve root that may take several days to a few months to resolve. The incidence of permanent symptoms is approximately 1 in 15 000.

Problems/special considerations

- *Other causes of nerve damage:* while it is perhaps natural to blame any lower limb neurological deficit on the neuraxial block that preceded it, nerve palsy is more likely to arise as a result of obstetric factors, as witnessed by patients with demonstrable permanent lesions despite not having had epidural or spinal procedures. The overall incidence of these complications is estimated to be around 1 in 2000 deliveries, and the causes and features are listed in Table 50.1. The potential for nerve damage during childbirth is apparent when one considers the anatomy of the nerves arising in the pelvis (Figure 10.6; p. 24).
- *Aetiology of nerve root damage:* a needle or catheter touching a nerve root is almost certain to cause paraesthesia in the awake patient, usually of a severe, lancinating quality and characteristically described as being like an electric shock in the distribution of the nerve root. Unless transient and mild, parasthesia should always prompt the anaesthetist to remove the needle or catheter and to reorientate it. Presence or absence of paraesthesia should always be recorded. If damage has occurred, symptoms are usually experienced in the same distribution (Table 50.2).
- *Central neurological lesions:* single nerve damage should be distinguished from the more serious central lesions that occur extremely rarely (see Chapter 51, Spinal cord lesions following regional anaesthesia, p. 130; Chapter 52, Arachnoiditis, p. 132; Chapter 53, Cauda equina syndrome, p. 134).

Management options

Prevention is the most important aspect of management. Blocks should be performed with the patient awake (not normally an issue in obstetric practice),

Table 50.1. Nerve lesions with non-anaesthetic, obstetric causes

Lesion	Presentation	Cause
Lumbosacral trunk	Foot drop Loss of sensation, esp. L4–5, S1	Pressure in pelvis from fetal head or forceps
Peroneal nerve	Foot drop	Pressure from lithotomy poles or prolonged squatting
Femoral nerve	Loss of sensation front of thigh Quadriceps weakness Reduced knee jerk	Hyperflexion of thighs, esp. squatting or lithotomy position
Lateral cutaneous nerve of thigh	Meralgia paraesthetica – altered sensation over anterolateral aspect of thigh	Antenatal weight gain $\pm$ lumbar lordosis
Conus of spinal cord	Anterior spinal artery syndrome – cauda equina/paraplegia	Obstruction of aberrant blood supply to conus by fetal head during prolonged labour

Table 50.2. Neurological deficit following nerve root trauma

Root	Sensory loss	Motor weakness
L2	Upper anterior thigh	Hip flexion
L3	Lower anterior & medial thigh	Thigh adduction
L4	Lateral thigh, knee & medial leg	Leg extension
L5	Lateral leg & dorsum of foot	Ankle dorsiflexion
S1	Lateral foot	Ankle plantar flexion

and care should be taken to ensure that the interspace chosen is below the level of termination of the spinal cord. Patients should be asked to indicate if they feel paraesthesia, and this should be a signal to the anaesthetist to remove the needle or catheter and start again. Spinal injections should only be given if there is free flow of cerebrospinal fluid, to ensure that the needle tip is not obstructed by nerve tissue. A note should always be made as to the presence or absence of paraesthesia during the procedure, as this information can be invaluable later.

Routine follow-up should be carried out assiduously, and midwives should be alerted to notify the anaesthetist if any mother shows signs of slow recovery of sensory or motor function. Careful mapping of the deficit should be carried out at the earliest opportunity to establish a baseline from which improvement can be measured. Other, non-anaesthetic, causes should be considered; the aetiology may be suggested by the distribution of the deficit and by other precipitating factors (see Table 50.1). The benign course of the vast majority of these lesions means that an explanation to the patient can include a reassuring prognosis. Generally neuro-praxias recover in three months though occasionally chronic pain may ensue, so postpartum follow-up should always be offered.

Except for minor and resolving lesions, further management should generally involve referral to a neurologist or neurophysiologist. Imaging of the lumbar region is rarely helpful but may be used to exclude coincidental causes such as a prolapsed intervertebral disc. Nerve conduction studies are often invaluable as they allow the site of the lesion to be identified and often help in determining prognosis.

Key points

- Paraesthesia should always be documented and is a sign to withdraw the needle, reorientate it and start again.
- Delayed recovery needs assiduous follow-up to detect neuraxial haematoma/abscess.
- Nerve palsy is usually a result of pregnancy/childbirth and unrelated to regional anaesthesia.

FURTHER READING

Dar AQ, Robinson APC, Lyons G. Postpartum neurological symptoms following regional blockade: a prospective study with case controls. *Int J Obstet Anesth* 2002; **11**: 85–90.

Loo CC, Dahlgren G, Irestedt L. Neurological complications in obstetric regional anaesthesia. *Int J Obstet Anesth* 2000; **9**: 99–124.

Wong CA. Neurological deficits and labor analgesia. *Reg Anesth Pain Med* 2004; **29**: 341–51.

51 SPINAL CORD LESIONS FOLLOWING REGIONAL ANAESTHESIA

Postpartum neurological lesions are often blamed on peripartum anaesthetic inter-ventions, even though non-anaesthetic causes are much more likely. Obstetric anaesthetists may therefore find themselves involved in the assessment and management of these problems. There are many causes of spinal cord lesions (Table 51.1).

Problems/special considerations

The initial problem is one of diagnosis. Different lesions may present in different ways that may overlap with each other and with other conditions (Table 51.1). Although cord lesions generally present with upper motor neurone signs and sensory impairment below the level of injury, and peripheral nerve injuries present with lower motor neurone signs, it may be surprisingly difficult to distinguish them clinically (see Chapter 50, Peripheral nerve lesions following regional

Table 51.1. Causes of postpartum spinal cord lesions

Mechanism	Condition	Comment
Compression	Epidural haematoma	May be associated with back pain
	Epidural abscess	Associated with back pain plus evidence of local and/or systemic infection; typically presents several days postpartum
	Prolapsed disc	Associated with back pain; may present de novo intra- or postpartum
	Tumour	May be associated with back pain
Ischaemia*	Severe hypotension	Not associated with back pain
	Anomalous arterial blood supply plus prolonged labour or hypotension	Includes arteriovenous malformations or a predominantly pelvic blood supply to the conus medularis and cauda equina
	Normal vascular supply and normotension	Has been reported in spinal stenosis following rapid injection of a large epidural bolus
Neurotoxicity	Injection of wrong solution	May be associated with back pain
Trauma	Back injury	Associated with back pain
	Direct damage during regional anaesthesia	May be associated with back pain although paraesthesia is more common

*N.B. compression results in local ischaemia.

anaesthesia, p. 128). Sinister signs such as pyrexia, severe back pain, bilateral distribution, or loss of bladder or bowel function are suggestive of a compressive lesion such as epidural or spinal haematoma/abscess. These conditions are very rare (less than 1 in 100 000) but may cause major, irreversible damage unless relieved within hours of presentation. Any suspicion should prompt immediate referral for a neurosurgical opinion. In the case of early lesions, some effects of spinal or epidural blockade may persist for several hours, occasionally over 12 hours (up to 48 hours has been reported after epidural blockade, with no apparent cause), obscuring the underlying pathology. Since regression of a block often occurs under observation by non-anaesthetic staff, there may be delay in appropriate medical input being requested. In the case of acute potentially reversible spinal cord damage, e.g. cord compression caused by haematoma, delay of more than 6–8 hours is associated with an increasing chance of permanent impairment.

Similarly, problems that present later, such as epidural abscess, may be missed if associated back pain is dismissed as trivial.

Management options

Anaesthetic-related problems may be reduced by attention to details such as:

- Assessing the coagulation status and pre-existing neurological status before performing regional techniques
- Aseptic technique
- Determining appropriate anatomical landmarks during the procedure and awareness of the risk of and from inserting the needle too high
- Removal of the needle if severe parasthesia or pain is experienced during a regional block
- Prevention and management of hypotension after anaesthesia.

Any unexpectedly dense or prolonged block should always be observed carefully, especially if other risk factors (e.g. heparin therapy) are present. A careful history and examination, and knowledge of the relevant anatomy, are vital to distinguish the various lesions from less severe conditions, and neurological referral is always advisable if there is any suspicion.

Individual conditions are managed as for non-pregnant patients, e.g. surgical decompression for cord compression, plus antibiotics for abscess.

Key points

- Anaesthetists may be involved in the assessment and management of postpartum spinal cord lesions.
- Knowledge of the appropriate anatomy is crucial.
- In acute spinal cord compression, delay in decompression beyond 6–8 hours may result in permanent disability.

FURTHER READING

Loo CC, Dahlgren G, Irestedt L. Neurological complications in obstetric regional anaesthesia. *Int J Obstet Anesth* 2000; **9**: 99–124.

Horlocker TT, Wedel DJ. Neurologic complications of spinal and epidural anesthesia. *Reg Anesth Pain Med* 2000; **25**: 83–98.

Reynolds F. Damage to the conus medullar is following spinal anaesthesia. *Anaesthesia* 2001; **56**: 238–47.

Wong CA. Neurological deficits and labor analgesia. *Reg Anesth Pain Med* 2004; **29**: 341–51.

52 ARACHNOIDITIS

Arachnoiditis is a rare condition comprising chronic radicular pain associated with radiologically diagnosed abnormalities, classically filling defects in the subarachnoid space, absence of spinal nerve root sleeves, arachnoid cysts and obstruction to flow of radio-opaque contrast medium. It is important to realise that radiological abnormalities may be present in asymptomatic patients, and a diagnosis of arachnoiditis should not be made on radiological criteria alone. It may occur spontaneously, although it has followed radiation and perispinal injection of irritant substances, e.g. oil-based contrast medium that used to be employed for myelography. Antiseptic solutions, powder from surgical gloves and preservatives in drug solutions (e.g. sodium metabisulphite) have been implicated, as have infection and traumatic bleeding.

Arachnoiditis may occasionally be confused with cauda equina syndrome; typical features of the two conditions are shown in Table 52.1.

Problems/special considerations

Chronic adhesive arachnoiditis typically develops several months or even years after the trigger, so it may be difficult to establish a causal link. Typically arachnoiditis presents with back pain, with or without leg pain parasthesia or weakness. It is usually steadily progressive and may follow neurological complications of regional anaesthesia.

Management options

Although obstetric regional analgesia and anaesthesia is considered to be extremely safe, it is important to maintain scrupulous attention to aseptic and atraumatic technique and to minimise the use of novel drugs and multiple combinations of drugs. Thus all solutions injected epidurally or spinally should be carefully checked first. Once the diagnosis is suspected, early involvement of a neurologist is mandatory with confirmation of the diagnosis by MRI scan. Detailed follow-up

Table 52.1. Typical features of arachnoiditis and cauda equina syndrome

	Aetiology	Features
Arachnoiditis	Inflammation of the arachnoid meningeal layer and subarachnoid space. Progressive fibrosis may cause spinal canal narrowing, ischaemia and permanent nerve damage	Meningeal irritation may occur early, although usually presents months or years later. May involve the cauda equina, presenting with similar features. Rarely extends cranially
Cauda equina syndrome	Damage to the lumbosacral nerve roots	Presents soon after regional anaesthesia, with numbness in corresponding dermatomes, weakness of corresponding myotomes, sphincter dysfunction

and possibly long-term support will be required. There is no specific treatment for arachnoiditis; steroids may be tried, although they are thought to be effective only in the very acute stage of the inflammatory process. Psychological support is important since the consequences of the condition may be catastrophic.

Key points

- Arachnoiditis is inflammation of the arachnoid and subarachnoid space; it typically occurs months or more after injury.
- Although rare, it may cause permanent neurological damage.

FURTHER READING

Aldrete JA. Neurologic deficits and arachnoiditis following neuroaxial anesthesia. *Acta Anaesthesiol Scand* 2003; **47**: 3–12.

Loo CC, Dahlgren G, Irestedt L. Neurological complications in obstetric regional anaesthesia. *Int J Obstet Anesth* 2000; **9**: 99–124.

Rice I, Wee MYK, Thompson K. Obstetric epidurals and chronic adhesive arachnoiditis. *Br J Anaesth* 2004: **92**: 109–20.

53   CAUDA EQUINA SYNDROME

Cauda equina syndrome is a rare condition that has been associated with ultra-fine spinal catheters, especially when hyperbaric lidocaine has been injected. It is thought that poor mixing of local anaesthetic in the cerebrospinal fluid results in pooling of anaesthetic in the terminal dural sac, especially if large doses are used to extend an inadequate block. Local anaesthetics are known to be directly neurotoxic in high concentrations, lidocaine more than bupivacaine. The cauda equina nerve fibres may be more vulnerable to damage than other structures because they lack protective sheaths.

Cauda equina syndrome may occasionally be confused with arachnoiditis (for typical features of the two conditions, see Chapter 52, Arachnoiditis, p. 132).

Problems/special considerations

Isolated areas of numbness on the leg and disturbances of perineal sensation are relatively common after delivery, making diagnosis difficult. Cauda equina syndrome may cause permanent neurological impairment.

Management options

Scrupulous attention to technique should be used when performing regional analgesia and anaesthesia. Special precautions should be taken when using continuous spinal blockade (e.g. avoiding lidocaine, especially in high concentrations, and not injecting large volumes of hyperbaric solutions). Once the diagnosis is suspected, early involvement of a neurologist is mandatory since detailed follow-up and possibly long-term support will be required. There is no specific treatment for cauda equina syndrome, although steroids may be tried. Psychological support is important since the consequences of the condition may be catastrophic.

Key points

- Cauda equina syndrome results from damage to the lumbosacral nerve roots; the condition occurs soon after the insult.
- Although rare, it may cause permanent neurological damage.

FURTHER READING

Loo CC, Dahlgren G, Irestedt L. Neurological complications in obstetric regional anaesthesia. *Int J Obstet Anesth* 2000; **9**: 99–124.

54   OPIOID-INDUCED PRURITUS

Itching can result from the administration of opioids by any route but is much more common following epidural and intrathecal opioids than with systemically administered opioids. The reported incidence of itching varies from 0 to 100% and it is sometimes only discovered as a result of observing the patient or asking direct questions. Severe itching is a problem in only a very small number of cases (possibly as low as 1%). The incidence of itching associated with opioids is higher in the obstetric population, probably due to an oestrogenic influence at the opioid receptors.

Facial itching predominates after epidural and intrathecal opioids. This is possibly due to migration of opioid in the cerebrospinal fluid to the trigeminal nucleus and the trigeminal nerve roots. More generalised itching occurs with systemically administered opioids and may be due to activation of peripheral opioid receptors and partly due to histamine release (especially with morphine). The mechanism of opioid-induced itching is still not completely understood.

Problems/special considerations

The incidence of pruritus varies considerably among different opioids, being highest with morphine and lowest with the most lipophilic drugs such as fentanyl and sufentanil. Mixed agonist–antagonist drugs such as buprenorphine and butorphanol have been used via the epidural route to reduce the incidence of itching without decreasing analgesia.

Itching following administration of intrathecal fentanyl for Caesarean section does not appear to predict that itching will also occur after epidural administration of diamorphine for postoperative analgesia.

Management options

No treatment is necessary for opioid-induced itching unless the mother is distressed. Simple antihistamines may be effective. Naloxone is an effective treatment for pruritus, but reduces the duration of analgesia obtained with neuraxial opioids, although a low-dose continuous infusion (0.4–0.6 mg/h) of naloxone is said to treat itching whilst maintaining analgesia from intrathecal morphine.

A variety of other treatments have been proposed, including intravenous droperidol, subhypnotic doses of propofol, ondansetron, nalbuphine and intramuscular promethazine. There is little evidence that any are effective.

Key points

- Itching can occur following the administration of any opioid drug by any route, but is most common following the epidural or intrathecal administration of morphine.
- Although the incidence of pruritus may exceed 90%, it is not often distressing for the mother and may not require any treatment other than reassurance.

FURTHER READING

Alhashemi JA, Crosby ET, Grodecki W, *et al.* Treatment of morphine-induced pruritus following caesarean section. *Can J Anaesth* 1997; **44**: 1060–5.

Szarvas S, Harmon D, Murphy D. Neuraxial opioid-induced pruritus: a review. *J Clin Anesth* 2003; **15**: 234–9.

Waxler B, Dadabhoy Z, Stojiljkovic L, Rabito S. Primer of postoperative pruritus for anesthesiologists. *Anesthesiology* 2005; **103**: 168–78.

55 SHIVERING

Although shivering may occur in about 10% of normal labours and following general anaesthesia, it is particularly associated with regional (especially epidural) anaesthesia and analgesia, during which it has been reported to occur in up to two-thirds of cases. The cause is uncertain, but evidence suggests the tremor is at least partly thermoregulatory and may be accompanied by vasoconstriction in the arms. It also appears that epidural blockade may inhibit the subjective feeling of being cold, even when the core temperature has fallen. Other postulated mechanisms include altered control of peripheral muscles and a central effect resulting from systemic absorption of local anaesthetic or its transport via the cerebrospinal fluid to the brain. In labour, the high levels of circulating catecholamines and general arousal may also be important. Finally, the tendency for maternal temperature to increase after prolonged epidural analgesia may contribute to shivering, although it has also been suggested that shivering may contribute to the increase in temperature.

Problems/special considerations

In most cases, shivering is mild and benign, although if severe it may increase maternal catecholamine concentrations and metabolic rate, interfere with fetal and maternal monitoring and be alarming to the mother. It also increases maternal oxygen consumption and carbon dioxide production, although this is rarely a problem in practice. Rarely, the mother may be unable to cooperate with medical and midwifery staff during examinations, etc.

Management options

If shivering is mild, simple reassurance is often all that is required. Measures that have been studied include warming of epidural and intravenous solutions and administration of intravenous opioids (pethidine 10–30 mg has been shown to be especially effective in the non-pregnant population). Epidural opioids may also reduce the incidence and severity of shivering. Other drugs shown to be effective after general anaesthesia outside of obstetrics include clonidine and doxapram, although these are infrequently used in the maternity suite.

Key points

- Shivering is common during epidural analgesia and anaesthesia.
- Simple reassurance is adequate treatment in most cases.

FURTHER READING

De Witte J, Sessler DI. Perioperative shivering: physiology and pharmacology. *Anesthesiology* 2002; **96**: 467–84.

Panzer O, Ghazanfari N, Sessler DI, *et al.* Shivering and shivering-like tremor during labor with and without epidural analgesia. *Anesthesiology* 1999; **90**: 1609–16.

56   ASPIRATION OF GASTRIC CONTENTS

Aspiration is one of the three factors consistently associated with maternal deaths related to obstetric general anaesthesia, the others being emergency operation and difficult tracheal intubation. Often, these three factors occur together.

Problems/special considerations

Several risk factors make the pregnant woman more prone to aspiration:
- Reduced efficacy of the lower oesophageal sphincter caused by progesterone
- Reduced gastric emptying if opioids have been given
- The physical effect of the gravid uterus on the stomach
- The presence of gastric contents if the mother has eaten, either as part of a liberal feeding policy in labour or as an attempt to stave off starvation in more rigidly prohibitive units by 'binge' feeding prior to hospitalisation (see Chapter 14, Gastric function and feeding in labour, p. 35).

Every mother in the third trimester should be considered at risk of aspiration, although the point during pregnancy at which increased risk occurs, and the point postpartum at which the risk returns to normal, are controversial. Many obstetric anaesthetists would consider 16–18 weeks of pregnancy as representing the onset of the 'at-risk' period, although an earlier cut-off point has also been suggested, especially if there are symptoms of gastroesophageal reflux, the mother is obese, or the procedure requires her to be positioned head-down. Similarly, although hormonal profiles alter dramatically within a few hours of delivery, studies of gastric emptying have not produced consistent results, although some have suggested as little as 4–8 hours postpartum as the time required for the risk to return to normal (longer if opioids have been administered). However, other general physiological changes of pregnancy may take several weeks to disappear.

Finally, it should not be forgotten that any pregnant woman with an obtunded level of consciousness may be at risk from aspiration, e.g. during or after convulsions, drug overdose, anaphylaxis, etc. Thus women identified as high risk may not only be those in whom surgical intervention is planned or expected.

Mortality or morbidity may be related to:
- Impairment of the view at laryngoscopy causing difficulty with intubation
- Obstruction of the upper airway by solid or semi-solid matter causing complete or partial airway obstruction and hypoventilation
- Chemical pneumonitis (Mendelson's syndrome), related to the pH and volume of the aspirated material. Extrapolation from animal work has suggested an increased risk of pneumonitis if the pH is less than 2.5 and the volume is more than 25 ml, although it is now generally accepted that there is a continuum of risk, such that smaller volumes are required if the pH is lower. The alveolar inflammatory reaction may be intense, with oedema, cellular infiltration and the features of acute lung injury. There may be associated hypotension and poor peripheral perfusion if large amounts of fluid have been transferred from the

intravascular space into the alveoli. Aspiration pneumonitis may also be caused by particulate antacids, e.g. magnesium trisilicate.

Management options

Prevention
- *Reduction of the volume and acidity of gastric contents*: this may be achieved by:
  - Withholding oral intake during labour
  - Administration of metoclopramide or other prokinetic drugs
  - Use of antacids or acid-reducing drugs such as H_2-antagonists and omeprazole
  - Emptying the stomach with a stomach tube before general anaesthesia or by inducing vomiting (rarely used although it has been suggested that a stomach tube should be routinely passed during general anaesthesia for emergency Caesarean section in order to reduce the risk of aspiration after extubation).

The first three measures are used to differing extents in different situations and countries. Thus, for example, all women in a particular unit might be given regular oral antacids and ranitidine throughout labour, whereas only women identified as being at high risk of intervention might be treated in another unit. Similarly, feeding in labour occurs to different degrees on different labour wards. Proponents of all-inclusive treatment point to the potentially devastating effect of aspiration, the relative cheapness of therapy and the difficulty of identifying women truly at risk of a general anaesthetic. Supporters of selective treatment cite the low incidence of aspiration overall, the relatively low incidence of general anaesthesia in modern obstetric practice and the cost of therapy compared with no therapy. In addition, the 'medicalisation' of normal labour may be resisted by many women and midwives.

A practical breakdown of commonly used pharmacological preventative measures might be as follows (although as already mentioned, the protocol in use may vary widely between units):
- Normal (i.e. low risk) labour: nil.
- High-risk labour (e.g. obstetric complications, multiple pregnancy etc.): regular oral ranitidine 150 mg 6-hourly in active labour; following administration of pethidine: ranitidine 50 mg intramuscularly 8-hourly.
- Emergency Caesarean section: ranitidine 50 mg $\pm$ metoclopramide 10 mg slowly intramuscularly or intravenously when the decision for surgery is made, 30 ml sodium citrate 0.3 M orally immediately before induction of general anaesthesia.
- Elective Caesarean section: oral ranitidine 150 mg the night before and repeated the morning of surgery, metoclopramide/sodium citrate as above.
- *Preventing regurgitation during general anaesthesia:* standard general anaes-thetic practice includes a rapid sequence induction with application of cricoid pressure, although the method of its application and the possibility that cricoid pressure might make laryngoscopy more difficult are controversial areas

(see Chapter 37, Cricoid pressure, p. 98). Tracheal extubation should be in the lateral position with the patient awake, following return of full protective reflexes.

- *Avoidance of general anaesthesia altogether by using regional anaesthesia for operative procedures:* this is generally thought to be a major factor in the reduction in maternal mortality associated with anaesthesia that occurred over the 1970s–90s, although there is no doubt that improvements in training in, and assistance and facilities for, general anaesthesia also occurred during this period.

Diagnosis

Regurgitation may be obvious, either during induction of anaesthesia or intra-/postoperatively. It may or may not be associated with aspiration. It is also possible for aspiration to occur without obvious, massive regurgitation, e.g. during induction or intraoperatively past the cuff of the tracheal tube. Features include bronchospasm, raised airway pressure, hypoxaemia, tachypnoea, tachycardia and pyrexia; these may present for the first time postoperatively following otherwise uneventful anaesthesia. A high index of suspicion is therefore required. If fluid is aspirated from the pharynx, larynx or tracheal tube, simple litmus paper is useful for identifying its acidity, although this may not always be reliable if antacid therapy has been used.

Treatment

Initial management comprises removing the regurgitated material from the airway by using pharyngeal, laryngeal and tracheal suction and maintaining oxygenation; tracheal intubation has the advantage of securing the airway and protecting it against further aspiration, as well as allowing ready access to the tracheobronchial tree for suction. Cricoid pressure may prevent further regurgitation during intubation. The head-down lateral position may be appropriate depending on the particular circumstances of the case, in order to encourage drainage of fluid from the upper airway and discourage further aspiration should regurgitation recur. Although popular in the past, the use of prophylactic steroid and antibiotic therapy in cases where aspiration is suspected is no longer advocated, since this approach has not been shown to reduce mortality and may even increase it. Solid particles may be removable via bronchoscopy; bronchoalveolar lavage may also be used to dilute the acidic fluid aspirated.

A chest X-ray may be useful to show the presence of large amounts of aspirated material (usually in the right lower lobe) and as a baseline, although a normal appearance does not exclude aspiration and indeed may exist in the presence of severe hypoxaemia. Patients suspected of having aspirated should be observed and monitored carefully for at least 12–24 hours since their condition may worsen considerably during this time.

> **Key points**
>
> - Aspiration of gastric contents is a major factor in maternal death associated with general anaesthesia, especially related to emergency Caesarean section and difficult tracheal intubation.
> - Prevention includes sensible policies on feeding in labour, use of pH-raising drugs and antacids, emptying the stomach, rapid-sequence induction when general anaesthesia is used and avoidance of general anaesthesia by encouraging regional anaesthetic techniques.
> - Diagnosis may not always be obvious.
> - Treatment includes general supportive measures; antibiotics and steroid therapy are no longer advocated.

FURTHER READING

Ng A, Smith G. Aspiration of gastric contents in anaesthesia. *Anesth Analg* 2001; **93**: 494–513.

57   AWARENESS

Awareness is a shorthand term referring to a state of inadequate general anaesthesia, which results in the patient remembering all or part of a surgical procedure. It is almost exclusively associated with techniques involving the use of neuromuscular blocking drugs, when the patient is unable to move or otherwise attract attention to her plight. Awareness is not an all-or-nothing phenomenon and may range from unpleasant 'dreams' via vague memories of painful stimuli to the extreme situation where the patient is fully conscious and alert but unable to move.

Problems/special considerations

Awareness is particularly associated with anaesthesia for Caesarean section. This probably results from the perceived need to protect the fetus from the sedative effects of the anaesthetic agent, coupled with an exaggerated fear of the adverse effects of volatile agents upon uterine contractility. Fortunately, pregnancy reduces anaesthetic requirements by as much as 40%, or complaints of awareness would probably be more common.

The incidence of awareness is dependent upon the anaesthetic technique being used. Before the early 1970s it was common practice to avoid volatile agents altogether and use a 50:50 mixture of nitrous oxide and oxygen; not surprisingly this led to maternal awareness in 12–26% of cases. The addition of a low concentration of a volatile agent (e.g. halothane 0.5%, isoflurane 1%) reduces this to less than 1%. The effect of these concentrations upon uterine contractility is minimal and, even at 1.5 minimum alveolar concentration (MAC), the uterus will respond normally to oxytocic drugs.

The need for adequate fetal oxygenation during Caesarean section has led to the use of higher inspired concentrations of oxygen (and therefore less nitrous oxide) than for other surgical procedures and this also has an impact on the depth of anaesthesia. There is little evidence to support the use of more than 30% oxygen for delivery of the unstressed fetus, but when fetal distress is present, 50% or even 100% oxygen has been advocated. The loss of the anaesthetic contribution of nitrous oxide and the second-gas effect mean that higher concentrations of volatile agent should be used throughout these cases, and the initial concentration should be higher still (overpressure) to drive up the alveolar concentration quickly.

One factor that contributed to the risk of awareness in the past was the perceived need to deliver the baby before it was affected by the anaesthetic drugs, which led to obstetricians starting to incise the abdomen while the alveolar concentration of the volatile agent was still low. There is no evidence to support this practice, which may even result in a baby that is maximally affected by the dose of induction agent, and such 'smash-and-grab' procedures should be discouraged.

The contribution of opioid drugs to the anaesthetic should not be ignored, and part of the explanation for the high incidence of awareness during obstetric anaesthesia lies in the common practice of withholding these drugs until after the baby is delivered. This also has adverse consequences for cardiovascular stability during tracheal intubation, and there is an increasing tendency to use a modest dose of a very short-acting drug such as alfentanil to obviate both of these problems.

Even minor degrees of awareness can lead to significant long-term psychological morbidity, typified by 'waking dreams', difficulty in sleeping, depression, and fear of hospitals and doctors. Full-blown post-traumatic stress disorder may also occur.

In addition to awareness, inadequate anaesthesia may result in release of catecholamines, which further decrease placental perfusion and promote fetal hypoxia.

Management options

Although some authorities recommend that patients undergoing general anaesthesia for a Caesarean section should be warned about the risk of awareness, this is not generally advocated. The low incidence with modern anaesthetic techniques, coupled with the risk of raising anxiety and actually increasing the likelihood of awareness, means that most practitioners would eschew such a warning. Because of the advisability of waking the mother before tracheal extubation after Caesarean section, it is wise to mention the possibility of waking up with 'a tube in the throat' to ensure that she does not mistake this for intraoperative awareness.

Most incidents of awareness in recent years can be clearly traced back to a technical problem with the anaesthetic apparatus, vaporiser faults being the most common. When checking the anaesthetic machine, correct seating of the chosen vaporiser on its mount and adequate filling should be ensured. The anaesthetist should be familiar with the breathing system and ventilator and understand how air or oxygen can be entrained into the system (e.g. a gas piston ventilator) and how the inspired concentration of volatile agent can be lower than that set on the vaporiser (e.g. a circle system). A volatile agent monitor is invaluable and it is rapidly becoming indefensible to be without one.

There is no guaranteed 'sleep' dose of an induction agent, and the drug must be titrated against the patient's response, bearing in mind that it will be responsible for maintaining anaesthesia throughout the onset of muscle relaxation and tracheal intubation. Thiopental is probably still the drug of choice for induction, and the anaesthetist should have 6 mg/kg available in the syringe. Suxamethonium has a very rapid onset of action and should not be given until after the eyelash reflex has been lost.

Volatile agents with a low lipid solubility will achieve alveolar-inspired equilibrium most quickly. Isoflurane is the best of the 'established' agents, but the rapid onset times of desflurane and sevoflurane suggest that they are particularly appropriate for Caesarean section. Concentrations representing at least 0.5 MAC should be used during the procedure and this should be higher if the inspired nitrous oxide concentration is to be less than 60%. An overpressure of 1.5–2 MAC should be employed in the first 2–3 minutes if a more soluble agent is being used.

The patient should be closely watched for signs of lightening anaesthesia (tears, sweating), and the monitors should be observed frequently for evidence of sympathetic overactivity (tachycardia, hypertension). Some practitioners advocate the use of specific monitors of anaesthetic depth, but none has so far been shown to be any more effective than simply watching vital signs (Table 57.1). A meticulous record should be kept, which should include vaporiser settings and end-tidal volatile concentrations, if available.

A generous dose of a suitable opioid drug should be given directly after cord clamping and the volatile agent left on until the skin is being sutured. It is better to wait a few minutes at the end of the operation rather than risk awareness.

All mothers undergoing general anaesthesia for Caesarean section should be followed up within 24 hours of delivery and questioned about dreaming or sensation during the operation. The psychological sequelae of awareness can be minimised by a sympathetic approach. Many such patients complain that the medical staff do not believe them when they first report that they have memories of the operation; this can exacerbate the degree of trauma, so all such complaints should be taken seriously and handled at a senior level. Midwives should be alert

Table 57.1. Methods for monitoring depth of anaesthesia

Clinical signs – PRST score (pressure, rate, sweating, tears)
Isolated forearm technique
Lower oesophageal contractility
Skin resistance
Evoked auditory/somatosensory potentials
Electroencephalogram
Cerebral function analysing monitor and derivations thereof (e.g. Bispectral Index; BIS)

to the possibility of awareness and ensure early referral to an anaesthetist. Early referral to a psychologist with experience of post-traumatic stress disorder is desirable.

Some patients will mistake their memory of awake extubation for true intra-operative awareness. This risk can be minimised by careful preoperative explanation, but any markers as to the timing of such memory should be sought in order to reassure the patient if possible. Just because true awareness did not occur does not mean that the patient will not be traumatised.

Key points

- Clinical signs are still the best indicator of awareness.
- A clinically effective concentration of volatile agent, suitably monitored, should be used at all times.
- Patients should be warned about awake extubation.
- Complaints of awareness should be treated seriously and sympathetically.

FURTHER READING

Lyons G, Macdonald R. Awareness during caesarean section. *Anaesthesia* 1991; **46**: 62–4.

58   AIR EMBOLISM

Subclinical entry of air into the circulation has been shown with Doppler techniques to occur in up to 60% of Caesarean sections (possibly more if the head-down position is used or if the uterus is exteriorised), although the significance of circulating microscopic bubbles is uncertain. It has been suggested that chest pain or S–T segment depression occurring during Caesarean section under regional anaesthesia may be related to air in the coronary circulation, although both are frequently unaccompanied by Doppler demonstration of bubbles. Large amounts of air may cause cardiovascular impairment, although this is less common (up to 2%); the mechanism is obstruction of right ventricular output by the presence of compressible gas within the contracting ventricle. In addition, bubbles may lodge in the pulmonary circulation, increasing dead space, whilst paradoxical embolism may occur there is a patent foramen ovale (a probe-patent foramen is found in about 30% of 'normal' hearts on routine autopsy) or other right-to-left shunt.

Although most cases are related to Caesarean section, it should not be forgotten that air embolism may occur whenever open veins are above the level of the heart, e.g. when central venous lines are manipulated with the patient in the sitting position or when the arm in which a peripheral venous cannula has just been placed is held aloft to prevent spillage of blood; both are more likely to occur when staff are inexperienced in the management of intravenous lines, as may (unfortunately) occur on the labour ward. Finally, the danger of accidental intravenous injection of air, e.g. when pressurising devices are used with air-containing bags of intravenous fluid or when bubbles are allowed into intravenous infusion lines, must not be forgotten. In patients with right-to-left shunts, even small bubbles may have disastrous systemic effects.

Problems/special considerations

- The diagnosis may not be clear, especially at first. Clinical features are fairly non-specific and include hypotension, tachycardia, reduced arterial saturation and reduced end-expiratory carbon dioxide concentration (during general anaesthesia), the latter firstly because of reduced cardiac output and hence return of carbon dioxide from the tissues and secondly because of increased pulmonary dead space. There may be an audible churning sound on cardiac auscultation, although this is usually only present in massive air embolism. Paradoxical embolism may result in systemic infarction of vital organs, especially heart and brain.

  Thus the differential diagnosis of air embolism is any cause of cardiovascular impairment or collapse, at least initially; a high level of awareness is required. In particular, amniotic fluid embolism or thromboembolism may cause the same initial right ventricular outflow obstruction. If it occurs during regional anaesthesia, it may mimic hypotension produced by anaesthesia-induced sympathetic blockade. Doppler or ultrasound detection is the gold standard in diagnosing air embolism, but most units do not have the necessary equipment to hand. It may be possible to aspirate bubbles from the right ventricle or atrium via a central venous catheter, but inability to do so does not exclude the diagnosis.

- Manoeuvres for preventing further embolism and managing the current embolism (as described below) may be difficult to carry out midway through a Caesarean section, especially if the patient is awake and distressed. In addition, some of the traditional advice concerning positioning of the patient is self-contradictory (head-up for prevention of further embolism; head-down for its management).

Management options

- Prevention of further embolism is important as soon as the diagnosis is considered. This includes immediately informing the obstetrician, who should return the uterus to the abdomen if possible, flood the surgical field with saline and look for open veins (the ability to do this will obviously depend to some extent on the stage of surgery). Positioning the patient head-up is generally suggested to raise the level of the heart and increase venous pressure in the pelvis and abdomen.

- Damage limitation is generally achieved by reducing the size of the bubble(s); this is done firstly by stopping any nitrous oxide that is being administered and secondly by attempting to remove air from the circulation, or more specifically from the right side of the heart. It may be possible to aspirate air from a routine central venous cannula or catheter; special wide-bore multi-perforated cannulae are manufactured specifically for this task but are not generally available on many labour wards. The head-down position is traditionally required for central venous cannulation, and the left lateral head-down position is advised for isolation of the bubbles away from the right ventricular outflow tract and easier aspiration of air. Both of these positions may compromise the advice given above, and moving to the left lateral position is at best awkward in the middle of surgery.

• Further management consists of general supportive treatment (increased concentration of inspired oxygen, vasopressor/inotropic drugs, intravenous fluids) and basic resuscitative measures as appropriate. If the baby has not yet been delivered, the cardiovascular effects of air embolism will be exacerbated by aortocaval compression; thus lateral displacement of the uterus is especially important and delivery should be expedited.

It has been suggested that Caesarean section should always be performed in the head-up position to reduce the incidence of air embolism; however, this has implications for the incidence and effects of hypotension following regional anaesthesia and for the spread of spinal blockade. It has also been suggested that Doppler or ultrasound monitoring (transthoracic or oesophageal) should always be available during Caesarean section, but this is hampered by the lack of equipment and expertise in its use.

Key points

- Air embolism occurs in up to 60% of Caesarean sections as detected by Doppler studies.
- Air embolism may cause cardiovascular collapse if large.
- Management includes general resuscitation, preventing further embolism and removal of air already in the circulation.

FURTHER READING

Fong J, Gadalla F, Druzin M. Venous emboli occurring during caesarean section: the effect of patient position. *Can J Anaesth* 1991; **38**: 191–5.

Lew TW, Tay DH, Thomas E. Venous air embolism during caesarean section: more common than previously thought. *Anesth Analg* 1993; **77**: 448–5.

Lowenwirt IP, Chi DS, Handwerker SM. Nonfatal venous air embolism during cesarean section: a case report and review of the literature. *Obstet Gynecol Surv* 1994; **49**: 72–6.

V Problems confined to obstetrics

59 INDUCTION AND AUGMENTATION OF LABOUR

Induction of labour (IOL) is the artificial commencement and stimulation of labour and involves the ripening of the cervix, artificial rupture of the membranes (ARM) and stimulation of uterine contractions. It is indicated when delivery of the baby before spontaneous labour occurs is in the best interests of the mother or fetus or both.

Augmentation of labour is used where the normal progression of labour is too slow.

Induction of labour

The indications for IOL are shown in Table 59.1.

Once the decision to induce labour has been made, the ease of induction is usually assessed by using the Bishop score, based on the result of pelvic examination. A low Bishop score indicates that the cervix is unfavourable and will need to be ripened. This is usually achieved by vaginal dinoprostone (PGE_2), which may

Table 59.1. Indications for induction of labour

Fetal reasons:	• Prolonged pregnancy
	• Intrauterine growth retardation
	• Multiple pregnancy
	• Unstable lie
	• Infection
	• Rhesus disease
	• Lethal fetal abnormality
	• Intrauterine death
Maternal reasons:	• Pregnancy-induced hypertension
	• Essential hypertension
	• Other maternal disease e.g. renal, malignant
	• Antepartum haemorrhage
	• Poor obstetric history e.g. previous stillbirth

Analgesia, Anaesthesia and Pregnancy: A Practical Guide Second Edition, ed. Steve Yentis, Anne May and Surbhi Malhotra. Published by Cambridge University Press. © Cambridge University Press 2007.

be repeated at intervals of 12–24 hours depending on the change in the Bishop score. This process may take more than 48 hours. Misoprostol has also been used to induce labour.

Surgical induction of labour is performed if the cervix is favourable or following cervical ripening with prostaglandins. It entails ARM. This stimulates labour and allows the colour of the liquor to be assessed and a fetal scalp clip electrode to be applied to monitor the fetal heart, both of which give useful information about the wellbeing of the fetus.

Oxytocics (Syntocinon) are usually an integral part of the management of IOL, and therapy is normally commenced after ARM has been performed.

Augmentation of labour

Augmentation of labour is used when labour is not proceeding at the standard rate (see Chapter 13, Normal labour, p. 33) or when there has been premature rupture of membranes without signs of labour after 12–24 hours. It is usually done by ARM (if intact) and/or oxytocics.

Problems/special considerations

- The most common complications of IOL are:
  - (i)   Prolapse of the cord
  - (ii) Abruption of the placenta
  - (iii) Acute fetal distress – particularly when ARM is performed in the presence of polyhydramnios
  - (iv) Hyperstimulation of uterine contractions – tetanic contraction may cause acute fetal distress
  - (v)   Postpartum haemorrhage associated with uterine atony.
- Complications of augmentation are as above; in addition, there is an increased risk of infection if the membranes have been ruptured for some time.
- Induction of labour is often prolonged and may be particularly tiring and painful; therefore epidural analgesia should be discussed as part of the labour management. Contractions augmented by oxytocic drugs are more painful. There may also be maternal or fetal reasons for the advisability of epidural analgesia, e.g. pregnancy-induced hypertension.
- Induction of labour may not be successful and since there has been a commitment to deliver the baby these women may need to be delivered by Caesarean section.

Key points

- Induction of labour is often associated with a high-risk pregnancy.
- Induction of labour increases the strength of the contractions, therefore they are more painful.
- There is an increased risk of precipitous labour and instrumental delivery.

FURTHER READING

Chamberlain G, Zander L. ABC of labour care: induction. *BMJ* 1999; **318**: 995–8.

60 OXYTOCIC AND TOCOLYTIC DRUGS

Oxytocic drugs are used to promote uterine contractions whereas tocolytic drugs relax the uterus. Both groups of drugs are widely used in obstetric practice.

Oxytocic drugs

These drugs may be given during labour to augment progress, at delivery and in the puerperium to reduce postpartum haemorrhage and aid expulsion of the placenta, and at earlier stages of pregnancy to help empty the uterus, e.g. following evacuation of retained products of conception or termination of pregnancy.

Although the third stage of labour can be managed without oxytocic drugs ('physiological management of the third stage'), it is common practice to give an oxytocic to all women at childbirth, usually on delivery of the anterior shoulder (vaginal delivery) or following delivery of the baby (Caesarean section). In most units, the drug used is either a mixture of oxytocin analogue and ergometrine (vaginal delivery) or oxytocin analogue alone (Caesarean section), although local practice varies.

- *Oxytocin analogue (Syntocinon):* its effects resemble those of natural oxytocin, released from the posterior pituitary gland. Oxytocin causes milk ejection from the lactating breast and acts directly on specific oxytocin receptors in the uterine myometrium, increasing the force and frequency of contractions. In early pregnancy, the uterine receptors are present in small numbers and their sensitivity is low; thus there is little value in giving the drug for operative procedures in early pregnancy, although this is commonly done. Syntocinon may cause vasodilatation and tachycardia; the latter is especially likely if the intravenous route is used, if large doses are given ($>5\,U$) by bolus injection and if other drugs causing tachycardia (e.g. ephedrine) are given concurrently. These effects can be disastrous in patients with fixed cardiac output states, e.g. aortic stenosis. A potential problem with prolonged Syntocinin therapy during labour is related to its antidiuretic effect, which may result in excessive water retention, compounded by excessive fluid administration if infused in weak solution over a long period of time. This has resulted in hyponatraemia and convulsions, hence the recommendation that oxytocin should be diluted in physiological saline rather than dextrose solutions. Oxytocin's half-life is approximately 10 minutes, another reason for giving it by infusion at Caesarean section.
- *Ergometrine:* this acts on smooth muscle generally; thus it may cause vasoconstriction and hypertension (both systemic and pulmonary) and increased central venous pressure. It may also cause severe vomiting, and bronchospasm has

been reported. It is therefore avoided in women with hypertensive disease and is less frequently given alone in routine use, especially intravenously, although it is commonly given intramuscularly together with oxytocin analogue (Syntometrine: 5 U Syntocinon and 500 µg ergometrine) at vaginal delivery. Intravenous administration (125–250 µg, repeated if necessary) may be useful in severe postpartum haemorrhage. It increases the force, frequency and duration of uterine contractions.

- *Prostaglandins:* gemeprost (PGE$_1$) is given vaginally to soften and ripen the cervix before termination of pregnancy or to induce abortion. Dinoprostone (PGE$_2$) has also been used for this purpose but is more commonly used to induce labour. Both may cause nausea, vomiting, pyrexia, diarrhoea, bronchospasm and hypertension (especially dinoprostone, which may also cause uterine hypertonus and fetal distress. The occurrence of bronchospasm and hypertension is despite PGE$_2$'s traditionally ascribed broncho- and vasodilator effects).

  Misoprostol has been used for medical termination of pregnancy, induction of labour and prevention of postpartum haemorrhage. The main side effects seen are shivering and pyrexia, although uterine hyperstimulation has been reported when used for induction.

  Carboprost (PGF$_2\alpha$) is used in postpartum haemorrhage associated with uterine atony if standard oxytocics are ineffective. It is given intramuscularly (250 µg) and has been injected directly into the myometrium; either route may still result in systemic effects as above. All the prostaglandins are more effective in late pregnancy, although this is thought to be related to increased sensitivity rather than increased number of receptors.

Tocolytic drugs

There are several different groups of drugs that have been used or studied as tocolytics. As with many areas of obstetric practice, their value (and even efficacy in some cases) is controversial.

- *β$_2$-Adrenergic agonists:* these act on uterine β$_2$-receptors causing relaxation of myometrium. Although the most commonly prescribed tocolytics for premature labour, improvement in outcome has not been conclusively proven. The emphasis of therapy has shifted away from long-term prolongation of pregnancy towards allowing enough time for steroids to promote fetal lung maturity before delivery. The most commonly used drugs are terbutaline, salbutamol and ritodrine and these may be given orally, subcutaneously or by intravenous infusion. They may cause tremor, restlessness, hypotension, tachycardia and pulmonary oedema. The last is thought to arise from fluid overload during the infusion, together with increased pulmonary blood flow resulting from β$_2$-receptor mediated pulmonary vasodilatation, often compounded by maternal steroid administration. Careful monitoring of blood pressure, pulse and arterial oxygen saturation is required during therapy. Metabolic effects include hypokalaemia and hyperglycaemia (thus they should be used with caution in diabetics).

Both regional and general anaesthesia may be used following β_2-agonist therapy; excessive fluid administration (e.g. during regional anaesthesia) should be avoided and drugs that may cause tachycardia (e.g. ephedrine) used with caution.

The drugs may also be given by intravenous bolus (salbutamol or terbutaline 100–250 µg) as part of intrauterine resuscitation of the fetus, e.g. in severe fetal distress.

- *Oxytocin antagonists (e.g. atosiban):* these bind competitively to uterine oxytocin receptors, causing dose-dependent reduction in contractions. Although shown to be comparable with β_2-agonists in preterm labour and to have fewer side effects, atosiban is expensive and usually reserved for cases at particular risk from the side effects of β_2-agonists (although it may cause nausea, vomiting, tachycardia and hypotension).
- *Glyceryl trinitrate (GTN):* this acts directly on uterine smooth muscle and has been given intravenously (50 µg boluses) or sublingually (200–400 µg) to produce acute but relatively brief uterine relaxation, e.g. in cases of uterine hypertonicity, retained placenta and uterine inversion and for external cephalic version. Similar doses have been used in severe fetal distress as above. Hypotension and headache are the main side effects.

  GTN delivered by dermal patch has been studied as a means of preventing premature labour following premature rupture of membranes.
- *Magnesium sulphate:* this acts directly on smooth muscle via calcium ion antagonism; it is rarely used as a tocolytic in the UK although it is more commonly given for this purpose elsewhere, e.g. the US. Anaesthetic considerations of magnesium therapy are discussed in Chapter 82, Magnesium sulphate (p. 196).
- *Others:* drugs studied as tocolytics but not widely accepted as standard therapy in the UK include calcium antagonists (e.g. nifedipine) and prostaglandin inhibitors (e.g. indometacin). Ethanol has been used in the past but has been largely abandoned because of its side effects.

Key points

- Oxytocic drugs are used routinely during labour, following delivery, in early pregnancy and in the emergency management of postpartum haemorrhage.
- Tocolytic drugs are used in premature labour and for intrauterine resuscitation of the fetus.
- Drugs of both groups may have implications for the anaesthetist because of their side effects.

FURTHER READING

Caponas G. Glyceryl trinitrate and acute uterine relaxation: a literature review. *Anaesth Intens Care* 2001; **29**: 163–77.

Goldenberg RL, Rouse DJ. Prevention of premature birth. *N Engl J Med* 1998; **339**: 313–20.

Gyetvai K, Hannah ME, Hodnett ED, Ohlsson A. Tocolytics for preterm labor: a systematic review. *Obstet Gynecol* 1999; **94**: 869–77.

Lamont RF. The development and introduction of anti-oxytocic tocolytics. *BJOG* 2003; **110** (Suppl 20): 108–12.

Royal College of Obstetricians & Gynaecologists. *Tocolytic drugs for women in preterm labour.* London : RCOG, 2002.

61   PREMATURE LABOUR, DELIVERY AND RUPTURE OF MEMBRANES

Labour or rupture of membranes is defined as preterm if it occurs at less than 37 completed weeks' gestation. Rupture of membranes is defined as premature if it occurs without being followed by spontaneous uterine contractions – the period of latency required before the diagnosis is made varies but is usually up to 8 hours. The term premature labour is often used interchangeably with preterm labour.

About 7% of deliveries are preterm in the UK, in about a third of cases without premature rupture of membranes (PROM) as the initiating event. Prematurity is a major cause of fetal and neonatal morbidity and accounts for the majority of infant deaths in the devloped world (Table 61.1). Many epidemiological studies have investigated neonatal morbidity and mortality according to birth weight instead of gestation, although there is evidence that the interplay of these two factors is more important than either one alone. For example, at a given gestation, heavier babies have less morbidity and mortality than lighter ones; similarly, at a given birth weight, mature babies do better than immature ones.

Although several risk factors for preterm delivery are recognised, about half of preterm deliveries have no obvious precipitating cause. Known risk factors include: a previous history of prematurity; young maternal age; maternal disease (especially infection), surgery or trauma; uterine abnormality; stress; smoking and use of recreational drugs; multiple gestation; placenta abnormality; and fetal disease.

Table 61.1. Approximate incidence of morbidity and mortality rates at different gestations

Gestation (weeks)	Incidence of RDS*	Incidence of major neurodevelopmental handicap	Mortality rate
23–24	80–100%	35–65%	70–85%
25–26		20–25%	35–55%
27–28	50–60%		
29–30		<10%	<10%
31–32	30–40%		
33–34	10–20%	<5%	<5%
35–36	<5%		

*RDS: respiratory distress syndrome

Problems/special considerations

- *Diagnosis:* careful obstetric assessment is required to establish the diagnosis of PROM since it is not always obvious. Amniotic fluid can be tested for by using special reagent sticks (nitrazine). The diagnosis of preterm labour is made according to gestation, the frequency of uterine contractions and changes in cervical dilatation or effacement. In some countries (not routinely in the UK) fetal maturity is assessed by the lecithin–sphingomyelin (LS) ratio, which increases as surfactant production increases and may indicate the likelihood of respiratory distress syndrome.
- *Maternal problems:* prolonged rupture of membranes may lead to chorioamnionitis with or without systemic features of infection. Thus there may be theoretical risks from regional anaesthesia (see Chapter 131, Pyrexia during labour, p. 295 and Chapter 137, Sepsis, p. 308).

  Administration of tocolytic drugs may result in tachycardia, fluid overload and pulmonary oedema (see Chapter 60, Oxytocic and tocolytic drugs, p. 149). Tachycardia may also be related to maternal sepsis and anxiety; the latter may be considerable because of the mother's fears for her baby.

  Any underlying cause of preterm labour or PROM (such as maternal disease) may have implications for the anaesthetic management.

  The best method of delivery is controversial, but operative delivery rate is higher than for term deliveries. Breech presentation is more common. Classical Caesarean section may be required if the lower uterine segment is poorly formed (uncommon after 26 weeks' gestation), with a greater risk of haemorrhage and other complications.
- *Neonatal problems:* the main problems for the neonate are respiratory distress, hypogylcaemia and intracranial haemorrhage. The last may be related to trauma during delivery, although it may also occur postpartum in severe respiratory distress. The neonate is more likely to require resuscitation. Necrotising enterocolitis and patent ductus arteriosus are also more common in premature neonates. If maternal infection is suspected, neonatal screening is performed since infection may also be present in the baby. It should be remembered that even with modern neonatal intensive care, the neonate has a greater risk of morbidity when born at 35–36 weeks than at 37–38 weeks.

Management options

Steroids are given to the mother to aid maturation of the fetal lungs. Since steroids require 24 hours to become optimally effective, delivery is usually delayed for this period if possible. Tocolytic drugs are commonly used in an attempt to prevent or stop labour but their use is controversial since the evidence for their efficacy is not conclusive. Antibiotics have been shown to reduce the incidence of preterm labour in women with PROM. Delivery is required in the presence of chorioamnionitis or fetal distress, although the precise mode of delivery is controversial. Since the preterm infant is more susceptible to intracranial haemorrhage, the need to prevent trauma during delivery often leads to Caesarean section, although the benefit of this is unproven.

Anaesthetic options are discussed more fully under the relevant related topics. In general, regional analgesia is often preferable in labour and is considered safe in the absence of systemic features of infection and if antibiotic cover has been provided, since it provides good conditions for a controlled delivery and can be readily extended for instrumental delivery. If Caesarean section is required, regional anaesthesia may offer the parents their only chance to see and hear their baby free of tubes etc. if the chance of neonatal survival is poor. In addition, neurobehavioural and physiological outcome is better in premature neonates when regional anaesthesia is used than with general anaesthesia. It is important to appreciate the dangers of concurrent tocolytic therapy with any anaesthetic technique. The preterm fetus is especially vulnerable to the adverse effects of maternal hypotension.

Key points

- 7% of deliveries in the UK are preterm.
- Potential maternal problems are those of fever and sepsis, use of tocolytic drugs and the increased requirement for instrumental delivery and anaesthetic intervention.
- Fetal and neonatal problems are those of prematurity, infection and the increased need for neonatal resuscitation.

FURTHER READING

Goldenberg RL. The management of preterm labor. *Obstet Gynecol* 2002; **100**: 1020–37.
Mercer BM. Preterm premature rupture of the membranes. *Obstet Gynecol* 2003; **101**: 178–93.
Simhan HN, Canavan TP. Preterm premature rupture of membranes: diagnosis, evaluation and management strategies. *BJOG* 2005; **112** (Suppl 1): 32–7.
Slattery MM, Morrison JJ. Preterm delivery. *Lancet* 2002; **360**: 1489–97.

---

62   MALPRESENTATIONS AND MALPOSITIONS

Definitions

- *Lie* – the relationship of the long axis of the fetus to that of the mother, e.g. longitudinal, transverse, oblique.
- *Presentation* – the part of the fetus that is foremost in the birth canal, e.g. cephalic, breech or compound.
- *Position* – the relationship of the presenting part of the fetus, using a reference point such as the occiput or sacrum, to the maternal pelvis, e.g. left occipito–anterior (LOA) or right sacral transverse (RST).

Approximately 85% of fetuses at term lie longitudinally, with a cephalic presentation in an occipito–anterior position. A malpresentation is anything that does not fulfil these criteria.

Problems/special considerations

The malpresenting fetus is less likely to deliver spontaneously, and instrumental or operative intervention is often required. Labour is often prolonged and particularly painful. Although it has been suggested that epidural analgesia may increase the likelihood of malpresentation, there is little, if any, evidence to support this view.

- *Occipito–posterior:* this is the commonest malpresentation, occurring in 10% of term pregnancies. Progress of labour may be slow, and the mother often experiences particularly severe pain in the back, which may be resistant to treatment by regional blockade. Manual or forceps rotation may be attempted to bring the head into a more favourable occipito–anterior position.
- *Breech presentation:* this occurs in 3–4% of term pregnancies and can be subdivided into frank (hips flexed and legs extended over abdominal wall), complete (hips and legs flexed) and footling (foot or knee presenting). The mother with a breech presentation may get the urge to 'push' before the cervix is fully dilated, thus running the risk of trapping the fetal head; this is a particular risk if the labour is preterm. It is becoming increasingly common for women with breech presentation to be delivered by elective Caesarean section, especially if primiparous as this reduces neonatal morbidity by two-thirds and mortality by three-quarters. External cephalic version (ECV) is becoming increasingly popular; in this manoeuvre, the obstetrician applies external pressure to rotate the fetus to a vertex presentation (see Chapter 63, External cephalic version, p. 156).
- *Transverse lie:* this occurs in 0.3% of term pregnancies and may be associated with placenta praevia, polyhydramnios and grand multiparity. Spontaneous delivery is impossible unless the lie is converted to longitudinal, which may be achieved by external version provided that placenta praevia has been excluded. Caesarean section is usually necessary, and a vertical uterine incision may be needed to prevent difficulty in delivering the fetus.
- *Face and brow presentations:* these are rare presentations, where the head is hyperextended. A face presentation may deliver vaginally, but Caesarean section is often needed.
- *Prolapsed cord:* cord prolapse occurs in 0.4% of cases when the vertex is presenting, but this incidence rises to 0.5% in frank breech, 4–6% in complete breech and 15–18% in footling presentations. It is generally more common when the fetus does not fully occlude the pelvic inlet, as in preterm labour, and may follow artificial rupture of the membranes with a high presenting part. If immediate vaginal delivery is not feasible, the presenting part is pushed and held out of the pelvis to prevent cord compression, often aided by steep head-down tilt, while the mother is transferred to theatre for immediate Caesarean section.

Management options

Good regional analgesia is desirable at an early stage since intervention is more likely to be required. If there is breakthrough pain, e.g. with an occipito–anterior position, addition of an epidural opioid such as fentanyl often improves pain relief, although more concentrated solutions of local anaesthetic than those used in 'low-dose' techniques may be required.

If vaginal delivery of a breech presentation is planned, epidural analgesia will help prevent premature 'pushing' and will enable controlled manipulation, extensive episiotomy and application of forceps to the aftercoming head.

For cord prolapse requiring Caesarean section, general anaesthesia is usually the quickest option, although extension of a pre-existing epidural block or institution of spinal anaesthesia is also possible (see Chapter 69, Prolapsed cord, p. 166).

Key points

- Regional analgesia is particularly indicated in malpresentation.
- Prolapsed cord is often associated with breech and transverse presentations and preterm delivery.
- Early multidisciplinary communication will help optimise management.

FURTHER READING

Hannah ME, Hannah WJ, Hewson SA, *et al*. Planned caesarean section versus planned vaginal birth for breech presentation at term: a randomised multicentre trial. *Lancet*. 2000; **356**: 1375–83.

63   EXTERNAL CEPHALIC VERSION

External cephalic version (ECV) is a procedure performed to convert a breech or shoulder presentation into a cephalic one by manipulating the fetus through the mother's abdominal wall and anterior wall of the uterus. Its success rate is 50–80%.

Problems/special considerations

ECV is usually attempted at 36–37 weeks' gestation; a fetus at earlier gestation is more likely to revert to a breech presentation subsequently since there is more room available to it, and since the procedure carries a risk of premature delivery a more mature gestation is preferable. On the other hand, the larger the fetus the more difficult it may be to achieve successful version, especially if the presenting part is engaged.

Contraindications include multiple pregnancy (although ECV is occasionally used to turn the second twin), antepartum haemorrhage, placenta praevia, ruptured membranes, fetal abnormalities and factors which indicate Caesarean section. Previous Caesarean section, intrauterine growth retardation, pre-eclampsia and obesity are controversial relative contraindications. The mother should be nil-by-mouth in case a complication occurs. The fetus is monitored continuously, and with the mother in the tilted supine position, talcum powder is applied to the abdominal wall and rotationary pressure applied to the fetus whilst attempting to lift the presenting part out of the pelvis. Tocolytic drugs, e.g. β_2-agonists, may be given. There may be considerable discomfort, particularly if the mother is especially tense, which reduces the chance of success. Various maneouvres have been used in an attempt to improve the success and tolerability of ECV, including sedation (e.g. with benzodiazepines) and epidural analgesia, although many obstetricians consider the degree of discomfort a useful indicator of when to stop the attempted procedure and prefer to avoid the use of adjuncts. In the UK, anaesthetists are rarely involved. A maximum of 10 minutes is usually allowed before considering the attempt at version unsuccessful.

Apart from discomfort, complications of ECV include maternal or fetal bradycardia, onset of labour and placental abruption (5–28% has been reported). It should also be remembered that breech presentation is more common in fetuses with other congenital abnormalities and in placenta praevia or uterine abnormalities.

Management options

From the anaesthetic viewpoint, awareness that ECV is being planned is usually the main issue, since anaesthetic input may be required at short notice. However, anecdotal experience suggests that most obstetricians perform ECV in clinics, wards or the delivery suite without routinely informing anaesthetists.

Key points

- External cephalic version has a success rate of 50–80%.
- Analgesia or sedation may occasionally be required.
- Complications include fetal distress, onset of labour and haemorrhage.

FURTHER READING

Hofmeyr GJ. Interventions to help external cephalic version for breech presentation at term. *Cochrane Database Syst Rev* 2004; (**1**): CD000184.

Myerscough P. The practice of external cephalic version. *Br J Obstet Gynaecol* 1998; **105**: 1043–5.

64   MULTIPLE PREGNANCY

The incidence of multiple pregnancy is increasing owing to an increase in assisted conception programmes, although twins, triplets and quadruplets also occur naturally. The incidence of twins is 1:80 pregnancies, triplets 1:8000 and quadruplets

1:800 000. The obstetric anaesthetist has an important part to play in the management of these deliveries.

Problems/special considerations

The mother carrying a multiple pregnancy experiences all the minor pregnancy complaints in excess. She will be more likely to be very uncomfortable and to suffer from backache, heartburn and varicose veins. Often she will be dyspnoeic at rest or on minor exertion and she may be unable to lie on her back because of supine hypotension; it is often difficult to relieve aortocaval compression except in the full lateral position. She is also more prone to the following complications:
- Anaemia (real and dilutional)
- Pregnancy-induced hypertension
- Intrauterine growth retardation
- Malpresentations
- Premature labour
- Prolonged labour
- Malpresentation of the second twin after delivery of the first twin
- Postpartum haemorrhage (because of uterine atony and the large placental site)
- Intrauterine death.

Management options

Twins may be delivered vaginally, although the labour and delivery may not be straightforward and the above factors should be considered. Epidural analgesia is recommended; firstly it will provide excellent analgesia for what may be a long labour requiring oxytocic drugs, and secondly – and most importantly – the epidural can be used if there are problems with the second twin. Malpresentation of the second twin may require external or internal version and/or operative delivery, including Caesarean section (which may be required in approximately 10%). The anaesthetist should be present for the delivery of twins to ensure that the epidural block is adequate for these manipulations. The second stage may be conducted in the operating theatre. If Caesarean section is indicated for the second twin, the anaesthetist must be able to extend the epidural block for the operation. Some anaesthetists advocate extending the epidural to produce a block suitable for Caesarean section in all cases of twins, in case surgery is required. In rare instances, general anaesthesia may be required for the delivery of the second twin.

Many twins and nearly all triplets and quadruplets are booked for delivery by elective Caesarean section, although because premature labour is more common, Caesarean section is often performed as a non-elective procedure. The indications for twins to be delivered by elective Caesarean section include malpresentation of the first twin, previous Caesarean section, poor obstetric history (which may include assisted conception) and maternal request.

Regional anaesthesia is considered preferable for Caesarean section in multiple pregnancy. Great care must be taken when performing regional anaesthesia in these women to ensure that supine hypotension is avoided. A Syntocinon infusion is usually set up post-delivery.

Key points

- Women with multiple pregnancies are an 'at-risk' group.
- The anaesthetist should be actively involved with the care of these women whether they are in labour or not.
- Special care is required to avoid aortocaval compression.
- There is increased likelihood of premature or prolonged labour, instrumental delivery and postpartum haemorrhage.

FURTHER READING

Wen SW, Demissie K, Yang Q, Walker MC. Maternal morbidity and obstetric complications in triplet pregnancies and quadruplet and higher-order multiple pregnancies. *Am J Obstet Gynecol* 2004; **191**: 254–8.

Wen SW, Fung KF, Oppenheimer L, *et al.* Occurrence and predictors of cesarean delivery for the second twin after vaginal delivery of the first twin. *Obstet Gynecol* 2004; **103**: 413–19.

65   TRIAL OF SCAR

Trial of scar is the term used for the trial of labour in a woman who has a scar on her uterus. The scar has usually resulted from a lower segment Caesarean section, but may also be from a hysterotomy or myomectomy. Traditionally, a previous classical Caesarean section has been considered a contraindication to a trial of scar, but there are many reports of this being done successfully. In the USA and increasingly in the UK, vaginal delivery after a lower segment Caesarean section is commonly called VBAC (vaginal birth after Caesarean).

Problems/special considerations

- A trial of scar would be considered if the reason for the scar was not a recurrent obstetric problem, such as cephalopelvic disproportion. The major anxiety is rupture of the uterine scar, particularly during strong uterine contractions. The incidence of uterine rupture is ~3–4 per 1000 cases. The risk is thought to be increased if prostaglandins are used for the induction of labour, although

Syntocinon, which is more controllable, is not usually considered contraindicated.

Features of uterine rupture are:

(i)   Fetal compromise

(ii) Hypotension and tachycardia

(iii) Intrapartum bleeding

(iv) Cessation of labour.

If uterine rupture occurs, urgent delivery is required.

- There is a 25–30% likelihood of a repeat Caesarean section if the reason for the previous Caesarean section is non-recurrent.
- There have been anxieties that epidural analgesia may mask the pain of uterine dehiscence. However, pain is not a constant feature of uterine rupture and may be absent in 10% of cases. In addition, severe pain may be present in the absence of uterine rupture. Finally, the pain of uterine rupture has been reported to 'break through' analgesia provided by modern, low-dose epidural techniques. In fact, many would consider epidural analgesia indicated in trial of scar since it may be readily converted to anaesthesia suitable for Caesarean section if required (unless there is uterine rupture, in which case there may not be time to extend the epidural).

Management options

Women undergoing trial of scar (and often, their obstetricians) should have the potential advantages and disadvantages of regional analgesia explained to them. Pain that breaks through low-dose epidural analgesia or is present between contractions should raise the possibility of uterine dehiscence.

Key points

- Uterine rupture is the most important complication of trial of scar and occurs in ~3–4 cases per 1000.
- Epidural analgesia has traditionally been considered to be contraindicated but may have advantages.
- Pain in the presence of a working epidural may be a warning of impending uterine rupture.

FURTHER READING

Kelly MC, Hill DA, Wilson DB. Low dose bupivacaine/fentanyl infusion does not mask uterine rupture. *Int J Obstet Anesth* 1997; **6**: 52–4.

Rageth JC, Juzi C, Grossenbacher H. Delivery after previous cesarean: a risk evaluation. Swiss Working Group of Obstetric and Gynecologic Institutions. *Obstet Gynecol* 1999; **93**: 332–7.

Smith GC, Pell JP, Pasupathy D, Dobbie R. Factors predisposing to perinatal death related to uterine rupture during attempted vaginal birth after caesarean section: retrospective cohort study. *BMJ* 2004; **329**: 375–7.

66 UNDER-AGE PREGNANCY AND ADVANCED MATERNAL AGE

Under-age pregnancy refers to pregnancy in girls under the age of consent (16 years in the UK). The term 'elderly' is applied to parturients over the age of 35. The UK has one of the highest teenage pregnancy rates in Europe, whereas the incidence of older women becoming pregnant is increasing in the developed world as a result of both maternal choice and infertility treatment.

Problems/special considerations

Under-age pregnancy

Those girls who are under-age when they present in pregnancy can be placed in the following groups:

- Those who have had normal antenatal care and have the full support of their family. This group usually have a parent available to give consent on behalf of the minor if that is felt appropriate, e.g. for epidural analgesia or for anaesthesia.
- Concealed pregnancy. This group may pose a problem with consent. Many will have had little or no antenatal care and may present to the hospital for the first time when they are in labour. Many present in advanced labour or to the Accident and Emergency Department with a life-threatening condition such as eclampsia, and there may not be time to find a parent or guardian before instituting treatment. Overall, this is an 'at-risk' group who often need considerable support, including epidural analgesia.

Hypertension, anaemia, premature labour and low birth weight are all more common in under-age mothers.

Advanced maternal age

Miscarriage, fetal chromosomal abnormalities, multiple pregnancy, hypertension, diabetes, instrumental delivery, neonatal mortality and postpartum haemorrhage are more common in elderly mothers, who feature disproportionately in the Reports on Confidential Enquiries into Maternal Deaths.

Management options

In under-age mothers, it is important to remember at all times that the minor is the patient and must be involved in the decision making. In line with the Children's Act, the child may make the decisions for her treatment. This may involve epidural analgesia and/or regional anaesthesia. Ideally, the support of a parent or guardian should be sought, although this may not be practical. If no adult support is available it is sensible to treat the person as an adult and therefore able to consent to her own treatment and to sign her own consent form, assuming she is able to understand what is involved.

Elderly mothers require no special management other than an appreciation of the increased risks associated with advanced age. These women too should be considered an 'at-risk' group.

Key points

- Both under-age and elderly mothers are at-risk groups and have a higher incidence of complications.
- For minors, parental consent should be obtained when possible; if none is available, treatment should not be denied.
- Elderly mothers should be managed as routine, but the increased risk of complications should be remembered.

FURTHER READING

Cleary-Goldman J, Malone FD, Vidaver J, *et al.* Impact of maternal age on obstetric outcome. *Obstet Gynecol* 2005; **105**: 983–90.

Jacobsson B, Ladfors L, Milsom I. Advanced maternal age and adverse perinatal outcome. *Obstet Gynecol* 2004; **104**: 727–33.

Jolly MC, Sebire N, Harris J, Robinson S, Regan L. Obstetric risks of pregnancy in women less than 18 years old. *Obstet Gynecol* 2000; **96**: 962–6.

Joseph KS, Allen AC, Dodds L, *et al.* The perinatal effects of delayed childbearing. *Obstet Gynecol* 2005; **105**: 1410–8.

67   PLACENTA PRAEVIA

The placenta usually implants in the fundus of the uterus. It is defined as low-lying when it comes to lie in the lower segment, or partial or total praevia when it partially or fully overlies the cervical os. The condition may also be graded on a four-point scale, where in Grade 1 the placenta is low lying; in Grade 2 it reaches the os; in Grade 3 it asymmetrically covers the os; and in Grade 4 it symmetrically covers the os. This classification is further subdivided into anterior or posterior.

A low-lying placenta is noted in about 5% of early ultrasound scans, but most of these have moved into the fundus by the third trimester, and this finding is thus only regarded as significant after 27 weeks' gestation. The incidence at term is around 0.5%. It occurs more frequently in mothers who have previously delivered by Caesarean section, and is also associated with increased parity, increasing maternal age and multiple gestation.

Problems/special considerations

- *Presentation:* placenta praevia usually presents as painless bleeding, with the first bleed commonly occurring at 27–32 weeks' gestation. Occasionally, bleeding may not be apparent until the mother goes into labour, which is more likely to be preterm. If there has been recurrent bleeding, the mother is usually kept in hospital, with cross-matched blood continuously available.
- *Diagnosis:* the mother who presents with late bleeding should undergo urgent ultrasonography to determine the position of the placenta. The differential diagnosis is of placental abruption, in which bleeding is normally accompanied by abdominal pain and tenderness. If there is uncertainty as to whether vaginal delivery is possible, then an examination in theatre may be performed with to a view to proceeding to immediate Caesarean section if necessary.
- *Placenta accreta:* when an anteriorly located placenta praevia presents in a mother who has a previous uterine scar the possibility of placenta accreta (where the placenta is firmly implanted into the old scar) should be considered. Placental separation may be difficult or even impossible to achieve, and torrential blood loss may occur, which can only be controlled by removing the uterus. The risk of placenta accreta increases with the number of previous Caesarean deliveries: from 9% for placenta praevia but no previous Caesarean section; 20–30% with one previous Caesarean section; to 40–50% with 2–3 previous Caesarean sections. Placenta increta (where the placenta invades the myometrium) and percreta (where placental tissue fully penetrates the uterine wall) are rarer and more severe variants.
- *Vasa praevia:* a rare cause of third trimester bleeding is where a velamentous insertion of the umbilical cord crosses the cervical os. It may present as abrupt onset of bleeding with rupture of the membranes and, since blood loss is entirely fetal, is associated with a high perinatal mortality.
- *Mode of delivery:* although lesser degrees of placenta praevia, where the placenta does not encroach on the os, may be managed conservatively, Caesarean section is the normal method of delivery. When the mother is actively bleeding, emergency Caesarean section and delivery of the placenta may be essential to preserve the life of the mother and the baby. Placenta praevia may interfere with the development of the usually thin lower uterine segment and thus increase blood loss. Occasionally it may be necessary for the obstetrician to divide an anterior placenta praevia in order to gain access to the fetus, and this is usually accompanied by very heavy blood loss.

Management options

Investigation

High-resolution ultrasound may define the degree of invasion of the placenta, although recent studies suggest that magnetic resonance and colour flow

Doppler imaging provide a more reliable indication of invasiveness, allowing surgery and anaesthesia (and supportive facilities) to be tailored to the individual patient.

Immediate resuscitation

Management of the bleeding mother should follow basic principles of resuscitation. Two large-bore peripheral cannulae should be inserted and blood taken for haemoglobin estimation and emergency cross-match. The possibility of disseminated intravascular coagulation should be borne in mind if blood loss is very heavy, and coagulation factors should be replaced (usually as fresh frozen plasma) according to local haematological guidelines for massive transfusion.

Anaesthesia for Caesarean section

Placenta praevia has commonly been regarded as an indication for general anaesthesia, because of the risk of heavy, uncontrolled bleeding. Regional anaesthesia has traditionally been contraindicated because of the perceived risk of vasodilating the patient who is, or is about to become, hypovolaemic.

However, in recent years, the use of epidural or spinal anaesthesia in these circumstances has become more acceptable, and many senior anaesthetists would choose a regional technique for Caesarean delivery. Points that would tend to favour this approach would be a posterior placenta that will not interfere with delivery (although bleeding from a posterior placental bed may be more difficult to control), no or little active bleeding, prior cardiovascular stability and low risk of placenta accreta (no previous sections). However, the mother and her partner should be informed that conversion to general anaesthesia may occur. The patient who is bleeding heavily, who has an anterior placenta, or with a history of previous Caesarean sections, may be best managed with general anaesthesia.

Whichever technique is used, delivery should be carried out by senior obstetric and anaesthetic staff and major blood loss should be anticipated. Occasionally, when there are signs of acute placental insufficiency, the risks to the fetus of waiting for cross-matched blood must be balanced against the risk to the mother of proceeding without it; these are decisions that must be taken coolly and rationally, with full consultation between the parties.

Key points

- The chances of placenta accreta increase with number of previous Caesarean sections.
- The risk of massive haemorrhage should be assessed when choosing an anaesthetic technique.
- Senior staff should be involved in obstetric and anaesthetic management.

FURTHER READING

Bonner SM, Haynes SR, Ryall D. The anaesthetic management of Caesarean section for placenta praevia: a questionnaire survey. *Anaesthesia* 1995; **50**: 992–4.

Miller DA, Chollet JA, Goodwin TM. Clinical risk factors for placenta previa-placenta accreta. *Am J Obstet Gynecol* 1997; **177**: 210–4.

Parekh N, Husaini SWU, Russell IF. Caesarean section for placenta praevia: a retrospective study of anaesthetic management. *Br J Anaesth* 2000; **80**: 725–73.

68   PLACENTAL ABRUPTION

Placental abruption is defined as premature placental separation and occurs in around 1–2% of pregnancies. Major degrees of abruption have an incidence of 0.2%, with a perinatal mortality of 50%.

Abruption is more common in mothers with an overdistended uterus (twins, polyhydramnios) or pre-eclampsia, increasing parity and a past history of abruption.

Problems/special considerations

- *Presentation:* the usual clinical picture is of bleeding in the third trimester which, unlike the differential diagnosis of placenta praevia, is associated with abdominal pain due to uterine distension. The uterus commonly starts contracting and this will exacerbate the underlying pain. The diagnosis of minor degrees of abruption may be made retrospectively after an uneventful delivery. Abruption that is retroplacental, as opposed to at the edge of the placenta, may be concealed; these patients may present with a hard, tense abdomen, hypovolaemic shock and even disseminated intravascular coagulation.
- *Blood loss:* it is easy to underestimate blood loss in abruption, especially if the membranes have not ruptured, since much of the bleeding will be concealed. Cardiovascular changes occur late, probably because of the sympathetic activity engendered by abdominal pain and because patients are generally young and fit.
- *Coagulopathy:* coagulopathy is an early development in placental abruption, since coagulation factors are rapidly consumed by the intrauterine clot. Where abruption is severe enough to cause fetal death, the risk is as high as 30%. The risk of amniotic fluid embolism is also increased, especially in severe cases.

Management options

Management is dependent upon whether the fetus is still alive at presentation and upon the wellbeing of the mother. If there is no evidence of placental insufficiency, then the mother may be allowed to labour, with careful fetal and maternal monitoring. Basic fluid resuscitation is essential, and platelet count, coagulation tests and fibrin degradation products should be measured on admission and at regular intervals. Regional analgesic techniques are not contraindicated, but normovolaemia and unimpaired coagulation are of paramount importance if they are to be used. Blood should be cross-matched and available. Early artificial rupture of the membranes may reduce the risk of coagulopathy and amniotic fluid embolism.

When the fetus has already died, then vaginal delivery is the technique of choice. Particular attention should be paid to the risk of coagulopathy.

Caesarean section

Caesarean section is indicated if signs of fetal distress occur or if there is any evidence of developing coagulopathy. As with placenta praevia, general anaesthesia is the method of choice in the mother with cardiovascular decompensation, and should also be used in the presence of clotting disorders. If an epidural catheter is already *in situ,* then this should be used to provide anaesthesia unless there are major contraindications. Unlike placenta praevia, where the mother may be put at risk if Caesarean section is carried out before blood is available, there are benefits for fetus *and* mother in operating without delay in the case of abruption; coagulopathy may be prevented and the risk of causing massive bleeding by having to cut through the placenta is not an issue.

After delivery

Postpartum haemorrhage is far more common following abruption. This may arise as a result of coagulopathy or because the uterus fills with blood and cannot contract (Couvelaire uterus).

Key points

- Blood loss may be underestimated in abruption.
- Coagulopathy is common.
- Caesarean section should not be delayed once the mother has been resuscitated.

69   PROLAPSED CORD

Cord prolapse occurs when the umbilical cord prolapses through the birth canal ahead of the presenting part, often before the cervix is fully dilated. It is generally more common when the fetus does not fully occlude the pelvic inlet and may follow artificial rupture of the membranes with a high presenting part. The incidence is 0.4% when the vertex is presenting, but this incidence rises to 0.5% in frank breech, 4–6% in complete breech and 15–18% in footling presentations.

Problems/special considerations

Prolapsed cord is a true obstetric emergency, since the almost invariable result is compression of the cord by the presenting part of the fetus, which effectively cuts off its own blood supply. Delivery must be achieved very rapidly to prevent hypoxic–ischaemic damage to the fetus, ideally within a few minutes of prolapse.

By definition, there is usually little, if any, warning of a cord prolapse. It usually occurs during procedures such as assessment of progress or artificial rupture of membranes, when it is detected by the appearance of the cord through the introitus, but it may present spontaneously as acute, severe fetal distress or the mother noticing 'something coming down'.

Management options

The successful management of prolapsed cord requires that there is a well-established mechanism for performing immediate Caesarean section with a minimum of notice. Guidelines should be established for handling emergencies of this nature. Regular simulated drills will highlight weak points in the process and ensure that all staff are familiar with their roles. Well-recognised areas of delay include transfer of the patient to the operating theatre, gathering the theatre team, and waiting for inappropriate investigations or cross-matched blood.

The other danger of the need for rapid delivery is that important preparations may be overlooked in the rush, for example anaesthetic assessment, antacid premedication and removal of dentures. Damage to the bladder may occur if it is not emptied preoperatively.

However rapidly delivery can be achieved, every effort should be made to relieve the occlusion of the umbilical cord by manually lifting the presenting part off the cord. This can be difficult, and may be helped by maintaining a steep head-down tilt until delivery is imminent. Rapid transfer of the patient in this position, especially with a midwife supporting the fetus with her hand inside the birth canal, can be very fraught indeed. Instillation of saline into the bladder via a catheter has been claimed to assist this manoeuvre.

General anaesthesia

Caesarean section in these circumstances is often best managed by induction of general anaesthesia. It is a fast and reliable technique, and the manoeuvres needed to relieve the pressure on the cord often preclude positioning the patient for a *de novo* regional block. Many practitioners recommend that drugs for anaesthetic induction (usually thiopental and suxamethonium) should be ready prepared and kept in the theatre refrigerator at all times for just such an emergency. Others argue that the risk of these drugs being wrongly labelled or used in error is such that it outweighs the time advantage obtained.

If general anaesthesia is to be used, a preoperative airway assessment is mandatory. If a problem with intubation is anticipated, the anaesthetist may have to make the difficult decision – in conjunction with the obstetrician – of whether the mother's life should be risked for the sake of the fetus. It is impossible to give general guidance for individual cases of this nature, but the main precept is that the mother should take priority.

Steps should always be taken to protect against aspiration of gastric contents (see Chapter 56, p. 138).

Regional anaesthesia

Prolapsed cord does not necessarily rule out a regional block for Caesarean section, especially if the mother already has a functioning epidural *in situ*. It is obviously better to avoid the risks of general anaesthesia in the unprepared patient if possible, and many mothers express a strong wish to be awake to witness the birth of their baby if its viability is in doubt. The obvious problem with using an epidural block is the time delay whilst it takes effect, but various recipes for rapid top-up have been described (see Chapter 34, Epidural anaesthesia for Caesarean section, p. 86). Even if this is not fully effective by the time the operation starts, the first 2–3 minutes of surgery before the peritoneum is manipulated can be managed with a relatively low block. It is important in these circumstances for the anaesthetist to constantly reassure the mother (and often the partner as well); good, sympathetic communication may mean the difference between failure and success.

Spinal anaesthesia is often ruled out because of the time factor and the need to maintain steep head-down tilt to protect the umbilical cord. The technique is not recommended for the inexperienced in these circumstances and, if it is attempted, a strict time limit should be applied and the clock watched by an independent observer. If a 3-minute cut-off point is used, and the mother is preoxygenated during the spinal attempt, then no time is lost if conversion to general anaesthesia is necessary. As with epidural anaesthesia, the mother may need support during the first few minutes before the block is fully established.

Key points

- The successful management of prolapsed cord depends on good communication and well-rehearsed guidelines.
- General anaesthesia may be the best option, but the risks to the mother should be borne in mind.
- Regional anaesthesia is often possible, but should not be allowed to delay delivery.

70   FETAL DISTRESS

Fetal distress is a loosely defined term used to indicate that the baby is compromised and in need of delivery. The diagnosis may be made before labour or in the intrapartum period.

Problems/special considerations

The main problem is that the diagnosis of fetal distress can be difficult and must take into account many clinical parameters, together with the woman's previous obstetric history and her age. Although cardiotocography (CTG) and the presence of meconium are most commonly used to indicate fetal distress, fetal heart rate changes and meconium do not always correlate with acidosis or hypoxia, and the sensitivity and specificity for predicting a poor neonatal outcome are relatively low. In particularly high-risk cases, these signs may be more significant; in such cases antenatal diagnosis of impending fetal distress may be possible, based on ultrasound scans, Doppler blood flow studies and CTG monitoring.

Fetal distress is often used as a label to hasten operative delivery. The difficulty associating intrapartum signs with outcome means that the allowable time before delivery is uncertain. At one end of the spectrum is the baby that needs to be delivered as soon as possible since there is immediate threat to the life of the fetus, e.g. placental abruption. At the other end of the spectrum the baby needs to be delivered soon but there is time to plan the delivery. Most units' guidelines call for a maximum of 15–30 minutes between decision to deliver by Caesarean section and delivery itself, for all cases of non-elective Caesarean section. However, these times are derived largely from animal experiments over 30 years ago and their relevance is arguable, especially since most cerebral palsy is now known to be related to factors arising before labour. In addition, most units find it difficult to meet these time limits.

Delivery of babies who are diagnosed as being 'distressed' before labour (see Chapter 19, Antenatal fetal monitoring, p. 46) often need the support of the neonatal unit; thus the time and place of delivery must also take account of neonatal cot availability. For women in labour, transfer to another unit is usually not possible.

For the above reasons, the term 'fetal distress' has fallen out of favour; for example, in UK national guidance on CTG monitoring, it is not used at all, and potentially abnormal CTG patterns are described as being 'non-reassuring', 'suspicious' or 'pathological'. In practice, though, the term is still often used to indicate a potentially compromised fetus.

Management options

It is most important that there is good communication between all members of the team, the mother and her partner. In particular, obstetricians should describe the clinical situation to their anaesthetic colleagues in more detail than just saying there is 'fetal distress' – and anaesthetists must be aware of the various signs that might indicate fetal compromise, so that they can put such descriptions into context. The choice of anaesthetic technique will depend on maternal factors and the degree of urgency of the case, the onus resting with the obstetrician to indicate the latter.

Given the uncertainty of the degree of 'distress' as outlined above, many apparently 'distressed' babies are born with good Apgar scores.

The ability to improve the fetus's condition whilst preparing for delivery is often forgotten. Intrauterine resuscitation includes ensuring the mother is in the left lateral position, giving her oxygen (although there is little hard evidence that this is beneficial) and treating any hypotension, stopping oxytocic drugs and giving tocolytic drugs such as salbutamol or terbutaline 100–250 µg intravenously or glyceryl trinitrate 50 µg intravenously or 200–400 µg sublingually.

Fetal distress is a descriptive label for a variety of diagnoses and clinical situations, but if the anaesthetist understands that all fetal distress is not a life-threatening emergency, the care of the mother will improve. There are few situations in which there is not time to institute or extend a regional block to provide regional anaesthesia. For extreme cases, general anaesthesia is often used; although not necessarily faster than a spinal anaesthetic, it is generally more reliable if more hazardous.

Key points

- 'Fetal distress' is an ill-defined term, often erroneously used.
- Signs of 'fetal distress' are poorly correlated with poor neonatal outcome.
- Degree of urgency of delivery is a useful guide for anaesthetists to plan the anaesthetic technique, although definitions are vague.
- Anaesthetists must communicate with their obstetric and midwifery colleagues.
- Intrauterine resuscitation should always be remembered.

FURTHER READING

James D. Caesarean section for fetal distress. *BMJ* 2001; **322**: 1316–17.

National Institute of Clinical Excellence. *The use of electronic fetal monitoring: the use and interpretation of cardiotocography in intrapartum fetal surveillance.* London: NICE, 2001.

Thurlow SL, Kinsella SM. Intrauterine resuscitation:active management of fetal distress. *Int J Obstet Anesth* 2002; **11**: 105–16.

Yentis SM. Whose distress is it anyway? 'Fetal distress' and the 30-minute rule. *Anaesthesia* 2003; **58**: 732–3.

71 INTRAUTERINE DEATH

Most pregnancy loss occurs during the first trimester, and it is estimated that after 20 weeks' gestation fewer than 1% of all pregnancies end with fetal death. Of these, approximately a third occur with no explicable fetal or maternal cause.

Problems/special considerations

- Intrauterine death may cause major obstetric as well as psychological sequelae. It is unusual in the UK for intrauterine death to remain undiagnosed for several days but if this situation arises it is potentially life threatening, since the mother is at risk of developing disseminated intravascular coagulation and sepsis.
- Fetal death occurring during the second half of pregnancy may be suspected by the mother when she fails to feel fetal movements. The diagnosis is confirmed

by an absent fetal heartbeat on ultrasonography. In the majority of cases, the pregnancy will have been progressing apparently normally until shortly before fetal death occurs, and the diagnosis is devastating for the mother and her partner. The psychological as well as the medical wellbeing of the parents must be considered.

- Labour will normally be induced at the earliest possible opportunity after diagnosis of intrauterine death, and adequate analgesia must be provided. Tissue thromboplastin, a trigger factor for disseminated intravascular coagulation, is not released from the fetus until 3–5 weeks after intrauterine death, but may be released from the placenta if there has been any placental separation. If there is intrauterine infection, this may also act as a trigger for developing a coagulopathy.
- All the potential complications of labour and delivery may occur, including slow progress in labour, difficulty with delivery and postpartum haemorrhage. Whilst the use of oxytocics is not limited by concerns about fetal welfare, the risk of overstimulating uterine contractions and causing uterine rupture must be considered, especially in the multiparous woman or the woman with a uterine scar. It may, very occasionally, be necessary for the obstetrician to perform destructive procedures to the fetus to achieve vaginal delivery, or alternatively to perform hysterotomy. Intrapartum care of the mother is stressful and traumatic for midwifery and medical staff.

Management options

Analgesia for labour should be discussed with the mother and her midwife before active labour begins. It is common for combinations of parenteral opioids (usually diamorphine) and phenothiazines (such as chlorpromazine or promazine) or benzodiazepines to be administered in relatively large doses, the aim being to sedate the mother heavily as well as providing her with analgesia. Whilst this may seem humane (and certainly renders the midwife's task less stressful), it is not necessarily the best analgesic option and may impede the grieving process. If opioid analgesia is used, consideration should be given to the use of patient-controlled analgesia.

Epidural analgesia can provide more effective pain relief without clouding maternal consciousness. Although this may appear distressing for the mother at the time, parents often appreciate memories of seeing and holding their baby. Epidural analgesia should not be instituted until the mother is in active labour, as the latent phase may be prolonged. However, women tolerate the discomfort and pain of the latent phase poorly, and it may be useful to administer intravenous diamorphine during this stage. Epidural analgesia is contraindicated if there is a coagulopathy, although disseminated intravascular coagulation is rarely seen and only after the fetus has been dead for at least 1–2 weeks. Units should have guidelines on the management of these women, including the need for coagulation studies.

The anaesthetist should be aware of the possible risks of uterine rupture and postpartum haemorrhage in multiparous women.

Following delivery, the parents are usually encouraged to see and hold their dead baby. Photographs of the baby should be taken and kept with the medical records even if the parents do not wish to see the baby. The obstetric and midwifery staff should ensure that help is available for registering the stillbirth, discussing post-mortem examination and making any funeral arrangements.

Intrauterine death of one twin is a recognised risk of monochorionic twin pregnancy. Recommended management is usually conservative, although there have been recent reports that early delivery (by hysterotomy) of the dead twin improves outcome for the remaining twin. The psychological sequelae for both the parents and the surviving twin may be particularly difficult to deal with and may persist into the surviving twin's adult life.

Key points

- Intrauterine death is devastating for the parents; it is often completely unexpected and occurs towards the end of an apparently normal pregnancy.
- Standard obstetric management is induction of labour, with the aim of achieving vaginal delivery whenever possible.
- The obstetric anaesthetist should be able to advise about suitable analgesia and be available to deal with any complications of vaginal delivery.
- The situation demands the highest standard of communication skills and sensitivity from all medical and midwifery staff.

---

72   UTERINE INVERSION

Uterine inversion is a rare but potentially lethal complication of pregnancy. It may be incomplete or complete, depending on whether the fundus is delivered through the cervix. Nearly all occur within 24 hours of birth, although subacute (up to 4 weeks) and chronic forms have also been described.

The incidence is said to be between 1 in 2000 and 1 in 50 000 deliveries; this variation is thought to relate to the management of the third stage of delivery. Uterine inversion is more likely to occur when vigorous fundal pressure or cord traction is exerted before adequate placental separation. Coughing and vomiting and fundal insertion of the placenta are all thought to contribute to the risk of uterine inversion.

Problems/special considerations

Uterine inversion is an obstetric emergency. The presentation of the uterus through the cervix, usually with the placenta still attached, causes pain and severe vagal shock, the most important manifestation of which is bradycardia. This is often followed by severe haemorrhage.

Management options

Initial treatment is aimed at basic resuscitation, including intravenous fluids (including blood), oxygen and atropine to treat the bradycardia when indicated.

Replacement of the uterus should take place as soon as possible, since oedema quickly develops in the extruded uterus, hampering efforts to return it to its correct position. Urgent manual replacement may be successful without general anaesthesia in the first few minutes after the patient has collapsed, but general anaesthesia is usually required and should not be delayed. In the absence of shock or haemorrhage, regional anaesthesia may be suitable. Manual replacement of the uterus may be facilitated by uterine relaxation (see Chapter 60, Oxytocic and tocolytic drugs, p. 149). Traditionally, deep halothane anaesthesia has been used but this may be associated with marked hypotension and prolonged uterine atony; more recently, glyceryl trinitrate or β-adrenergic agonists have been used.

If the above method is not successful, hydrostatic pressure may be considered. In this technique, warm isotonic fluid is allowed to run into the uterus. Up to 5 litres of fluid may be required; therefore there is a risk of systemic absorption. An open abdominal method of treatment has also been described but this is rarely required.

After the uterus has been replaced, oxytocic drugs are required straight away. It is important to remember that the relaxant effects of tocolytic drugs may persist for some time.

Key points

- Uterine inversion may present with collapse, severe bradycardia and haemorrhage.
- Anaesthesia is usually required for replacement of the uterus.
- Uterine relaxation may be required to enable its replacement.
- Good communication between anaesthetists and obstetricians is essential, with minimal delay in initiating treatment.

FURTHER READING

Beringer RM, Patteril M. Puerperal uterine inversion and shock. *Br J Anaesth* 2004; **92**: 439–41.
Dawson NJ, Gabbott DA. Use of sublingual glyceryl trinitrate as a supplement to volatile inhalational anaesthesia in a case of uterine inversion. *Int J Obstet Anesth* 1997; **6**: 135–7.

73   MAJOR OBSTETRIC HAEMORRHAGE

Successive Reports on Confidential Enquiries into Maternal Deaths/Maternal and Child Health have highlighted major obstetric haemorrhage as a significant direct cause of maternal mortality. In many cases, care is substandard: women at particular risk of haemorrhage are not identified beforehand, or else management is inadequate when bleeding does occur. A similar situation exists in other countries, especially developing ones, where haemorrhage is one of the leading causes of death, often related to a lack of resources.

Obstetric haemorrhage may be antepartum or postpartum. The most common causes of antepartum bleeding are placenta praevia and placental abruption. Postpartum haemorrhage is most commonly associated with uterine atony, trauma to the genital tract, ruptured uterus and Caesarean section.

Problems/special considerations

- The extent of bleeding may be underestimated because it is concealed, for example in the vagina or bedclothes, between the legs (at Caesarean section) or within the abdomen, or mistaken for bloodstained amniotic fluid.
- Pregnant women are generally healthy and tolerate blood loss well. The patient may therefore remain cardiovascularly stable even when there has been a significant decrease in her circulating blood volume. Consequently the presence of hypotension, tachycardia and vasoconstriction in an obstetric patient represents severe hypovolaemia.
- Apparently moderate bleeding in obstetric patients may rapidly progress to major haemorrhage.
- Coagulopathy may be an underlying cause of haemorrhage, but severe haemorrhage may result in dilutional coagulopathy or disseminated intravascular coagulation.

Management options

The anaesthetist's first priority is resuscitation of the patient, but the management of major haemorrhage must involve the whole delivery suite as a team. The diagnosis and treatment of the cause of bleeding should be carried out during the primary resuscitation. The blood lost must be replaced urgently, and time should not be wasted placing monitoring lines.

If a surgical procedure is required (e.g. examination under anaesthesia, removal of retained placenta, Caesarean section, hysterectomy etc.), the presence of hypovolaemia and the possibility that coagulopathy might develop (or already exist) usually precludes regional anaesthesia.

When major haemorrhage continues, aortic compression, uterine or internal iliac artery occlusion/ligation or hysterectomy (which may be life saving) should be considered. Embolisation of the uterine arteries under radiological control has been used, but this requires special expertise.

Blood products are given according to the condition and results of coagulation tests.

Intraoperative cell salvage is well described in non-obstetric practice, though experience in obstetrics is limited. The main concern is the risk of infusing amniotic fluid into the mother's circulation, although recent reports have suggested that amniotic fluid can be effectively separated from autotransfused red cells, by washing and filtering. Recently, use of recombinant activated factor VII (rFVIIa) in intractable haemorrhage has been reported.

Major haemorrhage guidelines must be available on all delivery suites and should be rehearsed regularly by all the delivery suite staff. Guidelines are published and recommended in the Confidential Enquiries reports, although they may be adapted for local use. The guidelines should be brief, easily understood, with standard abbreviations and restricted to one A4 sheet so that it can be readily referred to in an emergency (Table 73.1).

Table 73.1. Example of a major obstetric haemorrhage guideline

Aims:	To resuscitate the patient
	To treat the cause
Inform/summon:	Obstetrician (including senior staff)
	Anaesthetist (including senior staff)
	Midwives
	Anaesthetic assistants and porters
	Haematologist (including senior staff)
Initial resuscitation:	Airway/oxygenation
	Circulation (including $2 \times 14\,G$ intravenous cannulae)
Initial blood sample:	Full blood count
	Coagulation screen
	Cross-matching for at least six units of blood
Initial monitoring:	Pulse rate
	Blood pressure
	Pulse oximetry
Initial fluids:	Colloid usually recommended until blood ready
	In dire emergency, uncross-matched blood:
	Patient's own ABO and Rh group if possible
	Uncross-matched O Rh negative if immediate transfusion is required
Subsequent monitoring:	Central venous pressure
	Direct arterial blood pressure
	Arterial blood gas analysis
	Urine output
	Temperature
Specific obstetric management:	May require general anaesthesia
Subsequent blood samples:	As above, for assessment and guidance of therapy, e.g. to assess the need for fresh frozen plasma, platelet concentrates and cryoprecipitate
Subsequent fluids:	Blood/blood products according to condition. Fluids must be administered through warming equipment. A pressure bag is required for rapid infusion
Subsequent management:	Early transfer to an intensive care unit should be considered

It is good practice for a delivery suite to have all the equipment that may be needed for a sick patient collected together for easy access, preferably on a mobile trolley that can be quickly wheeled to the patient's bedside. This trolley should be regularly checked.

Key points

- Obstetric haemorrhage continues to be a major contributor to maternal mortality.
- Major haemorrhage guidelines should be in place in all delivery suites and should be regularly rehearsed.

FURTHER READING

Franchini M, Lippi G & Franchi, M. The use of recombinant activated factor VII in obstetric and gynaecological haemorrhage. *BJOG* 2007; **114**: 8–15.

74 POSTPARTUM HAEMORRHAGE

Placental separation involves the sudden exposure of a vascular bed receiving up to 20% of the maternal cardiac output. Prevention of potentially massive haemorrhage requires contraction of uterine and arteriolar muscle, activation of circulating and endothelial clotting factors and platelet aggregation and deposition.

Postpartum haemorrhage (PPH) occurs in 2% of deliveries and is defined as a blood loss of over 500 ml after delivery of the placenta. A PPH occurring within 24 hours of childbirth is termed a primary PPH. A secondary PPH occurs within the next 6 weeks and is due to retained products of conception and/or infection.

Postpartum haemorrhage can be one of the most frightening obstetric emergencies and may be associated with maternal mortality.

Problems/special considerations

- There are a number of different causes of PPH (Table 74.1). Although initial management is the same (i.e. resuscitation), subsequent management depends on the cause, which may be difficult to ascertain in the face of continuing haemorrhage.
- After a normal delivery, attention is often focused on the baby and thus moderate PPH may be unnoticed initially. This is compounded by the ability of normal pregnant women to compensate until hypovolaemia is severe (see Chapter 73, Major obstetric haemorrhage, p. 173).

Table 74.1. Causes of postpartum haemorrhage

Obstetric	• Uterine atony	Previous history of PPH
		Large placental site, e.g. multiple pregnancy
		Long or precipitous labour
		Prolonged oxytocic infusion
		Grandmultiparity
		Chorioamnionitis
		Retained products (placenta or membranes)
		Inverted or ruptured uterus
		Drugs, e.g. volatile anaesthetic agents, tocolytic drugs
	• Trauma to the cervix, birth canal or perineum	
Non-obstetric	• Primary coagulopathy, e.g. von Willebrand's disease	
	• Secondary coagulopathy, e.g. disseminated intravascular coagulopathy, HELLP syndrome, post-massive transfusion dilutional coagulopathy, drugs	

- There may be few medical and midwifery staff in close attendance if PPH occurs without warning. This may lead to delay in resuscitation unless staff are well versed in the emergency management of such cases.

Management options

The first priority of the anaesthetist called to a patient with PPH is resuscitation followed by urgent assessment of the cause of bleeding.

The extent of haemorrhage is often underestimated. Any woman who has an unexplained tachycardia or a hypotensive episode in the postpartum period should be treated as having had a major blood loss until proven otherwise.

The most common cause of PPH is uterine atony. It is routine practice to administer oxytocics at the delivery of the anterior shoulder of the baby (see Chapter 60, Oxytocic and tocolytic drugs, p. 149). This hastens placental separation and encourages uterine contraction in the third stage of labour. If the uterus fails to contract and bleeding continues, further oxytocic drugs may be given (Table 74.2), aided by manual rubbing of the uterus to stimulate contraction. If the uterus continues to relax, the possibility of retained products of conception should be considered, which necessitates exploration of the uterus. A retained placenta may involve the whole or part of the placenta, and manual removal of the placenta is indicated.

Genital tract trauma should be sought and this may require anaesthesia. Ideally, primary resuscitation of the patient, together with confirmation of preparation of blood for transfusion, should be established before anaesthesia is administered. It is often necessary to proceed to anaesthesia before the blood is available.

Table 74.2. Prevention and drug treatment of uterine atony causing postpartum haemorrhage (PPH)

Routine prophylaxis	Syntometrine (5 U Syntocinon with 0.5 mg ergometrine) intramuscularly at delivery of the anterior shoulder
PPH occurs	Syntocinon 5–10 U given slowly, intravenously, or an infusion containing 40–50 U Syntocinon/500 ml saline at a rate depending upon the clinical response but usually over a 4 h period
PPH persists	Ergometrine 125–250 µg intravenously, repeated as necessary
PPH unresponsive to the above	Carboprost (PGF2α) 250 µg given intramuscularly (may also be injected directly into the myometrium)
Various*	Misoprostol 200–800 µg depending on the route: oral, sublingual, vaginal, rectal and intrauterine administration has been described

N.B. consider retained placenta, genital tract trauma and other causes of haemorrhage.
*use of misoprostol may vary according to local protocols but it has been used to prevent as well as treat PPH.

If there is continued uterine bleeding, the abdomen needs to be opened. Hysterectomy may sometimes be avoided by packing the uterus or using an intra-uterine balloon, compression (B-Lynch) sutures, and ligation or embolisation of the uterine or internal iliac arteries or use of intravascular balloon catheters (depending on the expertise and proximity of the radiology department). Finally, infusion of recombinant activated factor VII (rFVIIa) has been described when PPH is complicated by coagulopathy uncorrected by clotting factors.

Key points

- Any postpartum haemorrhage must be seen as a potential major obstetric haemorrhage and should be treated early and aggressively.
- Postpartum haemorrhage should be taken seriously, and senior help should be sought at an early stage.
- Full resuscitation should not be regarded as being complete until the cause of the bleeding has been identified and treated.

FURTHER READING

Hofmeyr GJ, Walraven G, Gulmezoglu AM, et al. Misoprostol to treat postpartum haemorrhage: a systematic review. *Br J Obstet Gynaecol* 2005; **112**: 547–53.

Karalapillai D, Popham P. Recombinant factor VIIa in massive postpartum haemorrhage. *Int J Obstet Anesth*; **16**: 29–34.

Mousa HA, Alfirevic Z. Treatment for primary postpartum haemorrhage. *Cochrane Database Syst Rev* 2003; (1): CD003249.

75 COLLAPSE ON LABOUR WARD

Although uncommon, collapse of a mother in the delivery suite may represent serious underlying pathology and demands rapid treatment; the mother may also rapidly respond to relatively simple measures, thus avoiding disaster.

Problems/special considerations

Collapse on the labour ward may have several causes, some of which require specific investigation and/or management (Table 75.1). Typically, the labour ward staff are less familiar with emergency equipment and drugs than staff in the operating theatres, so continuous checking of equipment and education of staff is required; regular 'drills' have been recommended.

Management options

Initial resuscitation in the undelivered patient is influenced by the risk of aortocaval compression and aspiration and the fact that the fetus is at risk. Thus the airway should be secured, the lungs ventilated and the circulation supported with fluids, vasoactive drugs or cardiac massage as appropriate, with measures taken to displace the uterus or deliver the fetus if antepartum.

Concurrent with treatment is the need to determine the cause, with further management directed as appropriate.

All staff should be familiar with basic resuscitative techniques, and protocols should exist for the more important causes, e.g. pre-eclampsia and haemorrhage. Rapid delivery of relevant information about the collapsed mother to the medical staff resuscitating her is also crucial in directing management towards a particular

Table 75.1. Causes of collapse on the labour ward

Cardiovascular	• Haemorrhage (antenatal, e.g. placenta praevia, abruption; postnatal, e.g. splenic artery rupture)
	• Regional anaesthetic sympathetic block
	• Cardiac disease (congenital, acquired)
	• Embolism (amniotic fluid, air, thrombus)
	• Arrhythmias/vasovagal syncope
Neurological	• Convulsion (eclampsia, epilepsy, local anaesthetic toxicity)
	• Intracranial lesion (stroke, tumour)
Pharmacological	• Local anaesthetics (toxicity, sympathetic block, total spinal)
	• Opioids (systemic or especially spinal)
	• Other (magnesium, antihypertensives, other sedatives, cocaine abuse, etc.)
Other	• Anaphylaxis (drugs, latex)
	• Airway obstruction (anaphylaxis, oedema)
	• Sepsis

possible cause. This will be easier in delivery suites where there is good multi-professional communication about routine as well as problem cases.

Key points

- Collapse on the labour ward has many causes, including obstetric, anaesthetic and medical factors.
- Immediate management is as for the non-pregnant patient but with avoidance of aortocaval compression.

---

76   MATERNAL CARDIOPULMONARY RESUSCITATION

Although the basic principles of cardiopulmonary resuscitation (CPR) are the same as in the non-pregnant state, the underlying causes of collapse are generally different, and the presence of the fetus has major implications for management and outcome.

Problems/special considerations

- *General management:* because most mothers are healthy, cardiac arrest is rare in this group (estimated at 1:30 000) and thus resuscitative skills are easily forgotten, especially by those not regularly exposed to patients requiring cardiorespiratory support. There may be delay in recognising and responding to cardiorespiratory arrest. Midwives and obstetricians (and also anaesthetists) may be unfamiliar with protocols for life support and the drugs and equipment required, which may easily become faulty or out of date if not checked regularly. The maternity suite is often an unfamiliar place to the regular cardiac arrest team.
- *Cause of collapse:* in contrast to the situation in the non-pregnant population, most mothers are young and fit and thus unlikely to have ischaemic heart disease. However, the incidence of this condition is increasing as the effects of smoking in women are becoming apparent and more women are having children at older ages. In addition, cocaine abuse (especially problematic in the USA) may cause myocardial ischaemia. Most cases of peripartum cardiorespiratory arrest or collapse, however, will involve non-ischaemic causes (see Chapter 75, Collapse on labour ward, p. 179). Thus actual cardiac arrest requiring artificial ventilation and cardiac massage is much more likely to be caused by hypovolaemia, embolism (with thrombus, air or amniotic fluid) and other conditions such as sepsis, electrolyte disturbances, anaphylaxis, drug abuse, etc.
- *Presence of the fetus:* in late pregnancy, CPR is ineffective if the woman is supine, and many reports have shown that outcome is improved by taking steps to avoid aortocaval compression. As long as the fetus stays within the uterus, there will thus be a conflict between the requirement for a stable and relatively supine chest

in order to peform chest compressions effectively and the need to relieve aorto-caval compression in order to improve cardiac output.

Airway management may be difficult as for any pregnant woman, depending on the gestation and particular details of the case. The presence of a gravid uterus may hinder effective artificial ventilation and increase the risk of regurgitation by exerting pressure on the stomach. It may also increase the risk of injury to the liver, spleen and ribs because of the increased intra-abdominal pressure and altered shape of the chest. In addition, the fetus will consume oxygen and thus deprive the mother at a time when maternal oxygenation may be critical.

Management options

Some cases of cardiac arrest may be prevented by general training and drawing up of protocols in airway management and cardiovascular monitoring, identification of high-risk cases, good communication and organisation of facilities, equipment, etc.

All staff who work in the maternity suite must receive training and regular updates in CPR, including use of the defibrillator and other equipment. Drills have been shown to improve retention of skills, although they may be very disruptive to a busy unit.

Actual management of cardiac arrest is as for the non-pregnant patient, although the different causes of collapse should be considered. The hands should be placed higher up the sternum than in the non-pregnant state, but transthoracic impedance (and thus the energy required for DC cardioversion) is the same. Relief of aortocaval compression is paramount; methods include manual displacement of the gravid uterus, placing a wedge under the mother's hip (the 'Cardiff wedge' is a wooden wedge mounted on wheels for use in the delivery suite), an assistant kneeling on the floor and using his/her thighs as a 'human wedge' under the mother's back and delivery of the fetus by 'perimortem' Caesarean section if CPR is unsuccessful. There are many reported cases of return of spontaneous cardiac output and maternal survival once delivery has been achieved, in cases where CPR has failed initially. Neonatal outcome is usually poor, although this depends on the gestation, the cause of collapse, the delay before delivery and the effectiveness of CPR.

The risk of regurgitation and aspiration of gastric contents should be remembered and cricoid pressure applied, if hands are spare, until the trachea has been intubated.

Key points

- Ischaemic heart disease is unlikely in most mothers, and other causes (e.g. hypovolaemia, embolism) are more common.
- Regular training of staff and maintenance of equipment is required.
- Maternal cardiopulmonary resuscitation is impossible in late pregnancy unless aortocaval compression is relieved.

FURTHER READING

Goodwin AP, Pearce AJ. The human wedge: a manoeuvre to relieve aortocaval compression in resuscitation during late pregnancy. *Anaesthesia* 1992; **47**: 433–4.

International Liaison Committee on Resuscitation. International consensus on cardiopulmonary resuscitation and emergency cardiovascular care science with treatment recommendations. Part 4: advanced life support. *Resuscitation* 2005; **67**: 213–47.

Mallampalli A, Guy E. Cardiac arrest in pregnancy and somatic support after brain death. *Crit Care Med* 2005; **33**(10): S325–S331.

Morris S, Stacey M. Resuscitation in pregnancy. *BMJ* 2003; **327**: 1277–9.

77   AMNIOTIC FLUID EMBOLISM

Amniotic fluid embolism (AFE) has been estimated to occur in 1:8000–1:80 000 deliveries, the wide range reflecting the difficulty in its accurate diagnosis. Despite its rarity, AFE has been implicated in 10–12% of direct maternal deaths in the UK, making it one of the major causes of mortality.

The traditional explanation of AFE is that amniotic fluid enters the maternal circulation following forceful contractions, causing pulmonary vascular obstruction and thence right ventricular failure and cardiovascular collapse. However, more recent studies suggest a biphasic response, with initial transient pulmonary vasoconstriction and severe hypoxaemia followed by left ventricular failure. The mechanism now proposed is systemic release of inflammatory mediators causing cardiovascular collapse, although the trigger for mediator release is still disputed (amniotic fluid, meconium, fetal cells or other substances having all been suggested). The role of amniotic fluid itself is uncertain since infusion of amniotic fluid may be well tolerated experimentally. Similarly, the traditional opinion that AFE is more common in older, multiparous women experiencing forceful labour has also been challenged. Both traditional and current views suggest that AFE is more common in placental abruption. Although AFE is most common during labour, it may also occur during Caesarean section or even after delivery.

Problems/special considerations

Features of AFE include sweating, shivering, convulsions, fetal bradycardia, dyspnoea, cyanosis, cardiovascular collapse and disseminated intravascular coagulation (DIC). Collapse is typically profound, rapid and resistant to treatment. Thus the initial problem of AFE is its immediate management.

In addition, there are many causes of sudden collapse (see Chapter 75, Collapse on labour ward, p. 179) and it may be difficult to diagnose the underlying condition. Although the diagnosis of AFE is often based on the demonstration of fetal squames in the maternal circulation or lung, this has been shown to be neither a sensitive nor a specific test, since normal mothers may demonstrate circulating fetal squames whilst 'classic' cases of AFE may not.

A final problem – and one that hinders development of effective methods of prevention and treatment – is the debate over the nature of AFE itself, even whether it represents a separate entity at all (the term 'sudden obstetric collapse syndrome' has been suggested as being more appropriate). Since the mechanism is so poorly understood, the condition remains an enigma.

Management options

Management is supportive, with basic resuscitative manoeuvres and correction of DIC. Even with prompt and appropriate management, mortality of 60–80% has been traditionally been reported, with about 40% fetal loss. Two-thirds of mothers die within 5 hours of presentation. More recent reports suggest a lower mortality if resuscitation is prompt (~30%), suggesting a benefit of good supportive intensive care.

In the UK, a national register of suspected cases of AFE has been established, to include women who survive and are therefore not reported to the Confidential Enquiries. A similar scheme ran for 5 years in the USA and was reported on in 1995.

Key points

- Amniotic fluid embolism is probably a misnomer, but represents a catastrophic event on the labour ward.
- Features include convulsions, respiratory and cardiovascular collapse, and disseminated intravascular coagulation.
- There is no specific treatment and the prognosis is poor.

FURTHER READING

Davies S. Amniotic fluid embolus: a review of the literature. *Can J Anaesth* 2001; **48**: 88–98.

Moore J, Baldisseri MR. Amniotic fluid embolism. *Crit Care Med* 2005; **33** (10 Suppl): S279–S285.

Tufnell DJ. United Kingdom Amniotic Fluid Embolism Register. *BJOG* 2005; **112**: 1625–9.

Yentis SM. Sudden obstetric collapse syndrome. *Int J Obstet Anesth* 1999; **8**: 296.

78   CHOLESTASIS OF PREGNANCY (OBSTETRIC CHOLESTASIS)

Cholestasis of pregnancy (intrahepatic cholestasis of pregnancy) is thought to result from an exaggerated cholestatic effect of oestrogens. It occurs in approximately 0.2% of pregnancies (except in Scandinavia and South America, where incidences of up to 10% have been reported) and is associated with multiple pregnancy. Its presenting symptom is pruritus, caused by the deposition of bile acids in the skin. Symptoms usually occur during the third trimester and may be sufficiently distressing to necessitate induction of labour. The condition is specific to pregnancy, and patients are invariably completely asymptomatic within 1–2 weeks of delivery. The condition tends to recur in subsequent pregnancies.

Problems/special considerations

Although symptoms usually occur in the third trimester, the condition may present at any stage of pregnancy. There is a personal or family history of jaundice whilst using the oral contraceptive pill, or during a previous pregnancy, in about 50% of cases.

Jaundice occurs in up to 50% of cases if untreated or undelivered. Clinical examination is otherwise normal except for scratch marks owing to the severe itching. Fat malabsorption occurs, and the mother may complain of steatorrhoea. Malabsorption may result in vitamin K deficiency. Liver function tests reveal predominately conjugated bilirubinaemia, with markedly increased alkaline phosphatase and mildly increased transaminases.

There is an increased risk of preterm labour and fetal distress, presumed to be secondary to reduced placental blood flow or a direct effect of bile salts.

Management options

Treatment with cholestyramine, antihistamines or topical preparations has variable success. Corticosteroids have also been used, but most women are now treated with ursodeoxycholic acid, which has been shown to improve symptoms and reduce serum bile acid levels. Both the mother and the neonate should receive vitamin K therapy.

The mother's coagulation should be checked during the antenatal period and before considering insertion of an epidural or spinal needle, although coagulopathy is rare. If coagulation studies are within normal limits, the mother should be encouraged to have epidural analgesia for labour, since there is an increased incidence of Caesarean section in women with cholestasis of pregnancy.

Key points

- Cholestasis of pregnancy is a benign and self-limiting condition for the mother but is associated with an increased incidence of preterm labour, fetal distress and Caesarean delivery.
- Coagulopathy may occur secondary to vitamin K malabsorption.
- The only definitive treatment is delivery.
- Epidural analgesia should be encouraged unless contraindicated by coagulopathy.

FURTHER READING

Kenyon AP, Piercy CN, Girling J, *et al*. Obstetric cholestasis, outcome with active management: a series of 70 cases. *Br J Obstet Gynaecol* 2002; **109**: 282–8.

Milkiewicz P, Elias E, Williamson C, Weaver J. Obstetric cholestasis. *BMJ* 2002; **324**: 123–4.

79   ACUTE FATTY LIVER OF PREGNANCY

Acute fatty liver of pregnancy is an uncommon (estimated 1 in 9000–13 000 pregnancies) but serious complication of predominately primiparous women, especially those with multiple pregnancy. The condition was first reported in the literature in 1934 and traditionally the mortality for both mother and fetus has been reported to be as high as 75%. Current figures estimate maternal mortality to be about 20%, the improvement being attributed to earlier diagnosis and earlier delivery.

In some cases the condition may be associated with long-chain-3-hydroxyacyl-CoA dehydrogenase (LCHAD) deficiency, an abnormality of fatty-acid metabolism. Both parents have 50% of normal LCHAD activity and the fetus has no LCHAD activity, with the fetal liver dysfunction apparently causing fatty liver disease in the mother.

Symptoms usually present in the third trimester and tend to be non-specific: malaise, nausea and vomiting (which may be severe), headache and diffuse right upper quadrant or epigastric pain. Liver function may deteriorate rapidly, leading to acute liver failure. There is overlap between acute fatty liver and pre-eclampsia, and it has been suggested that acute fatty liver is a manifestation of pre-eclampsia, as is the HELLP (haemolysis, elevated liver enzymes and low platelet count) syndrome.

The only treatment for acute fatty liver of pregnancy is termination of the pregnancy. As with pre-eclampsia, there may be a time lag of several days between delivery and clinical improvement.

Recovery is usually complete, with no evidence of chronic liver disease. Recurrence in subsequent pregnancies is said to be uncommon, although there have not been a large number of documented pregnancies in survivors of acute fatty liver. In cases associated with LCHAD deficiency the risk of acute fatty liver is 25% in each pregnancy.

Problems/special considerations

The differential diagnoses at initial presentation include pre-eclampsia, acute viral hepatitis, drug-induced hepatitis, cholestasis of pregnancy and biliary tract disease. Pruritus is uncommon in acute fatty liver and is highly suggestive of cholestasis.

- *Clinical examination:* the mother is usually, but not invariably, jaundiced. Although she may complain of abdominal pain it is unusual to find marked liver tenderness on examination, and this finding is suggestive of viral hepatitis or HELLP syndrome. If presentation occurs late, all the stigmata of acute liver failure may be present, including hepatic encephalopathy, disseminated intravascular coagulation (DIC) and renal failure. The prognosis is poor if the disease presents in this advanced state.

- *Laboratory findings:* serum alanine and aspartate transaminases levels are increased, but not as high as in viral hepatitis. Bilirubin is increased. Platelet counts fall, and there may be giant platelet formation. Prothrombin time is prolonged, and the more severe the liver damage the more deranged the coagulation profile becomes. There are reduced levels of antithrombin III, and DIC with low fibrinogen levels and increased fibrin degradation products occurs in severe disease. Haemoconcentration may occur secondary to hypovolaemia. There is frequently an increased white cell count and increased uric acid concentration. Hypoglycaemia is common.
- *Other investigations:* liver biopsy provides confirmation of the diagnosis, but it may be contraindicated on clinical grounds. The findings are of fibrin deposition, haemorrhage and microvesicular fatty infiltration. Both computerised tomography and ultrasonography have been used with some success to demonstrate fatty infiltration of the liver.

Management options

Acute fatty liver of pregnancy is uncommon but has a high mortality if the diagnosis is delayed. A high index of clinical suspicion is needed for the non-specifically unwell mother with pre-eclampsia, especially if there is any indication that she may be jaundiced.

Once the diagnosis is confirmed the mother should be stabilised as necessary and delivered. Operative delivery is not indicated unless the obstetrician considers that successful vaginal delivery is unlikely to be achieved. Regional analgesia and anaesthesia are contraindicated in the presence of any coagulopathy.

Medical support is likely to include administration of glucose, blood, clotting factors and platelets. Hypertension associated with pre-eclampsia should be controlled. Analgesia for labour can be provided by using cautious doses of opioid drugs, preferably by a patient-controlled intravenous route. Adjuvant sedative drugs such as promazine and promethazine should not be given. Because of impaired metabolism, atracurium is the preferred neuromuscular blocking drug for general anaesthesia. Elimination of opioid drugs is likely to be prolonged.

If operative delivery is needed, persistent bleeding from surgical sites should be anticipated and prophylactic wound drains are advisable. Close observation is essential following delivery, and intensive care management including multiorgan support may be required. Less sick mothers should have a low protein diet and scrupulous fluid and electrolyte management until clinical and laboratory findings return to normal.

Key points

- Acute fatty liver of pregnancy occurs in about 1 in 10 000 pregnancies and potentially has a very high mortality unless diagnosed and treated promptly.
- Some cases are caused by long-chain-3-hydroxyacyl-CoA dehydrogenase (LCHAD) deficiency and have an increased risk of recurrence.
- Delivery of the fetus is the only definitive treatment.
- Acute liver failure and multiorgan derangement can occur rapidly. Regional analgesia and anaesthesia are usually contraindicated because of abnormal clotting studies.
- Pre-eclampsia frequently co-exists with acute fatty liver, and it is possible that acute fatty liver is a variant of pre-eclampsia.

FURTHER READING

Antognini JF, Andrews S. Anaesthesia for caesarean section in a patient with acute fatty liver of pregnancy. *Can J Anaesth* 1991; **38**: 904–7.

Holzman RS, Riley LE, Aron E, Fetherston J. Perioperative care of a patient with acute fatty liver of pregnancy. *Anesth Analg* 2001; **92**: 1268–70.

Rahman TM, Wendon J. Severe hepatic dysfunction in pregnancy. *QJM* 2002; **95**: 343–57.

80   HELLP SYNDROME

HELLP (haemolysis, elevated liver enzymes and low platelet count) syndrome is one of the presentations of pre-eclampsia and may occur before or soon after delivery. Severe HELLP syndrome is associated with disseminated intravascular coagulation (DIC) and placental abruption and may progress to multiorgan failure. It is associated with a high fetal and maternal morbidity and mortality.

Problems/special considerations

- The mother with HELLP syndrome may not necessarily have presented with symptoms or signs of pre-eclampsia. The main presenting feature may be abdominal pain, perhaps with nausea and vomiting, so a high index of suspicion is needed.
- Mild changes in liver function tests have been reported in up to 50% of women with pre-eclampsia, but more serious dysfunction may occur, including periportal haemorrhage and hepatic infarction. There have also been several reported cases of liver rupture associated with severe HELLP syndrome. Acute fatty liver of pregnancy is also considered by many authorities to be part of the spectrum of pre-eclampsia/eclampsia.
- Other complications of HELLP syndrome include renal failure, DIC, pulmonary oedema, pleural effusions, acute respiratory distress syndrome, retinal

detachment and cerebral oedema. About 16% of women who are undelivered and who develop HELLP syndrome present with placental abruption.

Management options

The treatment of HELLP syndrome is supportive; delivery of the placenta is the definitive treatment.

Women should be delivered as soon as the maternal condition has been optimised, usually by Caesarean section. Recommendations vary regarding pre- or perioperative platelet transfusion, with some centres suggesting platelet transfusion if the platelet count is below $50 \times 10^9/l$ and others not giving platelets until the count falls below $20 \times 10^9/l$.

The benefits of invasive pressure monitoring must be balanced against the potential hazards, and the antecubital fossa approach to the central veins is recommended if possible. Careful fluid balance is important, and bladder catheterisation is mandatory.

Regional anaesthesia is relatively contraindicated in the presence of thrombocytopenia, but ultimately the anaesthetist must choose the anaesthetic technique which he or she judges to be the safest in the circumstance. The choice of regional anaesthesia in a woman with a platelet count of less than $80 \times 10^9/l$ should be made only by an experienced consultant obstetric anaesthetist.

If general anaesthesia is used, attempts must be made to attenuate the hypertensive response to intubation, usually by use of an intravenous opioid as part of the induction sequence (see Chapter 81, hypertension, pre-eclampsia and eclampsia, p. 189). Tracheal intubation should be carried out as atraumatically as possible.

There is no specific treatment for HELLP syndrome other than symptomatic treatment of the associated complications, although there is some evidence to support steroid, therapy, e.g. two doses of dexamethasone 10 mg 12 hours apart followed by 5 mg at 24 and 36 hours. Plasma exchange has been reported to be useful anecdotally, although the evidence for it is weak. Women with HELLP syndrome should be managed in a high-dependency or intensive therapy environment. Postnatal management is entirely supportive.

Key points

- HELLP syndrome is part of the spectrum of pre-eclampsia/eclampsia and may present without prodromal symptoms and signs of pre-eclampsia.
- It may present before or after delivery and is associated with significant maternal and fetal morbidity and mortality.
- Epigastric pain, nausea and vomiting are common presenting features, and a high index of suspicion is essential in every pregnant woman presenting with abdominal pain.
- Treatment consists of delivery and supportive management of the associated complications.

FURTHER READING

Forster JG, Peltonen S, Kaaja R, Lampinen K, Pettila V. Plasma exchange in severe postpartum HELLP syndrome. *Acta Anaesthesiol Scand* 2002; **46**: 955–8.

Isler CM, Rinehart BK, Terrone DA, *et al.* Maternal mortality associated with HELLP (hemolysis, elevated liver enzymes, and low platelets) syndrome. *Am J Obstet Gynecol* 1999; **181**: 924–8.

Matchaba P, Moodley J. Corticosteroids for HELLP syndrome in pregnancy. *Cochrane Database Syst Rev* 2004; (1): CD002076.

Sibai BM. Diagnosis, controversies, and management of the syndrome of hemolysis, elevated liver enzymes, and low platelet count. *Obstet Gynecol* 2004; **103**: 981–91.

81   HYPERTENSION, PRE-ECLAMPSIA AND ECLAMPSIA

Hypertension in pregnancy is diagnosed either by raised absolute values of systolic or diastolic pressure (> 140 mmHg or > 90 mmHg respectively) or by increases in systolic or diastolic pressures above those at booking (> 30 mmHg or > 15 mmHg respectively). Pressures should be raised on two separate occasions using appropriate methods of measurement (see below).

Hypertensive disorders of pregnancy are divided into chronic hypertension, gestational hypertension and pre-eclampsia.

Chronic hypertension and gestational hypertension

Chronic hypertension occurs in 3–5% of pregnancies, although the incidence is increasing in the UK as maternal age increases. It is diagnosed by pre-existing hypertension or hypertension that occurs before 20 weeks' gestation, although the diagnosis may be masked by the normal slight fall in blood pressure that occurs in early pregnancy, and pre-eclampsia may rarely present earlier than 20 weeks. The risk of pre-eclampsia is approximately doubled, and there is also a greater risk of abruption and fetal growth restriction, but if the blood pressure is controlled women with chronic hypertension would be expected to have good outcomes.

Gestational hypertension describes hypertension after 20 weeks' gestation without any features of pre-eclampsia, and occurs in 6–7% of pregnancies. The risk of pre-eclampsia is increased slightly, this risk increasing the earlier the hypertension develops. Blood pressure usually returns to normal within 1–2 months of delivery.

Pre-eclampsia

Pre-eclampsia is usually defined as hypertension and proteinuria that develops after 20 weeks' gestation in a previously normotensive and non-proteinuric woman (oedema is now omitted from the definition, although it is often present).

It is possible to develop non-proteinuric pre-eclampsia and also to have eclamptic seizures with minimal or even no hypertension. Pre-eclampsia occurs in 5–6% of pregnancies overall (up to 25% in patients with pre-existing hypertension).

Pre-eclampsia/eclampsia is a major direct cause of maternal death worldwide. Pre-eclampsia is a multisystem disease with a variable clinical presentation. The pathophysiology of pre-eclampsia is still only partially understood, but it is known that failure of placentation occurs early in pregnancy and this leads to vascular endothelial cell damage and dysfunction. The endothelial cell damage is thought to lead to release of vasoactive substances, which promote generalised vasoconstriction and reduced organ perfusion. This is exacerbated by the increased sensitivity to circulating catecholamines found in the pre-eclamptic patient. Pre-eclamptic women demonstrate an imbalance of the normal thromboxane/prostacyclin ratio and increased free radical activity.

Pre-eclampsia encompasses HELLP (haemolysis, elevated liver enzymes and low platelets) syndrome, eclampsia and possibly acute fatty liver of pregnancy. Although the disease is progressive, a mother may be asymptomatic until she presents with an eclamptic fit, and although pre-eclampsia is a disease of pregnancy, terminated only by delivery, pre-eclampsia, HELLP syndrome and eclampsia may all present only after delivery.

There have been many attempts to prevent development of pre-eclampsia, e.g. with dietary vitamins, antioxidants and minerals, with no clear benefit found. The large international CLASP (Collaborative Low-dose Aspirin Study in Pregnancy) trial failed to show universal benefit from low-dose aspirin, suggesting instead that aspirin may be beneficial in selected high-risk women.

Problems/special considerations

- *Measurement:* blood pressure measurements should be made with the mother sitting (or on her side in late pregnancy) to avoid aortocaval compression. Most automated blood pressure measuring devices have not been validated in pregnancy and many tend to underread blood pressure, especially in pre-eclampsia, giving a false sense of security (though they can be used to monitor trends, so long as manual measurements are taken at intervals). If manual methods of measurement are used, it is now recommended that Korotkoff phase V sounds should be used to measure diastolic pressure, not phase IV, since the former are more reproducible and better correlated with true diastolic pressure in pregnancy.
- *Clinical features:* pre-eclampsia is frequently asymptomatic despite significant disease. Symptoms are often non-specific and include headache, visual disturbance and epigastric pain. The most commonly occurring signs are hypertension, oedema and hyperreflexia, although the latter is subjective and unreliable as a prognostic indicator (though sustained clonus is pathological). Women may also present with the clinical features of pulmonary oedema, cerebral haemorrhage, impaired liver function, placental abruption or coagulopathy. Oedema may also affect the airway. Investigations may reveal abnormal renal and hepatic function,

coagulation disorders and pleural and pericardial effusions. Occasionally the clinical presentation may be dramatic – ruptured liver has been reported.

- *Fetal effects:* chronic impairment of uteroplacental blood flow causes intrauterine growth retardation and this may be one of the first signs of pre-eclampsia. There is an increased risk of prematurity.
- *Haemodynamic changes:* the normal expansion of blood volume which takes place in early pregnancy fails to occur in pre-eclamptic women and there is therefore a relatively hypovolaemic state. This is exacerbated by leaky capillaries, which allow inappropriate fluid shifts between compartments. Colloid osmotic pressure is low in pre-eclamptic women, and any increased hydrostatic pressure due to iatrogenic fluid overload, impaired left ventricular function or postpartum fluid shifts may therefore readily precipitate pulmonary oedema.

   Results of the numerous studies (both invasive and non-invasive) of the haemodynamic changes occurring in pre-eclampsia are confusing. There is generalised vasoconstriction and therefore systemic vascular resistance is usually increased. Cardiac index and cardiac output may be high, low or normal but this is frequently a reflection of drug therapy. In severe pre-eclampsia, especially if there is pulmonary oedema, right atrial pressure may not accurately reflect pulmonary artery pressure, and central venous pressure monitoring may therefore be an unreliable guide to treatment.

- *Convulsions:* in the UK, approximately 1–2% of pre-eclamptic women develop eclampsia, though the incidence is higher in the developing countries. Forty per cent of eclamptic fits occur after delivery, most commonly within the first 3 days and rarely more than one week postpartum. In approximately a third of cases, there are minimal prodromal signs or symptoms. Recurrent seizures are associated with increased maternal morbidity and mortality. Twenty per cent of eclamptics experience pre-eclampsia in the next pregnancy, and 2% have eclampsia.

Management options

The management of chronic and gestational hypertension consists of anti-hypertensive drugs and close monitoring for development of pre-eclampsia or intra-uterine growth retardation.

The Report on Confidential Enquiries into Maternal Deaths in the United Kingdom strongly recommends that every obstetric unit should have written guidelines for the management of pre-eclampsia and eclampsia. There have also been recommendations that every obstetric unit should have an 'eclampsia pack' containing everything necessary to treat eclamptic women with magnesium.

Women with mild to moderate disease and without major fetal compromise are usually offered a trial of vaginal delivery, whilst those with severe pre-eclampsia (especially at less than 37 weeks' gestation) are likely to be delivered by Caesarean section (although some evidence exists to support expectant care). The anaesthetist should assess the mother, paying particular attention to any symptoms of pre-eclampsia, drug treatment, the airway, level of hypertension, results of haematological and biochemical investigations and proposed mode of delivery.

Hypertension

Treatment of hypertension does not modify the course of the underlying disease process but may reduce the morbidity and mortality attributable to uncontrolled hypertension. Whether treatment of mild hypertension during pregnancy is worth while is unclear.

The first-line treatment of hypertension is usually methyldopa, which has a long safety record for the fetus, although randomised controlled trials are few. Labetalol and nifedipine have both been used increasingly in recent years, either instead of, or in addition to, methyldopa. Patients already receiving angiotensin-converting enzyme inhibitors or anti-angiotensin receptor agents should have them withdrawn because of their fetotoxic effects.

Hydralazine is the most commonly used agent for management of acute hypertension. Administration of small repeated intravenous boluses (e.g. 5 mg) is preferable to continuous infusion. Hydralazine acts primarily as a vasodilator and should therefore be used with caution and preferably in conjunction with gentle volume replacement. Acute vasodilatation may cause an uncontrolled fall in blood pressure and thus provoke fetal distress. (Reduction in maternal blood pressure is associated with a significantly greater percentage reduction in uteroplacental perfusion.)

Labetalol (10 mg boluses) may be used parenterally in the acute situation, and oral nifedipine (5–10 mg) has also been used, acting within 15–30 minutes. Although there have been concerns over sublingual nifedipine and the risk of uncontrolled hypotension, particularly in combination with magnesium sulphate, this is not thought to be a common problem, especially with slow-release preparations.

Nitroprusside and glyceryl trinitrate have been used in North America for acute control of hypertension but are not commonly used in the UK.

Convulsions

Magnesium sulphate has been shown to reduce the incidence of eclampsia in pre-eclampsia by about half, although whether it should be offered routinely to pre-eclamptics is controversial since only 1–2% of the latter go on to develop pre-eclampsia and a significant proportion of eclamptics cannot be identified beforehand (see, Chapter 82, Magnesium sulphate, p. 196).

Magnesium sulphate reduces the incidence of recurrent convulsions in eclampsia, by about half compared with phenytoin and diazepam, and 'magnesium packs' should be available on every labour ward.

There is no place for clomethiazole or phenytoin in the prophylaxis or treatment of eclampsia. Diazepam is still used to terminate eclamptic fits, although magnesium sulphate is also effective, and it would seem logical to treat with a single agent rather than two. Some authorities claim that eclamptic fits are self-limiting and that no treatment other than initiation of the magnesium sulphate regimen is needed.

Analgesia for labour

Regional analgesia is the method of choice. Good analgesia prevents hypertensive episodes associated with contraction pain. Well-conducted epidural or combined epidural–spinal analgesia may be beneficial to the compromised fetus by improving uteroplacental perfusion. A combination of low-dose local anaesthetic and opioid may be given by continuous epidural infusion or intermittent boluses, and this can be supplemented as necessary should instrumental or operative delivery be required. A pre-epidural platelet count should be performed (if trends suggest that platelet numbers are decreasing significantly, a platelet count should be repeated immediately before epidural injection is commenced). Current opinion suggest that a platelet count of at least $80 \times 10^9/l$ is advisable before instituting central neural blockade, although any stated lower safe limit is entirely arbitrary, and the relative risks and benefits of regional analgesia and anaesthesia must be considered for each patient. Several studies have confirmed that if the platelet count is at least $100 \times 10^9/l$ there is no need to perform further coagulation studies. In some centres thromboelastography or similar techniques have been used to indicate the status of coagulation and fibrinolytic, but these are not widely available. Bleeding time has been suggested as a clinical tool for assessment of coagulation, but a normal range for bleeding time has not been established in pregnancy and there is considerable inter- and intraobserver variability in its measurement, so this is rarely used.

If epidural analgesia is contraindicated, it is important to control the blood pressure by using appropriate agents (hydralazine, nifedipine, labetalol) and to provide alternative analgesia. Patient-controlled intravenous opioids offer the mother the psychological benefit of being in control of her analgesia and are more predictable than intramuscular opioids.

Transcutaneous electrical nerve stimulation, Entonox and non-pharmacological methods of analgesia are not suitable for the pre-eclamptic mother in established labour. They do not provide reliable analgesia and increase the likelihood of general anaesthesia being used if emergency Caesarean section is required.

Anaesthesia for Caesarean section

Regional anaesthesia
Regional is preferable to general anaesthesia, both for the mother and for the fetus. There is vasoconstriction of the uteroplacental vasculature in pre-eclampsia and

this may be relieved by epidural anaesthesia. There is some evidence that addition of adrenaline to epidural bupivacaine negates this benefit.

Although the use of spinal anaesthesia in pre-eclampsia has traditionally been advised against because of the risk of severe hypotension, there is evidence that cardiovascular stability is maintained if the patient has been pre-treated with vasodilators and intravenous fluids. Further, there is evidence that uterine artery velocity and neonatal condition are unaffected by spinal anaesthesia if systolic arterial pressure remains at least 80% of baseline.

Combined spinal–epidural anaesthesia confers the benefits of dense anaesthesia (especially of the sacral nerve roots) with the flexibility of epidural anaesthesia and postoperative analgesia. Use of a smaller dose of intrathecal local anaesthetic and subsequent use of the epidural to extend the level of anaesthesia facilitates haemodynamic stability in the non-pretreated case.

The pre-eclamptic mother may exhibit greater sensitivity to ephedrine than the usually normotensive mother.

General anaesthesia

General anaesthesia may be necessary if there is great urgency to deliver the mother or if regional anaesthesia is contraindicated by coagulopathy or major haemorrhage. Extreme prematurity does not contraindicate regional anaesthesia and nor does eclampsia.

The additional risks of general anaesthesia for Caesarean section are compounded in the pre-eclamptic woman by the potential for a significantly compromised airway and the hypertensive response to intubation and extubation. There may also be potential drug interactions, especially between magnesium sulphate and neuromuscular blocking agents.

Laryngeal oedema is uncommon but may be sufficient to obscure all normal anatomy at laryngoscopy. Each obstetric theatre should include microlaryngeal tracheal tubes on the intubation trolley for this eventuality.

Uncontrolled hypertension in response to tracheal intubation may provoke cardiac arrhythmias, myocardial ischaemia or cerebrovascular catastrophe. Numerous agents have been used to attenuate this response but the most commonly used agents in the UK are fentanyl 1–4 µg/kg or alfentanil 7–10 µg/kg and labetalol 10–20 mg. Other opioids, β-blockers and lidocaine may be used; magnesium sulphate 30 mg/kg also appears to be effective.

Monitoring and fluid therapy

All women with moderate or severe pre-eclampsia should have continuous electronic fetal monitoring. There is a trend towards more invasive maternal monitoring, and the use of central venous pressure catheters provides useful guidance for fluid administration during regional anaesthesia, although this is still less common in the UK than in the USA. Access via the antecubital fossa rather than via neck veins is recommended, especially in the undelivered mother. Direct arterial pressure monitoring is more accurate than non-invasive methods, because of the inaccuracy of most non-invasive monitors. The relative benefits of intra-arterial monitoring must be balanced against the familiarity of midwifery staff with its use. The need for pulmonary artery catheterisation is an indication for transfer to an intensive care unit, and it is important to remember that pulmonary artery catheters are associated with morbidity and mortality.

All pre-eclamptic women should have a urinary catheter inserted and an accurate hourly fluid balance recorded. Fluid management is controversial. The risks of volume overload and iatrogenic pulmonary oedema must be balanced against the risk of hypotension if vasodilators are given without concomitant volume replacement. In general, the emphasis has shifted away from liberal use of fluids in order to encourage urine output, towards careful restriction, since long-term problems from renal failure are rare whereas deaths from pulmonary oedema are well reported.

Postoperative management

The risks of deterioration in blood pressure control, of HELLP syndrome and of eclampsia do not end immediately with delivery of the placenta. Women with moderate and severe pre-eclampsia should be monitored in a high-dependency environment for at least 48 hours after delivery. Invasive monitoring and antihypertensive treatment should be continued during this time.

Key points

- Hypertensive disorders of pregnancy are divided into chronic hypertension, gestational hypertension and pre-eclampsia.
- Pre-eclampsia and eclampsia are a major cause of maternal death in the UK.
- Pre-eclampsia can only be effectively treated by delivery of the placenta, although symptomatic treatment attenuates maternal morbidity.
- Effective control of hypertension in pre-eclampsia reduces cardiovascular and cerebrovascular morbidity and mortality.
- HELLP syndrome is part of the spectrum of pre-eclampsia and may not be preceded by significant pre-eclampsia.
- Eclampsia may occur without premonitory symptoms or signs, and 40% of eclamptic fits occur after delivery.
- Although the classic presentation of the disease is hypertension, proteinuria and oedema occurring after 20 weeks of pregnancy, pre-eclampsia is a multisystem disease and may present atypically.

FURTHER READING

Duley L, Henderson-Smart DJ. *Drugs for treatment of very high blood pressure during pregnancy (Cochrane Review)*. In *The Cochrane Library*, Issue 2, 2004. Chichester, UK: John Wiley & Sons, Ltd.

Engelhardt T, MacLennan FM. Fluid management in pre-eclampsia. *Int J Obstet Anesth* 1999; **8**: 235–9.

James PR, Nelson-Piercy C. Management of hypertension before, during, and after pregnancy. *Heart* 2004; **90**: 1499–504.

Sibai BM. Diagnosis, prevention, and management of eclampsia. *Obstet Gynecol* 2005; **105**: 402–10.

Vidaeff AC, Carroll MA, Ramin SM. Acute hypertensive emergencies in pregnancy. *Crit Care Med* 2005; **33** (10 Suppl): S307–S312.

Walker JJ. Pre-eclampsia. *Lancet* 2000; **356**: 1260–5.

82   MAGNESIUM SULPHATE

Magnesium was first reported to be effective in preventing further fits in eclamptic women in 1925. The Collaborative Eclampsia Trial, reporting in 1995, confirmed that magnesium sulphate is significantly more effective than either diazepam or phenytoin in preventing recurrence of fits in eclamptic women.

The MAGPIE Trial, reporting in 2002, showed that magnesium sulphate was also effective in reducing (by about half) the incidence of eclampsia when given to pre-eclamptic women. However, since the incidence of eclampsia in the UK is low (~1–2% of pre-eclamptic cases), the number needed to treat in order to prevent a single woman having a convulsion is ~110 in the UK. This has led to controversy about whether magnesium should be routinely given to all pre-eclamptics in the UK, especially since there was no overall effect on maternal and neonatal morbidity and mortality in the trial. In populations in which the incidence is higher, e.g. the African subcontinent, or in those with severe pre-eclampsia, the number needed to treat is lower, so administration to such cases is less controversial. Even in these cases, however, it is impossible to predict which women will go on to suffer eclampsia.

These two studies have changed clinical practice around the world but especially in the UK, where magnesium used to be infrequently given in pre-eclampsia/eclampsia.

Magnesium sulphate is widely used in the USA as a tocolytic agent in preterm labour but randomised trials have failed to confirm its efficacy for this purpose.

Site of action

Magnesium is essential for potassium and calcium metabolism. It acts as a calcium antagonist, probably reducing systemic and cerebral vasospasm via action at calcium channels and intracellular sites. It is a cofactor in the sodium–potassium–ATPase system and is also an n-methyl d-aspartate (NMDA) receptor antagonist, and it is thought that its anticonvulsant action is mediated through these systems.

Production of endothelial prostacyclin is increased by magnesium and this may help to restore the thromboxane–prostacyclin imbalance that occurs in pre-eclampsia.

Magnesium sulphate relieves the cerebral vasospasm associated with pre-eclampsia and eclampsia; transcranial Doppler studies have demonstrated an increase in cerebral blood flow.

Side effects

Magnesium sulphate has widespread effects, not all of which are beneficial. Its use has been associated with increased obstetric haemorrhage (presumably due to generalised vasodilatation and uterine atony), increased length of labour and increased rate of Caesarean section. Prophylactic use of magnesium sulphate before induction of general anaesthesia for Caesarean section can prolong the effects of neuromuscular blocking agents; use of a peripheral nerve stimulator is mandatory.

Toxicity is possible during infusion, although this is unlikely in usual dosage unless there is concomitant renal impairment. Symptoms/signs of toxicity occur as blood levels increase (see Table 82.1). Magnesium toxicity is reversed by intravenous calcium gluconate (10 ml of 10% solution, given by slow intravenous injection), and calcium should always be available when magnesium therapy is given.

Dose

The Collaborative Eclampsia Trial and MAGPIE Trial used an intravenous loading dose of 4–5 g magnesium sulphate (given over 5–15 minutes) followed by either 5 g intramuscularly into each buttock and a further 5 g intramuscularly every 4 hours for 24 hours, or an intravenous infusion of 1–2 g/h after the intravenous loading dose.

There is controversy about whether an intravenous maintenance infusion of 1 g/h produces adequate plasma levels, with some studies suggesting that 3 g/h is required to guarantee therapeutic levels. The Collaborative

Table 82.1. Signs and symptoms of magnesium toxity at various blood levels

Symptoms	Magnesium level	
	mg/dl	mmol/l
Normal adult levels	1.7–2.4	0.7–1.1
Therapeutic range	4–8	2–4
Loss of patellar reflexes,warmth, flushing, somnolence	9.5–12	4.2–5
Respiratory depression	12–16	5–6.5
Muscle paralysis	15–17	6.2–7
Cardiac conduction defects	>18	>7.5
Cardiac arrest	30–35	12.5–14.5

Eclampsia group has stated that use of higher doses would increase the risk of toxicity without conferring proven benefit, and in the MAGPIE Trial side effects occurred in a quarter of cases.

Monitoring

If the regimen used in the two above trials is followed, clinical monitoring is considered to be adequate. Quarter-hourly measurement of respiratory rate, assessment of patellar tendon reflexes and hourly monitoring of urine output should be performed. Monitoring of plasma levels is advisable if larger doses of magnesium sulphate are used, if there is impaired renal function, if symptoms/signs of toxicity occur or a convulsion occurs despite therapy.

Key points

- Magnesium sulphate is the only drug proven to be effective in preventing recurrence of fits in eclampsia.
- Magnesium sulphate reduces the incidence of eclamptic fits before they occur but its use for this purpose is controversial because there is no reliable method of predicting eclampsia.
- Both intramuscular and intravenous regimens are effective, and clinical monitoring is adequate.
- Calcium gluconate should be available at the bedside of every woman receiving magnesium sulphate.

FURTHER READING

The Eclampsia Trial Collaborative Group. Which anticonvulsant for women with eclampsia? Evidence from the Collaborative Eclampsia Trial. *Lancet* 1995; **345**: 1455–63.

The Magpie Trial Collaborative Group. Do women with pre-eclampsia, and their babies, benefit from magnesium sulphate? The Magpie Trial: a randomised placebo-controlled trial. *Lancet* 2002; **359**: 1877–91.

Sibai BM. Magnesium sulphate prophylaxis in preeclampsia. Lessons learnt from recent trials. *Am J Obstet Gynecol* 2004; **190**: 1520–6.

Yentis SM. The Magpie has landed: preeclampsia, magnesium sulphate and rational decisions. *Int J Obstet Anesth* 2002; **11**: 238–41.

83   HYPEREMESIS GRAVIDARUM

Nausea and vomiting during early pregnancy occur in about 75% of women, although in most cases this is not severe and has diminished by the mid-second trimester. Rarely, though, severe vomiting continues throughout pregnancy and may require hospitalisation in about 3–10 per 1000 women. It is more common in first pregnancies and with younger maternal age, obesity and multiple pregnancy. The aetiology is unknown but hormonal (particularly oestrogen and human chorionic gonadotrophin), metabolic and psychological factors have been implicated.

Anaesthetists may be asked to advise on antiemetic therapy or to assist in establishing peripheral or central venous access for fluid replacement and/or nutrition. They may also be involved in providing analgesia or anaesthesia for delivery or, rarely, for termination of pregnancy if hyperemesis is very severe.

Problems/special considerations

There may be evidence of malnutrition and/or dehydration, with associated biochemical and metabolic derangement including renal and particularly hepatic impairment and mineral/vitamin deficiency, e.g. Wernicke's encephalopathy. The muscle bulk is virtually always reduced in severe cases and there may be fetal growth retardation. Because of the importance of psychological factors, these patients may need psychological/psychiatric support, which may be difficult in the maternity suite; in early pregnancy they are often managed on general gynaecological wards.

Management options

Diagnosis
The diagnosis of hyperemesis gravidarum should be one of exclusion since there are other conditions that should be considered in severe vomiting in pregnancy (Table 83.1).

Treatment
Initially, non-pharmacological methods of management are usually proffered, such as frequent small snacks (e.g. dry crackers), ginger root tea, hypnosis and use of acupressure bands or acupuncture to stimulate an area on the ventral surface of the wrist between the long flexor tendons. The evidence for the more esoteric treatments is somewhat mixed, although probably strongest for acupressure or acupuncture for its general (as opposed to obstetric) antiemetic effect. Psychological support is generally advocated.

Standard antiemetics such as metoclopramide, prochlorperazine and cyclizine are usually tried first; many obstetricians favour promazine, more for traditional than for scientific reasons. Ondansetron and related drugs are increasingly used with apparent success, although randomised trials are few and far between in this area, largely because of the rarity of severe cases and the potential involvement of so many factors in the aetiology of nausea and vomiting. It should be remembered that the effects of these drugs on the fetus are unclear and that few are licensed for use in pregnancy.

There has been much enthusiasm recently for steroids as treatment (e.g. prednisolone 50–75 mg/day, reduced to 20–40 mg/day within 1–2 weeks if possible)

Table 83.1. Causes of vomiting in pregnancy

Infective
  Gastroenteritis
  Urinary tract infection
  Hepatitis
Surgical
  Intra-abdominal pathology
Primary gastrointestinal
  Severe reflux oesophagitis
Neurological
  Increased intracranial pressure
  Migraine
Metabolic
  Diabetes
  Hypercalcaemia
  Uraemia
  Acute fatty liver of pregnancy
Drug-related
  Antibiotics
  Analgesics
  Alcohol
Psychogenic

but the results of proper trials are awaited. Individual reports of success with infusions of midazolam and propofol exist, but experience is limited.

In cases where dehydration is apparent, intravenous rehydration (and occasionally resuscitation) is required; use of glucose-containing solutions may provide a small amount of calorific intake but excessive administration may result in hyponatraemia. Vitamin and mineral supplementation is advisable, especially with thiamine. Enteral nasogastric nutrition has been used. In very severe cases, parenteral nutrition may be required; in fact, use of parenteral nutrition has been advocated as a treatment in its own right and there are several reports of its apparent success, occasionally more than once throughout the same pregnancy.

Oesophagitis may be severe and is treated by using standard methods.

Key points

- Nausea and vomiting occur in about 75% of pregnancies.
- Hospitalisation is required in about 3–10 per 1000 women.
- Urea and electrolyte disturbances and hepatic impairment may occur.
- There are few randomised controlled trials of therapy but many different non-pharmacological and pharmacological therapies have been used.

FURTHER READING

Jewell D, Young G. Interventions for nausea and vomiting in early pregnancy. *Cochrane Database Syst Rev* 2003; (4): CD000145.

Kuscu NK, Koyuncu F. Hyperemesis gravidarum: current concepts and management. *Postgrad Med J* 2002; **78**: 76–9.

Philip B. Hyperemesis gravidarum: literature review. *WMJ* 2003; **102**: 46–51.

Yost NP, McIntire DD, Wians FH Jr, *et al.* A randomized, placebo-controlled trial of corticosteroids for hyperemesis due to pregnancy. *Obstet Gynecol* 2003; **102**: 1250–4.

84   MATERNAL MORTALITY

There has been continuous audit of maternal deaths in England and Wales since 1952, the results of which have been published every 3 years as the Report on Confidential Enquiries into Maternal Deaths (CEMD, more recently, as the report 'Why Mothers Die' published by the Confidential Enquiry into Maternal and Child Health; CEMACH (part of the National Patient Safety Agency)). Since 1984 the published reports have included audit of maternal deaths from the whole of the UK.

Maternal mortality in 2000–2 was 13.1 per 100 000 maternities, a rate that has changed very little since 1982 but compares with a rate of approximately 70 per 100 000 maternities in the early 1950s.

The leading direct causes of maternal death in the UK in 2000–2 were:

- Cardiac disease (44 cases)
- Thromboembolic disease (30 cases)
- Haemorrhage (17 cases)
- Psychiatric disease (16 cases)
- Deaths in early pregnancy (15 cases).

Although maternal death is, fortunately, an uncommon tragedy in the UK compared with many other countries, when under-reporting is taken into account it is estimated that there is a maternal death nearly every other day somewhere in the UK.

Definitions and data collection

A maternal death is any death occurring during or within 42 days of the pregnancy ending. The enquiry into any maternal death is initiated by local CEMACH reporters in each unit and organised by CEMACH regional offices. Each death is assessed by regional obstetric anaesthetic, midwifery and pathology assessors where appropriate, before being reviewed by central assessors.

Maternal deaths are classified as:

- Direct (resulting from obstetric complications of pregnancy) – 27% of reported cases in 2000–2

- Indirect (deaths resulting from previous existing disease or disease that developed during pregnancy and that was not due to direct obstetric causes but was aggravated by the physiological effects of pregnancy) – 40% of reported maternal deaths in 2000–2
- Late (occurring after 42 days and within one year of the pregnancy ending) – 24% of deaths in 2000–2
- Coincidental (from unrelated causes, such as road traffic accident) – 9% of deaths in 2000–2.

Deaths may be associated with substandard care. This term is used not only to denote failure of clinical care, but may also indicate failure of the woman to take responsibility for her own health (such as refusal of blood transfusion or refusal to be admitted) and inadequate resources for staffing, intensive care and back-up services. The CEMACH report makes recommendations for improved care.

Anaesthetic deaths

Although anaesthesia is no longer one of the three leading causes of maternal death, the number of deaths associated with anaesthesia rose in 2000–2 (six deaths and one late death) compared with the previous triennium, when there were only three deaths. The direct deaths due to anaesthesia in this triennium were all associated with general anaesthesia, two of the deaths and the late death being as a result of intubation. In addition, there were 20 deaths that were related to poor perioperative management.

The 2000–2 CEMACH report emphasised the need to identify and refer high-risk patients, particularly obese patients, to the anaesthetist at an early stage in order that an appropriate management plan is established. In addition, the report recommended that obstetric anaesthetic training should ensure competent airway management, including complications e.g. oesophageal intubation. Lack of intensive care facilities was also identified as a cause of substandard care.

The quality of anaesthetic record keeping was poor in some cases.

Key points

- Obstetric anaesthesia is high-risk anaesthesia.
- The severity of coexisting medical disease is easily underestimated.
- Adequate monitoring equipment and trained anaesthetic assistance are required for obstetric anaesthesia.
- Intensive care facilities may be required.
- The anaesthetic record is a legal document and is essential for adequate evaluation of morbidity and mortality.

FURTHER READING

Clyburn PA. Early thoughts on 'Why Mothers Die 2000–2002'. *Anaesthesia* 2004; **59**: 1157–9.

Cooper GM, McClure JH. Maternal deaths from anaesthesia. An extract from Why Mothers Die 2000–2002, the Confidential Enquiries into Maternal Deaths in the United Kingdom: Chapter 9: Anaesthesia. *Br J Anaesth* 2005; **94**: 417–23.

McClure J, Cooper G. Fifty years of confidential enquiries into maternal deaths in the United Kingdom: should anaesthesia celebrate or not? *Int J Obstet Anesth* 2005; **14**: 87–9.

Report on Confidential Enquiries into Maternal Deaths in the United Kingdom 2000–02. London: The Stationery Office, 2004.

VI   Problems not confined to obstetrics

85   ALLERGIC REACTIONS

Patients may be mildly allergic to many substances and this may become better or worse during pregnancy. Severe reactions, however, are rare on the labour ward. Most severe reactions are either anaphylactic or anaphylactoid. Anaphylactic reactions involve release of histamine and other inflammatory mediators from mast cells via cross-linkage of IgE molecules on the cell surface by the antigen molecule; this process requires prior exposure to the antigen. Anaphylactoid reactions involve direct release of mediators from mast cells via interaction of molecules (e.g. drugs) with the cell surface in a different way; this does not require prior exposure. The difference is largely academic since the clinical presentation is identical. Less commonly, direct complement activation may be involved.

Most severe reactions on the labour ward are caused by drugs, especially anti-biotics, intravenous anaesthetic drugs (particularly suxamethonium) and oxytocin. Some well-recognised cross-reactions exist, e.g. up to 10% of individuals with true penicillin allergy are also allergic to cephalosporins. Allergy to amide local anaesthetic drugs is rare but has been reported, as has allergy to preservatives used in local anaesthetic and other drug preparations. Non-steroidal anti-inflammatory drugs and paracetamol often cause rashes but these are usually mild following brief oral/rectal courses, although severe reactions have been reported following intravenous administration. Reactions may also follow admin-istration of gelatine intravenous fluids and blood. Latex allergy has become an increasing problem amongst both medical staff and patients, driven by an increase in the wearing of gloves because of concern about transmission of blood-borne infection and the ubiquitous use of latex in home and work environments. Latex allergy is more common in subjects with multiple exposures to latex such as med-ical or nursing staff, cleaners, those with neurological disease requiring repeated bladder catheterisation, e.g. spina bifida, and those with allergy to certain food-stuffs, including avocados, bananas, kiwi fruit and chestnuts. Finally, other condi-tions not primarily allergic may also present in a similar way, e.g. amniotic fluid embolism.

Analgesia, Anaesthesia and Pregnancy: A Practical Guide Second Edition, ed. Steve Yentis, Anne May and Surbhi Malhotra. Published by Cambridge University Press. © Cambridge University Press 2007.

Patients may have a history of previous allergic reactions to drugs or other substances, although many patients who give only a vague history are not truly allergic.

Problems/special considerations

Features range from mild skin rashes to severe urticaria, hypotension, bronchospasm, abdominal pain, diarrhoea, a 'feeling of impending doom' and cardiovascular collapse. Initial hypotension is largely related to profound vasodilation, which is followed by leakage of intravascular fluid into the interstitium. Cardiac depression (thought to be caused by circulating inflammatory mediators) may also contribute to hypotension. The cardiovascular effects are exacerbated by aortocaval compression.

Features usually occur within a few seconds or minutes of exposure to the allergen. In Caesarean section in latex allergic subjects, anaphylaxis typically occurs 10–15 minutes after induction of anaesthesia and once surgery has started, since the most provocative stimulus is exposure via mucous membranes.

Since clinical features may develop at a time of great physiological change, e.g. during Caesarean section or during/after delivery, it may be difficult to assess the situation and determine what has happened. Administration of many different drugs together or within a short time is common and this may hinder the diagnosis (and is suspected of increasing the risk of a reaction).

Management options

Immediate management of severe reactions consists of intravenous adrenaline 100 µg boluses and fluids, with management of the airway and administration of oxygen. Aortocaval compression must be avoided at all times. Any potential for adrenaline to cause uteroplacental vasoconstriction and uterine hypotony is outweighed by the restoration of cardiac output. Intravenous chlorphenamine 10 mg and hydrocortisone 200 mg may be given to reduce the effects of subsequent inflammatory mediator release. For less severe reactions (e.g. urticaria only), chlorphenamine alone may suffice.

In an acute reaction, blood should be taken for tryptase levels at 1 and 6–24 hours. The enzyme is normally present in mast cells and in miniscule amounts in the plasma; an increase in plasma concentration therefore represents mast cell degranulation (but does not distinguish between anaphylactic and anaphylactoid reactions). Immunoglobulin and complement levels may be suggestive, but not diagnostic, of an allergic response. If a severe reaction is suspected, the patient should be referred for testing at least 4–6 weeks later; normally this will involve skin tests (prick testing ±intradermal testing). Further tests may be performed on plasma (e.g. radioallergoabsorbent test (RAST) looking for concentrations of specific antibody, e.g. to latex) or occasionally basophils or other cellular components, if skin testing is not diagnostic. The patient should be advised to obtain a 'Medi-alert' bracelet and given written details of all the drugs tested and the results, in case she should require a subsequent anaesthetic. A copy of the letter should also be sent to her general practitioner.

It is important that mothers with a previous history of severe allergic reactions are identified antenatally. Wherever possible, the previous anaesthetic record should be obtained and a plan for her care documented. Management of the known allergic case includes a general state of readiness and awareness as well as the obvious avoidance of any known allergens. Latex allergic patients may be identified from the history in most cases by asking about food allergies and skin reactions after exposure, e.g. rubber gloves, condoms, etc. If patients have had a previous severe reaction where the allergen is unknown, pretreatment with H_1- and H_2-antagonists $\pm$ steroids should be considered, although whether this should be routinely done if the allergen is known and can be avoided is controversial. Routine screening of all women by using skin or blood testing is generally not indicated, since precautions should be taken on the basis of a strong history even if testing produces negative results.

Key points

- In severe allergic reactions, immediate management is with oxygen, adrenaline and intravenous fluids.
- Hydrocortisone and chlorphenamine are second-line drugs.
- Blood should be taken for mast cell tryptase levels as early as possible.
- Subsequent testing should include skin testing.
- Latex allergy is an increasingly common problem.

FURTHER READING

Dakin MJ, Yentis SM. Latex allergy: a strategy for management. *Anaesthesia* 1998; **53**: 774–81.

Fisher MM, Bowey CJ. Intradermal compared with prick testing in the diagnosis of anaesthetic allergy. *Br J Anaesth* 1997; **79**: 59–63.

Mertes PM, Laxenaire MC. Allergic reactions occurring during anaesthesia. *Eur J Anaesthesiol* 2002; **19**: 240–62.

86 CARDIOVASCULAR DISEASE

Cardiac disease is the second most common cause of maternal death in the UK after psychiatric causes. The spectrum of pre-existing cardiac disease affecting pregnant women has changed in the UK as rheumatic heart disease has become less common (though it is still a major problem in other parts of the world) and congenital heart disease more common, partly related to the improved survival of girls with congenital heart disease who undergo surgery during infancy and childhood.

The most common acquired heart disease in the UK is ischaemic heart disease. Possible epidemiological factors include an increased prevalence of risk factors, e.g. smoking amongst younger women, increased age and obesity.

Problems/special considerations

Although different sorts of cardiac disease require different management, there are general principles that are applicable to this heterogeneous group. Many of these have been highlighted in recent Reports on Confidential Enquiries into Maternal Deaths/Maternal and Child Health, which have found the following:

- There is a general failure fully to understand the impact of the normal physiological changes of pregnancy on pre-existing cardiovascular pathology (see Chapter 11, Physiology of pregnancy; p. 27).
- Management of women with cardiac disease is often undertaken by inappropriately experienced medical staff. Consultants should be involved in management from early pregnancy onwards and should be prepared to seek advice from (and if necessary to refer patients onwards to) specialist cardiological units.
- There may be failure to carry out essential investigations such as chest radiography, whereas the radiation risks to the fetus are minimal but the information gained from the investigation may be life saving.
- There may be failure to communicate with other specialties involved in a woman's care and failure to organise clear written plans for management of labour and delivery.
- The severity of the mother's condition may be underestimated, either because of the above or because symptoms are mild or absent, or because they are mistaken for those of pregnancy.

Management options

The pregnant woman with cardiac disease, whether congenital or acquired, should be seen as early as possible in her pregnancy. Ideally she should be seen for preconceptual counselling when her risks (Table 86.1) and those of her baby can be fully discussed.

A full history and examination should be performed during the first trimester of pregnancy, and baseline cardiological investigations should be arranged. These may include electrocardiography, chest X-ray, echocardiography and possibly cardiac catheterisation. Severity of cardiac disease is frequently assessed by using the New York Heart Association (NYHA) classification, which although originally described for heart failure is a useful overall measure of severity:

- NYHA I: no limitation of physical activity and no objective evidence of cardiovascular disease
- NHYA II: slight limitation of normal physical activity and objective evidence of minimal disease

Table 86.1. Risk of death or severe morbidity resulting from certain cardiac lesions in pregnancy

Low risk (mortality 0.1–1.0%)	• Most repaired lesions • Uncomplicated left-to-right shunts • Mitral valve prolapse; bicuspid aortic valve; aortic regurgitation; mitral regurgitation; pulmonary stenosis; pulmonary regurgitation
Intermediate risk (mortality 1–5%)	• Metal valves • Single ventricles • Systemic right ventricle; switch procedure • Unrepaired cyanotic lesions • Mitral stenosis; aortic stensosis; severe pulmonary stenosis
High risk (mortality 5–30%)	• NYHA III or IV • Severe systemic ventricular dysfunction • Severe aortic stenosis • Marfan's syndrome with aortic valve lesion or aortic dilatation • Pulmonary hypertension (N.B. mortality 30–50%)

- NYHA III: marked limitation of physical activity and objective evidence of moderately severe disease
- NYHA IV: severe limitation of activity including symptoms at rest and objective evidence of severe disease.

Women with cardiovascular disease graded NYHA I and II usually tolerate the physiological changes of pregnancy well, though it should be remembered that certain conditions (e.g. mitral and aortic stenosis, pulmonary hypertension and complex lesions) may be dangerous even in the absence of symptoms.

Consideration should be given to the appropriate place for both subsequent antenatal management and delivery. Referral to a local teaching hospital with facilities for cardiac surgery may be indicated, and in some cases it may be in the woman's best interests to be referred to a supraregional unit.

Routine antenatal care is not adequate for women with cardiac disease. Antenatal appointments need to be more frequent; there must be clear communication with the general practitioner and the community midwife and also with the woman herself, who should receive instructions about symptoms that demand immediate medical attention. Serial investigations and careful documentation of symptoms should alert medical staff to any deterioration in cardiac health, and it may be useful to admit women with cardiac disease for 24–48 hours towards the end of the second trimester of pregnancy in order to repeat investigations and arrange multidisciplinary review. Women require careful monitoring for development of pre-eclampsia, since it may be poorly tolerated in the presence of cardiac disease.

Elective admission to hospital in the third or even second trimester may be useful to ensure the mother can rest, with due attention to antithrombotic prophylaxis and regular assessments. Continuous oxygen therapy may also be given if required.

As a general rule, operative delivery should only be carried out if indicated for obstetric reasons or deteriorating maternal condition, and not just because the mother has cardiac disease. Regional analgesia and anaesthesia can be safely provided for the majority of women with cardiac disease, even in those with fixed cardiac output (although this is more controversial), although this may be precluded by anticoagulation in certain cases. Analgesia and anaesthesia should only be carried out in units familiar with the management of such high-risk patients. The risk of endocarditis should be remembered and antibiotics given as appropriate.

The puerperium is a time of high risk for many women with cardiac disease, and vigilance should be maintained. The mother with cardiac disease should be nursed on the delivery suite or high-dependency unit until all medical staff involved in her care agree that she can be safely returned to the general postnatal ward. Haemodynamic parameters have usually returned to normal within 3–5 days but may take longer in severe cases, and rarely may never return to pre-pregnancy values.

Key points

- Women with cardiovascular disease should be identified and assessed early in pregnancy, and referred to specialist units when necessary.
- Good communication between specialties is mandatory.
- Clear management plans should be written.
- Vigilance should be maintained into the puerperium.

FURTHER READING

Dob DP, Yentis SM. UK Registry of High-risk Obstetric Anaesthesia: report on cardiorespiratory disease. *Int J Obstet Anesth* 2001; **10**: 267–72.

European Society of Cardiology Task Force. Expert consensus document on management of cardiovascular diseases during pregnancy. *Eur Heart J* 2003; **24**: 761–81.

Siu SC, Sermer M, Colman JM, *et al.* Prospective multicenter study of pregnancy outcomes in women with heart disease. *Circulation* 2001; **104**: 515–21.

Thorne SA. Pregnancy in heart disease. *Heart* 2004; **90**: 450–6.

87 ARRHYTHMIAS

During pregnancy there is an increased incidence of both benign arrhythmias and arrhythmias associated with cardiac disease. If the abnormal rhythm causes haemodynamic instability, there is potential for fetal compromise and treatment should be instituted.

Problems/special considerations

- Sinus tachycardia is normal during pregnancy. Superimposed supraventricular ectopic beats occur commonly, particularly in association with caffeine and alcohol consumption, and may cause palpitations and anxiety. Underlying organic disease is extremely unlikely in these women, and they should be reassured and given advice about avoiding likely precipitators of the arrhythmia.
- Paroxysmal supraventricular tachycardia is more common in pregnancy and rarely indicates underlying organic disease. Palpitations, dizziness and syncope may occur, and although attacks may terminate spontaneously with rest, persistent tachycardia should be treated acutely with either suitable antiarrhythmic agents (adenosine or verapamil) or with DC cardioversion. In persistent cases, His bundle studies and subsequent ablation of abnormal conduction pathways may be indicated, although it is usual to wait until after delivery for such management.
- Atrial fibrillation is usually associated with mitral valve disease and less commonly with cardiomyopathy. The major risks from atrial fibrillation in pregnancy are thromboembolic disease and pulmonary oedema. Prophylactic anticoagulants should be used, and it may be necessary to consider full anticoagulation in some situations, such as during and immediately following DC cardioversion. Pregnancy does not alter medical management of atrial fibrillation. It is particularly important to confirm that therapeutic plasma levels of antiarrhythmic agents are achieved throughout the pregnancy.
- Ventricular ectopic beats are relatively common during pregnancy and may be either asymptomatic or noticed by the patient as palpitations. No treatment is necessary other than reassurance that there is no sinister underlying cause.
- Ventricular tachycardia or fibrillation may occur in association with severe organic cardiac disease, such as myocardial infarction. In such situations, pregnancy is of secondary concern, since the arrhythmia is usually life threatening, and the primary goal of treatment is termination of the arrhythmia by whatever means is effective.
- Conduction disorders require referral for cardiological opinion, since some cardiologists recommend aggressive management (permanent pacing) of even first-degree heart block during pregnancy, although this is disputed.

Management options

In general, pregnant women with cardiac arrhythmias should be assessed and treated in the same way as those who are not pregnant. During an acute episode, it is especially important to avoid aortocaval compression since this will exacerbate any circulatory embarrassment.

All commonly used antiarrhythmics cross the placenta (and indeed may be administered to the mother to treat a fetal arrhythmia). There are published case reports of the use of most antiarrhythmic drugs during pregnancy but few well-designed controlled studies. Previous anxieties that β-blocking drugs caused intra-uterine growth retardation appear to have been largely discounted, but maternal β-blockade may cause fetal bradycardia and make interpretation of the fetal heart rate trace difficult. Consensus opinion recommends using the smallest dose of the most well-established drug that will achieve a therapeutic effect.

If DC cardioversion is performed during pregnancy, it is important to safeguard the airway and to remember the risks of aortocaval compression. In practice, this means using rapid sequence induction of general anaesthesia and tracheal intubation, together with uterine displacement off the great vessels for women in the second half of pregnancy. Prophylactic anticoagulation should be considered during and after DC cardioversion because of the increased risk of thromboembolic disease during pregnancy.

Agents that are associated with increased heart rate (e.g. oxytocin, ephedrine) should be avoided, or used very cautiously if needed, in women at risk of tachyarrhythmias.

Key points

- No antiarrhythmic drug is considered completely safe for use in pregnancy, but any cardiac arrhythmia compromising haemodynamic stability requires urgent treatment.
- Use of older and well-established antiarrhythmics is generally recommended for first-line management, but newer drugs should not be withheld if other means are unsuccessful.
- Relief of aortocaval compression is essential.

FURTHER READING

Ferrero S, Colombo BM, Ragni N. Maternal arrhythmias during pregnancy. *Arch Gynecol Obstet* 2004; **269**: 244–53.

Gowda RM, Khan IA, Mehta NJ, Vasavada BC, Sacchi TJ. Cardiac arrhythmias in pregnancy: clinical and therapeutic considerations. *Int J Cardiol* 2003; **88**: 129–33.

Lewis N, Dob DP, Yentis SM. UK Registry of High-risk Obstetric Anaesthesia: arrhythmias, cardiomyopathy, aortic stenosis, transposition of the great arteries and Marfan's syndrome. *Int J Obstet Anesth* 2003; **12**: 28–34.

88 PULMONARY OEDEMA

The pregnant mother may be at increased risk of developing pulmonary oedema because her cardiac output and blood volume are increased considerably compared with pre-pregnancy values. This increase is greater in the mother with multiple pregnancy. Colloid osmotic pressure is also reduced in pregnancy.

Problems/special considerations

- Acute pulmonary oedema in the pregnant woman may mimic an acute asthmatic attack. Attempts to treat the latter will tend to exacerbate the former.
- There are multiple aetiologies of pulmonary oedema in pregnancy, but a careful history will usually provide a diagnosis of the underlying cause. Pulmonary oedema may occur:
  - (i) As a complication of coexisting cardiac disease
  - (ii) Secondary to complications of pregnancy, e.g. pre-eclampsia, major obstetric haemorrhage, intrauterine fetal death, amniotic fluid embolism, peripartum cardiomyopathy
  - (iii) Secondary to aspiration of gastric contents
  - (iv) Secondary to major sepsis
  - (v) Following therapeutic or recreational drug administration, e.g. β-adrenergic agonists, glucocorticoids, oxytocics, cocaine
  - (vi) Following excessive administration of intravenous fluid.
- Hypoxaemia caused by oedema is exacerbated by the increased oxygen demand of pregnancy and the reduced functional residual capacity and oxygen reserve.

Management options

Women who are known to be at increased risk of developing cardiac failure should receive antenatal and intrapartum care in an obstetric unit with high-dependency and intensive care facilities on site. Pulse oximetry is particularly useful since a fall in saturation may be an early sign of pulmonary oedema.

Women receiving β-adrenergic agonists must have fluid balance and electrolytes monitored rigorously, and supplementary oxygen therapy should be considered. Invasive monitoring of central venous pressure should be considered if regional analgesia or anaesthesia is used in a woman who has been receiving β-agonists.

Appropriate investigations should be performed, including chest radiography, since this carries negligible risk to the fetus.

In the absence of any obvious cause for cardiac failure, it is important to consider the use of illicit drugs.

Invasive cardiovascular monitoring will guide diagnosis and treatment, and the mother should be transferred to a high-dependency or intensive care unit at the earliest possible opportunity.

Oxygen therapy is invariably beneficial. Delivery of the fetus reduces oxygen demand and relieves the physical effect of the gravid uterus on the diaphragm and lungs. Dexamethasone, given to improve neonatal respiratory function, may worsen fluid retention.

Key points

- Pulmonary oedema is uncommon in pregnancy but may be fatal.
- Chest radiography should not be withheld.
- Delivery of the fetus may be indicated.
- The mother should be managed in a high-dependency or intensive care unit.

89 CARDIOMYOPATHY

Pregnant women may have a pre-existing cardiomyopathy or may develop cardiomyopathy of pregnancy (peripartum cardiomyopathy – PPCM).

- The causes of pre-existing cardiomyopathy are diverse and include infection, systemic disease such as sarcoidosis, infiltrative disease such as amyloid, toxins such as alcohol and cocaine, ischaemic heart disease and congenital cardiomyopathies. Of this group, the most commonly encountered in the antenatal clinic are the congenital hypertrophic obstructive cardiomyopathies (HOCMs).
- The aetiology of PPCM is unknown but viral or autoimmune myocarditis, or an exaggerated response to the haemodynamic stresses of pregnancy, has been suggested. The classic criteria for diagnosis of PPCM are:
  (i) Development of cardiac failure in the last month of pregnancy or within 5 months of delivery
  (ii) Absence of other aetiology for cardiac failure
  (iii) Absence of cardiac disease prior to the last month of pregnancy.

  It has been suggested that the definition should be extended to include cardiac failure developing within the third trimester of pregnancy for which no other cause can be found, and echocardiographical evidence of left ventricular dysfunction. The incidence of PPCM is estimated to be 1 in 3000 pregnancies.

Functionally, patients with HOCM have an obstructive cardiomyopathy, whilst those with PPCM have a dilated cardiomyopathy.

Problems/special considerations

- Patients with obstructive cardiomyopathy have a hypertrophied left ventricle and interventricular septum. Mitral regurgitation is often present. Any factors that increase myocardial contractility (β-agonists, circulating catecholamines) or decrease preload or afterload (vasodilatation, hypovolaemia) will cause an increase in left ventricular outflow obstruction. Tachycardias reduce the time for diastolic filling, and atrial arrhythmias are particularly poorly tolerated.

The obstructive component of HOCM varies considerably. Women with minimal obstruction usually tolerate pregnancy well, although the more severe the degree of left ventricular hypertrophy the greater the risk of myocardial ischaemia, particularly in response to the stress of pregnancy and delivery.

- Patients with dilated cardiomyopathy have reduced myocardial contractility. The left ventricle is hypokinetic, ejection fraction is less than 0.4 and there is usually mitral and/or tricuspid regurgitation. Pressures in the right side of the heart are raised, and cardiac or pulmonary artery catheterisation usually confirms pulmonary hypertension. Any factors that depress myocardial contractility or increase afterload will further compromise cardiovascular stability.

Women with PPCM present with the classic signs of left ventricular or congestive cardiac failure. There is a high associated risk of embolic phenomena.

Management options

Obstructive cardiomyopathy

Women with HOCM have usually been diagnosed before pregnancy, and baseline cardiological investigations should be available. If β-blocking drugs are being used, these should be continued during pregnancy.

Serial cardiological investigations (electrocardiography (ECG), echocardiography) should be performed during pregnancy. Tachycardias should be treated with suitable β-blockers. Esmolol has been recommended for use in this situation. Cardioversion may be required to terminate supraventricular tachycardia; amiodarone is recommended for ventricular tachycardias. Nitrates should not be used to treat angina because the consequent vasodilatation and afterload reduction further aggravates left ventricular outflow obstruction.

There is no indication to deliver women by Caesarean section unless there are obstetric reasons to do so or unless the maternal condition deteriorates. Continuous ECG and arterial blood pressure monitoring should be used throughout labour and delivery and continued into the early postnatal period.

Traditionally, regional analgesia has been considered contraindicated because of the risk of acute reduction in afterload. However, provision of high quality analgesia is obviously beneficial, particularly for preventing pain-induced tachycardia. Intrathecal opioid analgesia is not accompanied by sympathetic blockade but is of limited efficacy in advanced labour. Combined spinal–epidural analgesia, using low-dose (<0.1% bupivacaine) local anaesthetic in the epidural space, offers good analgesia with minimum haemodynamic disturbance.

Maintenance of adequate hydration – intravenously if necessary – is important. Phenylephrine is preferable to ephedrine for treatment of hypotension because the α effects of phenylephrine have less effect on myocardial contractility and heart rate than the mixed α and β effects of ephedrine.

Dilated cardiomyopathy/PPCM

The majority of cases of PPCM present in the peripartum or immediate postpartum period. Treatment includes use of positive inotropes such as digoxin (and parenteral inotropes such as dopamine and dobutamine in the acute situation), oxygen and diuretics, vasodilators to reduce afterload (but not angiotensin-converting enzyme inhibitors because of the risk of fetal renal agenesis), bed rest and anticoagulants (because of the risk of thromboembolic disease). Heart or heart–lung transplantation may be needed in severe cases that fail to respond to maximal medical therapy.

If PPCM presents antenatally, delivery is indicated as soon as the woman's condition has been optimised. Caesarean section may be necessary unless conditions are favourable for induction of labour.

Regional analgesia and anaesthesia are theoretically beneficial for the patient with dilated cardiomyopathy, since the cardiodepressant effects of most general anaesthetic drugs are avoided, and afterload is beneficially reduced. However, there is little published experience of this. Hypotension should be treated with drugs with predominantly β activity, which stimulate myocardial contractility (ephedrine) rather than pure α-agonists (phenylephrine) which increase systemic vascular resistance.

PPCM has a high recurrence rate, and some authorities consider further pregnancies to be contraindicated following PPCM. Others suggest that another pregnancy can be considered if there is no residual cardiomegaly by 6 months postpartum. Case series suggest that if left ventricular function is still impaired one year after delivery there is a ~20% risk of death in the next pregnancy.

Key points

- Hypertrophic obstructive cardiomyopathy is usually inherited, and presents with variable left ventricular outflow obstruction.
- Treatment is directed at reduction of myocardial contractility and increasing preload and afterload.
- Tachyarrhythmias and myocardial ischaemia are particular hazards.
- Peripartum cardiomyopathy usually presents in the peripartum or early postpartum period.
- Treatment is symptomatic and is directed at maintaining myocardial contractility and reducing afterload.

FURTHER READING

Lewis N, Dob DP, Yentis SM. UK Registry of High-risk Obstetric Anaesthesia: arrhythmias, cardiomyopathy, aortic stenosis, transposition of the great arteries and Marfan's syndrome. *Int J Obstet Anesth* 2003; **12**: 28–34.

Murali S, Baldisseri MR. Peripartum cardiomyopathy. *Crit Care Med* 2005; **33**(10 Suppl): S340–S346.

Sliwa K, Fett J, Elkayam U. Peripartum cardiomyopathy. *Lancet* 2006; **368**: 687–93.

Whitehead SJ, Berg CJ, Chang J. Pregnancy-related mortality due to cardiomyopathy: United States, 1991–1997. *Obstet Gynecol* 2003; **102**: 1326–31.

90   COARCTATION OF THE AORTA

Coarctation of the aorta occurs in approximately 5% of patients with congenital heart disease and may occur as an isolated lesion or in association with other cardiovascular defects. Preductal coarctation is associated with patent ductus arteriosus, ventricular septal defect, bicuspid aortic valve and (in about 10% of cases) transposition of the great vessels. The majority of cases of preductal coarctation present with congestive cardiac failure in the neonatal period and are diagnosed and corrected surgically in infancy.

Postductal coarctation of the aorta may not be diagnosed until adolescence or adult life. There are associated berry aneurysms of the circle of Willis in approximately 10% of cases, and bicuspid aortic valve in 50% of patients.

Problems/special considerations

- Undiagnosed coarctation may present for the first time in pregnancy. There is invariably hypertension and this may be accompanied by congestive cardiac failure, caused by inability to compensate for the increased blood volume and cardiac output which occurs during pregnancy. The generalised peripheral vasodilatation and consequent reduction in systemic vascular resistance that occur in pregnancy may also precipitate cardiac failure.
- Pregnancy in women with an uncorrected aortic coarctation is associated with a maternal mortality of 3–9%, and a fetal mortality of up to 20%. Pregnancy or labour may be complicated by aortic dissection or rupture. Corrected coarctation is considered a low-risk lesion in pregnancy unless there are associated abnormalities such as those described above, or aortic dilatation.
- There is a risk of aortic rupture or dissection if blood pressure increases acutely, e.g. because of severe pain or following use of certain drugs e.g. ergometrine, vasopressors. Increased shearing forces associated with swings in blood pressure may also be dangerous.
- Hypertension is limited to the arms, and blood pressure may be reduced in the legs; palpation of the peripheral pulses frequently reveals absent foot pulses and radiofemoral delay. An aortic systolic murmur is heard on auscultation of the chest, and there may also be audible bruits over the intercostal and internal mammary vessels, which carry collateral flow to the lower limbs. A chest X-ray may show rib notching caused by the collateral vessels, and left ventricular hypertrophy.

Management options

Women with corrected coarctation should be assessed early in pregnancy, and any associated abnormalities noted.

There is no proven benefit of operative delivery for women with uncorrected coarctation, although anxiety about undiagnosed aneurysms of the circle of Willis may lead to recommendations for epidural analgesia and elective instrumental delivery. There is also no evidence that allowing the woman to labour increases her risks of aortic dissection or rupture. Minimising haemodynamic disturbance is the main aim of management of delivery. Cardiac output is relatively fixed; tachycardia secondary to uncontrolled pain may precipitate cardiac failure, but bradycardia and acute reduction in systemic vascular resistance are also hazardous. Hypovolaemia leads to compromised left ventricular filling.

Invasive systemic arterial pressure monitoring allows close attention to changes in blood pressure and facilitates analgesic and anaesthetic management. Central venous pressure monitoring may also be useful. Epidural or combined epidural–spinal techniques can provide safe and effective pain relief in labour. Although the main risk is from hypertension, it is also important to avoid hypotension.

For Caesarean section, neither regional nor general anaesthesia has obvious advantages over the other, although many practitioners would consider it advisable to avoid single-shot spinal anaesthesia because of the risk of uncontrolled hypotension. Combined spinal–epidural, continuous spinal or epidural techniques allow gradual extension of the anaesthetic level cephalad and minimise the risks of rapid onset of profound hypotension. If general anaesthesia is used, steps should be taken to prevent the hypertensive response to tracheal intubation.

Postoperative management in a high-dependency environment is essential; invasive monitoring should be continued postoperatively and adequate analgesia should be ensured by using either the epidural route or patient-controlled intravenous analgesia.

Key points

- Women with corrected coarctation do not pose any particular problem in pregnancy, although there may be other associated cardiovascular abnormalities.
- Uncorrected coarctation may be associated with aortic dissection or rupture.
- Both general and regional anaesthesia are acceptable options but both may be hazardous.
- Invasive arterial $\pm$ central venous pressure monitoring is recommended.

FURTHER READING

European Society of Cardiology Task Force. Expert consensus document on management of cardiovascular diseases during pregnancy. *Eur Heart J* 2003; **24**: 761–81.

Thorne SA. Pregnancy in heart disease. *Heart* 2004; **90**: 450–6.

Walker E, Malins AF. Anaesthetic management of aortic coarctation in pregnancy. *Int J Obstet Anesth* 2004; **13**: 266–70.

91   PROSTHETIC HEART VALVES

Most women with a prosthetic heart valve presenting to a UK antenatal clinic will have had the valve inserted because of congenital heart disease, although immigrants from the Indian subcontinent and some parts of eastern Europe still have a high incidence of acquired valve disease.

Women with corrected congenital heart disease and a prosthetic heart valve have increased morbidity in pregnancy, especially if they are anticoagulated.

Problems/special considerations

The relative risk of pregnancy in women with prosthetic heart valves is dependent not only on the underlying cardiac abnormality and residual impairment of cardiac function but also on the type of valve replacement used. Prosthetic heart valves may be mechanical, porcine or human allograft (homograft). Women with valves inserted before the end of the 1970s are almost certain to have mechanical valves. Homograft valves have only been widely available since the end of the 1980s.

*   Mechanical valves: the most important risks for women with mechanical valves are the risks associated with anticoagulation during pregnancy and the risk of endocarditis. Both warfarin and heparin therapy are associated with significant maternal morbidity and fetal morbidity and mortality; warfarin is better for maternal health but worse for the fetus, while heparin is better for the fetus and worse for the mother.

    Warfarin is teratogenic, causing mental retardation, short stature and multiple facial abnormalities. Its use in the second trimester of pregnancy is associated with fetal blindness, microcephaly and mental retardation. There is also an increased risk of fetal internal haemorrhage. Spontaneous abortion, maternal haemorrhage and stillbirth are also increased in women receiving warfarin.

    Although less common, administration of heparin during pregnancy is also associated with increased rates of spontaneous abortion, fetal and maternal haemorrhage and stillbirth. Prolonged use of heparin may also cause maternal osteoporosis, and women may present with acute severe back pain due to vertebral crush fractures. However, the main risk with heparin is thromboembolism involving the heart valves, increasing maternal morbidity and mortality. Traditionally, British practice has been to convert women to heparin for the first trimester of pregnancy and then maintain them on warfarin before reverting to heparin for the last few weeks of pregnancy and for delivery, while practice in the USA has been to heparinise women throughout pregnancy. In particular high-risk cases, low-dose aspirin may be added to heparin therapy in an attempt to improve maternal outcome.

- Porcine valves: the major risks of porcine valves are thromboembolic events and valve failure. The rate of valve degeneration at 10 years is estimated at 50–60%. There is some evidence that pregnancy accelerates the degeneration of porcine valves, and it is therefore imperative to follow these women closely during pregnancy and immediately to investigate any possibility of deteriorating cardiac function.

  Although the advantage of porcine compared with mechanical valves is that anticoagulation is not needed routinely, women with atrial fibrillation or a history of a thromboembolic event are likely to require full anticoagulation, with its attendant risks.

- Homograft valves: these valves are used primarily for aortic replacement, and the available evidence suggests that they are associated with a significantly lower pregnancy morbidity than either porcine or mechanical valves. There is no need for anticoagulant therapy and there do not appear to be the same risks of degenerative change as with porcine valves.

Women with aortic valve replacement tolerate the physiological changes of pregnancy relatively well, but those with mitral valve replacement have a relatively fixed cardiac output and are at risk of developing cardiac failure during pregnancy. They also have an increased risk of atrial fibrillation; if this occurs it should be treated promptly, by cardioversion if necessary.

Management options

Pre-pregnancy counselling should be offered to women with prosthetic valves, firstly to advise those with congenital heart disease of the increased risks of congenital heart disease in their offspring, and secondly to advise those who are dependent on anticoagulants of the risks of such therapy in pregnancy. Valve function and cardiac status should also be assessed before pregnancy if possible.

All women with prosthetic heart valves should be regarded as having high-risk pregnancies and should be delivered in large maternity units, preferably in or near to centres with facilities for cardiac surgery. Cardiac function should be assessed early in the first trimester of pregnancy and at regular intervals throughout the pregnancy. It is particularly important for women with prosthetic valves to receive regular dental care during pregnancy, and any dental treatment should be preceded by prophylactic antibiotics. Similarly, any intercurrent infection during pregnancy should be aggressively treated.

The presence of a prosthetic heart valve is not in itself an indication for operative delivery. There are obvious advantages in planned induction of labour in the anticoagulated woman, since she can be converted to prophylactic rather than therapeutic doses of heparin over the period of induction and delivery. This enables regional analgesic and anaesthetic techniques to be used (following laboratory assessment of coagulation status) if appropriate. If regional analgesia is contraindicated, patient-controlled intravenous opioid analgesia is the most appropriate alternative for labour and also for provision of postoperative analgesia if general anaesthesia has been used for Caesarean section.

Prophylactic antibiotics should be used to cover delivery in all women with prosthetic heart valves.

In general, management and monitoring will depend on the severity of residual cardiac disease and the underlying lesion, and the requirements of each woman must be determined on an individual basis.

Key points

- Women with prosthetic heart valves are not a homogeneous group. They differ in their underlying cardiac disease, degree of impairment of cardiac function and type of prosthetic valve.
- Pre-pregnancy counselling is recommended whenever possible.
- Antenatal care and delivery should be undertaken in a hospital with facilities for high-dependency care.
- Regular assessment of cardiac function during pregnancy is important.

FURTHER READING

Bates SM, Greer IA, Hirsh J, Ginsberg JS. Use of antithrombotic agents during pregnancy: the Seventh ACCP Conference on Antithrombotic and Thrombolytic Therapy. *Chest* 2004; **126** (Suppl): 627S–644S.

Chan WS, Anand S, Ginsberg JS. Anticoagulation of pregnant women with mechanical heart valves. *Arch Intern Med* 2000; **160**: 191–6.

European Society of Cardiology Task Force. Expert consensus document on management of cardiovascular diseases during pregnancy. *Eur Heart J* 2003; **24**: 761–81.

Leyh RT, Fischer S, Ruhparwar A, Haverich A. Anticoagulant therapy in pregnant women with mechanical heart valves. *Arch Gynecol Obstet* 2003; **268**: 1–4.

Thorne SA. Pregnancy in heart disease. *Heart* 2004; **90**: 450–6.

92   CONGENITAL HEART DISEASE

About 70–80% of children with congenital heart disease (CHD) now reach adult life (16 years and over) and thus reproductive age. Unfortunately, there is still a significant mortality rate amongst young adults with corrected CHD. In the pregnant population, cyanotic CHD is associated with a higher maternal morbidity and mortality than non-cyanotic disease, but both groups of women should be regarded as high-risk patients.

Problems/special considerations

- Patients primarily with disorders of cardiac output may experience cardiac failure as pregnancy progresses, because of the increased demands placed on the cardiovascular system and the increased oxygen demand. Patients with cyanotic (or potentially cyanotic) disorders may experience worsening cyanosis as the decreasing systemic vascular resistance encourages shunting of blood across the heart; this is compounded by increased oxygen demand. Both types of patients are prone to arrhythmias and and venous thromboembolism, and tolerate hypovolaemia poorly.
- Maternal haematocrit of greater than 60%, arterial oxygen saturation of less than 80%, right ventricular hypertrophy and episodes of syncope are all considered poor prognostic factors. Women with cyanotic disease have higher rates of spontaneous abortion and these are said to correlate with haematocrit.
- Conditions associated with particularly high risk in pregnancy are:
  - (i) Pulmonary hypertension (residual or primary)
  - (ii) Systemic right ventricle
  - (iii) Moderate and severe aortic stenosis
  - (iv) Marfan's syndrome with aortic dilatation
  - (v) Complex surgery such as Fontan or Mustard procedures.

  Women with corrected septal defects are usually asymptomatic but some may have conduction disorders and there may still be residual pulmonary hypertension. A large Canadian study found that the presence of more than one of the following predictors was associated with an estimated risk of pulmonary oedema, arrhythmia, stroke, cardiac arrest or cardiac death of 75%: New York Heart Association classification >2 or cyanosis; previous cardiac event or arrhythmia; left heart obstruction; and left ventricular systolic dysfunction.
- Regardless of the maternal cardiac condition, the fetus of the mother with CHD has an increased risk of CHD (Table 92.1).
- Bolus doses of Syntocinon cause a transient but sometimes profound fall in arterial blood pressure; the drug should be given by intravenous infusion if

Table 92.1. Risk of neonatal cardiac lesions when at least one parent has congenital heart disease

Tetralogy of Fallot	2–3%
Persistent ductus arteriosus; aortic coarctation	4%
Atrial septal defect	5–11%
Pulmonary stenosis	6–7%
Ventricular or atrioventricular septal defect	10–16%
Aortic stenosis	15–18%
Marfan's/Di George's syndrome	50%

at all. Ergometrine causes a sharp rise in arterial, central venous and intracranial pressures and should generally be avoided in women with CHD, although it may be preferable to Syntocinon in certain fixed output states without pulmonary hypertension. If Caesarean section is performed, the need for oxytocics may be avoided by performing a brace suture through the uterus to provide mechanical, rather than pharmacological, uterine compression.

- Women may be receiving therapeutic doses of anticoagulants. Regional analgesia and anaesthesia are usually contraindicated in such women.

Management options

Women with CHD must be identified early in pregnancy (preferably seen for pre-conception counselling) and managed jointly by the obstetrician, cardiologist and obstetric anaesthetist. Appropriate investigations and plans should be instituted (see Chapter 86, Cardiovascular disease, p. 206).

Caesarean section is not indicated for women with CHD unless there are obstetric indications or worsening maternal condition. Planned induction of labour may appear to have obvious benefits, but carries the risk of an increased likelihood of obstetric intervention.

Invasive arterial and/or central venous pressure monitoring is generally recommended except for mild conditions; the use of pulmonary artery catheters is controversial and usually impractical outside the intensive care unit.

Cautious use of low-dose epidural bupivacaine (0.1% or less) in combination with an opioid (usually 2.0–2.5 μg/ml fentanyl) provides optimal analgesia for women with CHD. Intrathecal opioids and continuous spinal analgesia have also been used. The use of high concentrations of bupivacaine (0.25–0.5%) in labour is contraindicated because of the risk of rapid and uncontrolled decrease in cardiac output.

Elective instrumental delivery avoids the fall in cardiac output that accompanies pushing and should be recommended for most cases, although a maximum of 15–30 minutes' pushing can be allowed for mild cases.

Anaesthesia for Caesarean delivery in women with CHD carries high risks. The options are for slow induction of regional anaesthesia (e.g. epidural, continuous spinal or combined spinal–epidural with a very small spinal component) or for a 'cardiac' general anaesthetic (which usually necessitates some hours of postoperative ventilatory support). There are no absolute rules; the relative risks and benefits in each individual case must be considered. A consultant anaesthetist with expertise in the management of high-risk pregnancy should be involved in the decision making.

Management of intrapartum anticoagulation should be discussed with both the haematologist and cardiologist. Prophylactic antibiotic cover for labour is important and usually consists of amoxycillin and gentamicin. All drug therapy should be discussed with a cardiologist with expertise in the management of CHD.

Key points

- Cyanotic congenital heart disease is associated with high maternal and fetal morbidity and mortality.
- Multidisciplinary antenatal and intrapartum care is essential.
- Regional analgesia for labour is usually beneficial; choice of anaesthetic technique for Caesarean section is controversial.

FURTHER READING

European Society of Cardiology Task Force. Expert consensus document on management of cardiovascular diseases during pregnancy. *Eur Heart J* 2003; **24**: 761–81.

Iserin L. Management of pregnancy in women with congenital heart disease. *Heart* 2001; **85**: 493–4.

Sermer M, Colman J, Siu S. Pregnancy complicated by heart disease: a review of Canadian experience. *J Obstet Gynaecol* 2003; **23**: 540–4.

Thorne SA. Pregnancy in heart disease. *Heart* 2004; **90**: 450–6.

93 PULMONARY HYPERTENSION AND EISENMENGER'S SYNDROME

Primary pulmonary hypertension is associated with an extremely high maternal mortality (40–60%) and is one of the few remaining maternal conditions in which pregnancy is considered absolutely contraindicated.

Secondary pulmonary hypertension may occur as a result of chronic pulmonary disease, e.g. connective tissue disease, or congenital heart disease such as severe aortic/mitral stenosis, or more usually, chronic left-to-right shunt. These conditions are also associated with high maternal mortality, particularly left-to-right shunt leading to Eisenmenger's syndrome (reversal of the shunt when pulmonary pressures exceed systemic pressures).

Although women are advised against pregnancy, many do not heed this advice.

Problems/special considerations

- Pulmonary artery pressures may be close to systemic arterial pressures and are associated with a high pulmonary vascular resistance. There is right ventricular hypertrophy and a relatively fixed low cardiac output. Increases in pulmonary vascular resistance, decreases in systemic vascular resistance or fall in cardiac output can all have catastrophic, and potentially fatal, consequences. In Eisenmenger's syndrome, peripheral vasodilatation increases shunt across the heart and thus worsens hypoxaemia.
- The increased cardiac output that occurs during pregnancy is poorly tolerated, since it causes further increase in pulmonary artery and right ventricular pressures, and volume overload. Right ventricular dilatation and tricuspid

regurgitation may occur, and left ventricular function and cardiac output may become increasingly impaired. The major haemodynamic changes occurring during parturition and the puerperium can prove fatal. Major haemorrhage causing hypovolaemia, or autotransfusion with the third stage of labour causing volume overload, are both poorly tolerated.

Management options

Close antenatal monitoring is essential, and women with pulmonary hypertension are frequently admitted for inpatient care in the third trimester of pregnancy or even earlier – most women resting more in hospital than is possible at home. Prophylactic anticoagulation is controversial, but low-dose heparin is often given in addition to simple anti-thromboembolism measures such as graduated compression stockings. Care must be taken to avoid prolonged immobility in hospital. The risks of aortocaval compression if women adopt supine or semi-supine positions are not confined to labour, and the lateral position should be adopted for any antenatal examinations of mother or fetus.

Pulmonary hypertension itself is not considered an indication for Caesarean section, though it may be required should maternal condition deteriorate or if there is fetal compromise. Continuous oxygen therapy may be beneficial for both mother and fetus. The mother may describe 'funny spells' and these should be taken seriously as potential indicators of episodes of severe pulmonary hypertension. Induction of labour is an option if the cervix is favourable but is associated with a higher rate of operative delivery than spontaneous labour.

For delivery, maternal monitoring should include electrocardiography and invasive right atrial and arterial blood pressure measurement. Use of a pulmonary artery catheter is more controversial and has been associated with a fatal outcome in Eisenmenger's syndrome. Scrupulous care must be taken to avoid inadvertent injection of air because of the risk of embolism in women with shunts.

Oxygen is a readily available and easily administered pulmonary vasodilator and should be given continuously throughout labour and delivery. Hypoxia, hypercarbia and acidosis all tend to increase pulmonary artery pressure and pulmonary vascular resistance. Prolonged labour, use of systemic opioids and inadequate hydration are all, therefore, risk factors for these women.

Regional analgesia has been used successfully; epidural infusions or intermittent boluses of low concentrations of local anaesthetic and opioid (0.0625–0.1% bupivacaine with fentanyl 2.0–2.5 µg/ml; alternatively opioid alone) provide good analgesia without compromising haemodynamic stability. Combined spinal–epidural analgesia is a suitable alternative but offers little advantage over low-dose epidural analgesia, except possibly more profound analgesia if opioids alone are used. There are theoretical advantages to using saline rather than air to identify the epidural space because of the risks of air embolism.

Although general anaesthesia has traditionally been recommended for women with pulmonary hypertension, regional anaesthesia has been successfully used for both Eisenmenger's syndrome and primary pulmonary hypertension. It is imperative to use a slow titration technique and invasive central monitoring if regional anaesthesia is chosen.

General anaesthesia offers potentially greater haemodynamic stability, and the opportunity to minimise oxygen consumption by eliminating the work of breathing and maximise arterial oxygen saturation. It is also easier to administer inhaled pulmonary vasodilators such as 100% oxygen, nebulised prostacyclin or nitric oxide; use of the latter two has been described although their place is still uncertain. However, the cardiodepressant effects of general anaesthesia with associated reduction in cardiac output are still hazards for these women, as is the potentially increased risk of thromboembolism. A high-dose opioid 'cardiac' general anaesthetic provides maximal haemodynamic stability. There is no particular advantage in elective ventilation postoperatively, but high-dependency or intensive care nursing is mandatory.

Postoperative and post-delivery analgesia can be provided by patient-controlled intravenous opioids or by epidural or intrathecal opioids. Invasive monitoring must be continued for several days; women with pulmonary hypertension are frequently successfully delivered, only to die during the first 2 weeks after delivery.

Key points

- Pregnancy is extremely hazardous for women with pulmonary hypertension.
- Maternal mortality may be as high as 60%.
- The physiological changes of normal pregnancy are poorly tolerated by women with pulmonary hypertension.
- Hypovolaemia and any increase in pulmonary vascular resistance must be avoided.
- Cautious use of regional analgesia for vaginal delivery with full invasive cardiovascular monitoring is recommended.
- Both general and epidural anaesthesia have been used for operative delivery; both have significant risks.

FURTHER READING

Bildirici I, Shumway JB. Intravenous and inhaled epoprostenol for primary pulmonary hypertension during pregnancy and delivery. *Obstet Gynecol* 2004; **103**: 1102–5.

Bonnin M, Mercier FJ, Sitbon O, *et al.* Severe pulmonary hypertension during pregnancy: mode of delivery and anesthetic management of 15 consecutive cases. *Anesthesiology* 2005; **102**: 1133–7.

Duggan AB, Katz SG. Combined spinal and epidural anaesthesia for caesarean section in a parturient with severe primary pulmonary hypertension. *Anaesth Intens Care* 2003; **31**: 565–9.

Lam GK, Stafford RE, Thorp J, Moise KJ Jr, Cairns BA. Inhaled nitric oxide for primary pulmonary hypertension in pregnancy. *Obstet Gynecol* 2001; **98**: 895–8.

Monnery L, Nanson J, Charlton G. Primary pulmonary hypertension in pregnancy; a role for novel vasodilators. *Br J Anaesth* 2001; **87**: 295–8.

94   ISCHAEMIC HEART DISEASE

Myocardial infarction (MI) during pregnancy is uncommon, with a reported incidence of 1 in 10 000 to 1 in 35 000 pregnancies. There have been an increasing number of case reports of MI during pregnancy and delivery, and it is possible that the incidence is now higher. Ischaemic heart disease in the antenatal population is frequently related to smoking and obesity but may also be associated with the use of illegal drugs, particularly crack cocaine. Postpartum MI has been reported as a complication of pre-eclampsia. Women who have had previous MI, with or without previous coronary artery bypass grafting, may also present to the obstetrician and obstetric anaesthetist.

Problems/special considerations

- A high index of suspicion is necessary. Myocardial ischaemia may not be considered in the differential diagnoses of a pregnant woman presenting with chest pain, and the presentation may be atypical. The woman who has been using cocaine is frequently an unreliable historian, and may conceal or deny her drug abuse. Clinical examination and investigations may be difficult to interpret; a systolic murmur is common during pregnancy, and changes in axis and ST, T and Q waves may all be found in the electrocardiogram of a healthy pregnant woman. Cardiac troponin I is a useful investigation since it is unaffected by pregnancy, labour and delivery.
- Maternal mortality of acute MI during pregnancy is reported to be as high as 30–50%, with the highest mortality associated with MI during the third trimester of pregnancy. Recent studies suggest a lower mortality rate of under 10%.
- Myocardial ischaemia and infarction caused by cocaine are associated with a high incidence of cardiac arrhythmias.
- Antenatal considerations include the use of anticoagulants; planning of place, time and mode of delivery; use of intrapartum invasive monitoring; and choice of analgesia and anaesthesia for delivery.

Management options

These women should be managed by a multidisciplinary team. Reported treatments include the use of intra-aortic balloon counterpulsation and percutaneous transluminal coronary angioplasty.

Mode of delivery

There is no consensus of opinion in the literature about the preferred mode of delivery of a woman who has had antenatal MI, nor about the method of anaesthesia. Vaginal delivery eliminates the stress of surgery and the need to provide anaesthesia. The risk of peripartum thromboembolism is also reduced, as is the potential for obstetric haemorrhage. However, induction of labour carries an increased risk of further obstetric intervention, whereas allowing spontaneous onset of labour is unpredictable. Caesarean delivery can be optimally timed to permit senior staff from all concerned specialties to be involved. There is adequate time to institute full invasive monitoring and to organise cardiovascular support, but surgical intervention increases the risks of complications.

Monitoring

Most authorities suggest using intra-arterial pressure monitoring, pulse oximetry and continuous electrocardiographic monitoring. The use of pulmonary artery pressure monitoring is more controversial and is associated with significant risks that may outweigh potential benefits.

Analgesia and anaesthesia

For analgesia in labour, epidural analgesia minimises haemodynamic instability caused by the pain and stress of labour. Use of low-dose local anaesthetic and opioid infusions or boluses avoids the risk of hypotension. Combined spinal–epidural analgesia would also be a suitable alternative.

Both 'cardiac' (high-dose opioid) general anaesthesia and epidural anaesthesia have been used successfully for Caesarean section. The major concerns with general anaesthesia are uncontrolled hypertensive response to tracheal intubation, risks of potentially life-threatening arrhythmias (particularly in cocaine users) and need for postoperative ventilatory support because of the high doses of opioids used.

The major concern with regional anaesthesia is haemodynamic instability caused by rapid onset of sympathetic blockade. For this reason, single-shot spinal anaesthesia is not recommended; if a regional technique is chosen a slow incremental epidural technique should be used (continuous spinal and combined spinal–epidural anaesthesia have also been used successfully).

Oxytocic drugs

Ergometrine causes acute hypertension and is contraindicated in women with ischaemic heart disease. Large intravenous boluses (> 5 U) of Syntocinon cause transient hypotension and may compromise coronary filling; it is therefore preferable to use an intravenous infusion of Syntocinon during management of the third stage of labour.

Puerperium

The fluid shifts that occur during the early postpartum period contribute to potential haemodynamic instability at this time. High-dependency nursing and medical care is mandatory; intensive cardiovascular monitoring should be maintained for at least 48 hours after delivery. Epidural opioids are recommended for provision of postoperative analgesia. The use of prophylactic anticoagulants should be considered for 3–6 months post-delivery.

Key points

- Myocardial infarction during pregnancy has high maternal mortality.
- The association between myocardial infarction and cocaine consumption should be considered.
- Management of labour and delivery is based on maintaining haemodynamic stability and minimising myocardial oxygen consumption.

FURTHER READING

Cuthill JA, Young S, Greer IA, Oldroyd K. Anaesthetic considerations in a parturient with critical coronary artery disease and a drug-eluting stent presenting for caesarean section. *Int J Obstet Anesth* 2005; **14**: 167–71.

Ladner HE, Danielsen B, Gilbert WM. Acute myocardial infarction in pregnancy and the puerperium: a population-based study. *Obstet Gynecol* 2005; **105**: 480–4.

Soderlin MK, Purhonen S, Haring P, *et al.* Myocardial infarction in a parturient. A case report with emphasis on medication and management. *Anaesthesia* 1994; **49**: 870–2.

Spencer J, Gadalla F, Wagner W, Blake J. Caesarean section in a diabetic patient with a recent myocardial infarction. *Can J Anaesth* 1994; **41**: 516–18.

95 ENDOCRINE DISEASE

The most common endocrine disorder affecting pregnancy is diabetes mellitus, which is considered separately. Although there are several other conditions that may have obstetric implications, most have little specific obstetric anaesthetic relevance over and above considerations applicable to the non-pregnant state.

Special considerations/management options

- *Thyroid disease:* anaesthetic implications are as for non-pregnant patients. Goitre may increase in size in pregnancy. Acute hyperthyroidism ('thyroid storm') may cause premature labour and fetal loss (and rarely, fetal hyperthyroidism). Rarely, the fetus may be affected by anti-thyroid treatment; goitre has been reported. Neonatal encephalopathy is more common if the mother has thyroid disease.
- *Adrenal disease:* hypoadrenalism is a rare cause of collapse on the labour ward. Patients receiving steroid therapy may require extra dosage peripartum (see Chapter 138, Steroid therapy, p. 310).

   Phaeochromocytoma is a rare but well-recognised cause of hypertension in pregnancy. Medical management is classically with α-blockade first and then β-blockade; it is important to ensure adequate fluid replacement. Magnesium therapy has also been used to control pre- and intraoperative hypertension. Regional anaesthesia has been safely used for labour and vaginal delivery.

Combined Caesarean section and excision of the tumour has been reported using both regional and general anaesthesia, with appropriate monitoring. More recently there have been reports of an elective two-step procedure being used whereby patients are treated medically first, followed by Caesarean section and then the tumour is excised. Phaeochromocytoma may be a part of the multiple endocrine neoplasia syndrome.

- *Neurological endocrine disease:* most of the anaesthetic implications relate to the effects of any intracranial space-occupying lesion. Specific hormonal conditions are managed as for non-pregnant patients. Sheehan's syndrome is pituitary infarction caused by severe hypotension ('pituitary apoplexy'), originally described in association with placental abruption. Pregnant women are thought to be particularly susceptible to this phenomenon because the pituitary gland enlarges during pregnancy and its blood supply is consequently more critical.
- *Other conditions:* these are managed as for non-pregnant patients.

Key points

- Diabetes mellitus is the most common and important endocrine disease in pregnancy.
- General management of endocrine disease is as for non-pregnant patients

FURTHER READING

Karabinas CD, Tolis GJ. Thyroid disorders in pregnancy. *J Obstet Gynecol* 1998; **18**: 509–15.
Chandraharan EA, Arulkumaran SB. Pituitary and adrenal disorders complicating pregnancy. *Curr Opin Obstet Gynecol* 2003; **15**: 101–7.

96   DIABETES MELLITUS

In the general population, diabetes mellitus (DM) is present in about 2% of individuals, in about half of them undiagnosed. In pregnancy, insulin requirements increase as peripheral sensitivity to insulin decreases (thought to be caused by the opposing action of placental hormones); thus known diabetics may become unstable, and otherwise normal subjects may reveal themselves as having gestational diabetes if they cannot meet the increased demands (the latter occurs in up to 3% of pregnancies). Most gestational diabetics recover after pregnancy, although most relapse in subsequent pregnancies at an earlier gestational age, and there is a 50% risk of developing type 2 DM in later life. Gestational diabetes is associated with older age, ethnicity, obesity, a family history of DM and poor previous obstetric history.

Screening of pregnant women for gestational diabetes is controversial and even amongst those that advocate it, there is disagreement about the cut-off points and definitions used. Most programmes involve initial random blood glucose testing with referral for a mini-glucose tolerance test (GTT) typically at 26 weeks' gestation if abnormal. The mini GTT involves a challenge of 50 g oral glucose followed by a blood glucose estimation one hour later; a concentration of ≥ 7.8 mmol/l constitutes abnormality. The full GTT includes a 75 g glucose challenge and has more specific divisions into normal/gestational diabetes/diabetes subgroups depending on fasting and GTT results.

Problems/special considerations

- *Effect of DM on the mother:* diabetes has many effects on most organ systems, the most immediately important being renal impairment, cardiovascular disease and central and peripheral neurological disease. Women with long-standing type 1 DM, depending on their overall glycaemic control, may already manifest these complications whereas those women with gestational DM or type 2 DM are usually younger than 40–45 years and systemic effects tend to be less common.
- *Control of blood sugar:* this is important during pregnancy since poor control is associated with increased incidence of fetal abnormalities (see below). In pregnancy, insulin requirements increase by up to 50% at term.

  During labour, it is important to avoid hyper- or hypoglycaemia, the former because it results in maternal and fetal acidosis and the latter because of the risk of impaired neurological function. Insulin requirements may decrease in the first stage but increase in the second stage, although this may depend on other factors such as length of labour, pre-labour state, etc.
- *Effect of DM on pregnancy:* diabetics have an increased incidence of pregnancy-induced hypertension, polyhydramnios, Caesarean section and preterm labour (the latter may not hold for gestational DM). There is also an increased incidence of neonatal hypoglycaemia and hyperbilirubinaemia. In type 1 DM, there is a 5–10-fold incidence of congenital malformation if glycaemic control during pregnancy is poor, with a 5-fold increase in stillbirth rate and 4–5-fold increase in perinatal death rate. Good glycaemic control reduces the incidence of congenital malformation to 2%, about twice the normal. Macrosomia occurs about 4–6 times as commonly in diabetics as non-diabetics, depending on the definition used; it is thought to be caused by reactive fetal insulin secretion in response to maternal hyperglycaemia and/or transfer of maternal insulin to the fetus. It may result in obstructed labour.

Management options

Before conception, known diabetics should be counselled and their care optimised (ideally, glycosylated haemoglobin concentration $< 7\%$).

During pregnancy, careful dietary advice $\pm$ pharmacological intervention aim to maintain normal blood glucose concentrations. Close follow-up of pregnant diabetics is required, with monitoring of glycaemic control as well as screening

Table 96.1. Sample sliding scale for insulin during labour in diabetics

Blood glucose concentration (mmol/l)	<3.9	4.0–5.9	6.0–8.9	9.0–11.9	12.0–14.9	15.0–17.9	>18
Insulin infusion rate (U soluble insulin/h)	0.5	1	2	3	4	5	6

for infections, since diabetic ketoacidosis may be precipitated by infection as in the non-pregnant state. Monitoring of fetal wellbeing and growth is also important. Increasing insulin requirements in pregnancy may reflect reduced placental function and may be an indication for induction of labour. Women with absent warning signs of hypoglycaemia should be advised against driving (pregnancy may alter awareness of hypoglycaemia).

During labour, most authorities advocate continuous glucose/insulin infusions; a suitable regimen comprises a 5% glucose infusion plus 20 mmol/l potassium chloride with a continuous insulin infusion using a sliding scale according to regular (30–60 minute) blood glucose concentration monitoring (Table 96.1). The aim is to maintain blood glucose concentration at 4–6 mmol/l; if this cannot be achieved the entire insulin infusion scale is increased by 1 U/h. If blood glucose concentration repeatedly falls below 4 mmol/l the 5% dextrose may be changed for 10% glucose. Urine should be tested, e.g. 4-hourly for glucose and ketones. Avoidance of glucose during labour has been popular previously but leads to maternal and fetal acidosis. Most authorities advise continuous fetal monitoring throughout labour, and a paediatrician should attend all deliveries, with neonatal unit admission prepared. For elective Caesarean section, the same intravenous regimen is started in the morning, the patient having been nil by mouth since midnight and having omitted her usual morning insulin.

Insulin requirements fall rapidly once delivery has occurred, and the infusion rate should be halved once the baby has been born. Most gestational diabetics do not need insulin at all postpartum; insulin-dependent diabetics may be given a subcutaneous dose of soluble insulin (e.g. 5 U) when ready to eat and drink and the infusion stopped 60 minutes later.

Management as far as regional or general anaesthesia is concerned is along standard lines, although the former is especially desirable. In labour, regional analgesia is thought to be beneficial by reducing catecholamine levels and thus avoiding their anti-insulin effects and the propensity for acidosis. Care should be taken to assess the mother for the complications of DM as above. In addition, of especial relevance to general anaesthesia, autonomic neuropathy may be associated with reduced gastric emptying, and a syndrome of stiff joints has been described in which difficult tracheal intubation has featured. The syndrome is suggested by the 'prayer sign' in which the patient is unable to lay the palmar surfaces of her index fingers fully flat against one another when pressing her palms together as if praying; when viewed from the side there is a space between the proximal phalangeal joints. The syndrome has also been implicated in causing reduced compliance of the epidural space, which may result in spinal cord ischaemia when large volumes are injected epidurally.

Fluid therapy should be separate from intravenous dextrose/insulin; thus two intravenous cannulae are usually required if anaesthetic intervention is needed. Hartmann's solution may result in a small increase in blood glucose concentration caused by gluconeogenesis from lactate metabolism, although this is rarely a problem in practice. Patients should receive adequate diabetic follow-up postpartum.

Key points

- Diabetes mellitus is associated with increased incidence of fetal malformations, macrosomia and death, especially if diabetic control is poor.
- Pregnant diabetics should be closely followed throughout pregnancy and peripartum.
- Regional analgesia and anaesthesia are especially desirable.
- Insulin and glucose infusions are used in labour.
- Insulin requirements fall rapidly after delivery.

FURTHER READING

Carroll MA, Yeomans ER. Diabetic ketoacidosis in pregnancy. *Criti Care Med* 2005; **33** (10 Suppl): S347–S353.

Kjos SL, Buchanan TA. Current concepts: gestational diabetes mellitus. *N Engl J Med* 1999; **341**: 1749–56.

Simmons D. Persistently poor pregnancy outcomes in women with insulin dependent diabetes. *BMJ* 1997; **315**: 263–4.

97 ANAEMIA AND POLYCYTHAEMIA

Pregnancy is associated with an increase in red cell mass and a greater increase in plasma volume. Circulating plasma volume can increase by about 50% in single pregnancies but may double in multiple pregnancies. Red cell mass increases by 20–30%. There is therefore a physiological dilutional 'anaemia'. This increase in red cell mass and the needs of the developing fetus increase requirement for iron and folate, which often need to be supplemented. Normal iron absorption is around 1–2 mg a day; however, requirements in pregnancy may be as high as 6.6 mg a day. Many women start pregnancy with depleted iron stores and a low haemoglobin concentration and the likelihood of this increases with subsequent pregnancies. In some cases of extreme iron deficiency, parenteral iron may be required.

Polycythaemia in pregnancy is rare and is usually secondary to other disease processes such as cyanotic heart disease. The underlying problem is usually more significant than the haemoglobin concentration itself. Primary polycythaemia (rubra vera) is a neoplastic disease more usually seen in older patients than in the childbearing population.

Problems/special considerations

Anaemia

Normal vaginal delivery of a single fetus is associated with a blood loss of around 500 ml, but this may double with twin deliveries. Caesarean section is associated with a blood loss of 1000 ml. Following delivery, there is a fall in plasma volume caused by diuresis; this partially compensates for the drop in haemoglobin concentration resulting from blood loss.

Mothers who are already anaemic have less reserve than normal and may thus be more susceptible to the effects of haemorrhage. Since they rely on an even greater increase in cardiac output than normal to maintain oxygen delivery, cardiac depression (e.g. caused by general anaesthesia) may have profound effects on maternal and fetal oxygenation. Maternal myocardial ischaemia is also more common. Haemorrhage in Jehovah's Witnesses is a particular problem and an important cause of maternal death.

Pernicious anaemia is extremely rare in pregnancy but the presence of a macrocytic anaemia may prompt investigation. Folate and B_{12} deficiency may cause congenital malformations in the neonate, abruption and haemorrhage. Maternal complications include neurological complications such as subacute combined degeneration of the cord. Aplastic anaemia has been reported in pregnancy and in some cases has resolved following delivery.

Polycythaemia

There have been few published cases of polycythaemia complicating pregnancy. There may be associated thrombocytopenia or thrombocythaemia. Thrombocytopenia may be dilutional and may not reflect function. Thrombotic events (arterial and venous) do occur and prophylactic aspirin and heparin have been given to prevent them.

In cyanotic heart disease, a haemoglobin concentration greater than 16 g/dl is associated with poor fetal outcome; this probably represents both a marker of severity of the underlying disease and impairment of uteroplacental oxygenation resulting from increased blood viscosity.

Coagulation times may be artefactually prolonged in severe polycythaemia.

Management options

As long as the above potential problems are considered, anaesthetic management in general is routine. In anaemia, the threshold for transfusion should be lower than normal. New formulations of parenteral iron (iron-sucrose) have been used postpartum to restore haemoglobin concentration more rapidly than oral iron, and are associated with few adverse reactions, unlike iron-dextran and sodium ferric gluconate preparations. Erythropoeitin has been used in Jehovah's Witnesses – management of whom must include senior staff.

In polycythaemia, regional analgesia and anaesthesia may be precluded by recent administration of heparin, although the benefits usually outweigh the risk of epidural haematoma.

Key points

- A drop in haemoglobin concentration during pregnancy is normal.
- Postpartum diuresis partially compensates for peripartum blood loss.
- Polycythaemia in pregnancy is usually secondary to underlying disease.

FURTHER READING

Management of anaesthesia for Jehovah's Witnesses. London: The Association of Anaesthetists of Great Britain and Ireland, 1999.

Steer P, Alam MA, Wadsworth J, Welch A. Relation between maternal haemoglobin concentration and birth weight in different ethnic groups. *BMJ* 1995; **310**: 489–91.

98   DEEP-VEIN THROMBOSIS AND PULMONARY EMBOLISM

Venous thromboembolism occurs in under 0.1% pregnancies but is the most common direct cause of death in pregnancy. It kills 15–22 women per million maternities and was responsible for 30 deaths in the last Report on Confidential Enquiries into Maternal and Child Health (CEMACH), 25 from pulmonary embolism and 5 from cerebral vein thrombosis. Key factors predisposing to thromboembolic events are bed rest, dehydration, coincident thrombophilia, pre-eclampsia, greater maternal age, patient/family history, obesity and Caesarean section (the last increasing the risk by up to eight times).

Untreated calf vein thrombosis is fatal in 15% of cases. Iliofemoral thrombosis (which is more common in pregnancy) may be associated with an even greater mortality. Untreated pulmonary embolus (PE) in pregnancy may recur and is associated with a mortality of 25%.

Problems/special considerations

- Physiological changes in pregnancy favour coagulation. In addition, obesity and the gravid uterus may cause venous stasis whilst supine, encouraging thrombus formation. Pregnant women are therefore 6–10 times more likely to develop thromboembolism than non-pregnant women.
- Diagnosis of deep-vein thrombosis (DVT) in pregnancy may be difficult; however, mortality audits have identified patients with classic symptoms and signs who

were not treated effectively. Not only is the diagnosis often not considered in pregnancy, but women may be denied appropriate investigation because of their pregnant state.

Management options

Treatment of thromboembolism in pregnancy

Suspected DVT in pregnancy should be investigated with duplex ultrasonography and venography if necessary. A raised concentration of d-dimers or other fibrin degradation products may help to confirm the diagnosis. Suspected PE in pregnancy should be investigated with chest radiography, arterial blood gas analysis and electrocardiography, followed by a ventilation/perfusion scan. Increasingly, non-invasive imaging technique such as spiral computerised tomography, magnetic resonance imaging and specialised echocardiography are being used to diagnose PE.

Treatment of thromboembolism is with intravenous heparin initially (although subcutaneous low-molecular weight heparins (LMWHs) are increasingly used) and should not be delayed whilst awaiting investigation. Warfarin is associated with fetal abnormalities and in particular should be avoided in the first trimester and after 36 weeks' gestation. Acute treatment is followed by subcutaneous prophylactic heparin. It had been thought that prophylactic heparin caused stillbirth, prematurity and haemorrhage but more recent reviews controlling for maternal comorbidity have cast doubt on this assertion. Prophylaxis with LMWHs is now recommended because their use is associated with a lower incidence of osteoporosis and thrombocytopenia than unfractionated heparin, they require less monitoring, and they may be given as a once daily dosage. However, LMWHs have a prolonged action and are only partially reversible with protamine, meaning that LMWH prophylaxis may delay administration of regional analgesia (see Chapter 100, Coagulopathy, p. 240) and can be a problem where pregnancy is complicated by ante- or postpartum bleeding.

Massive PE may require dispersion under radiological control or open embolectomy. Administration of potent intravenous fibrinolytic drugs may result in massive obstetric haemorrhage.

The use of vena caval filters in pregnancy is felt by many authors to be contraindicated though they have been used.

Thromboprophylaxis in pregnancy

Increasing numbers of women are being given prophylaxis against arterial or venous thrombosis in pregnancy. Some women have a hereditary or acquired thrombophilia or a past medical history of thrombosis. In addition, some obstetricians treat women with a strong history of stillbirth, intrauterine death and miscarriage with prophylactic doses of antithrombotics such as aspirin, heparin or both. Other women require continuation of pre-pregnancy therapeutic doses of antithrombotics, such as those with prosthetic heart valves.

Warfarin is teratogenic when used in the first trimester and may also lead to fetal cerebral haemorrhage; it is now rarely used in pregnancy apart from in women with metal heart valves who are at particular risk of valve thrombosis.

Thromboprophylaxis following Caesarean section

A significant proportion of fatal PEs occur 2–6 weeks postpartum and Caesarean section (especially emergency) is known to be an important risk factor. A working party of the Royal College of Obstetricians and Gynaecologists recently reviewed prophylaxis of venous thromboembolism following Caesarean section (Table 98.1). In some units, heparin is given to all women having Caesarean section in order not to miss those who are at high risk.

Increased doses of heparin are required in pregnancy. Neither warfarin nor heparin is excreted in breast milk.

Table 98.1. Royal College of Obstetricians and Gynaecologists guidelines for prophylaxis of thromboembolism following Caesarean section

Low risk: early mobilisation and hydration	Elective Caesarean section, uncomplicated pregnancy and no other risk factors
Moderate risk: prophylactic heparin or mechanical measures	Age > 35 years Obesity (> 80 kg) Four or more previous children Labour longer than 12 hours Gross varicose veins Current infection Pre-eclampsia Immobility prior to surgery (> 4 days) Major current illness, e.g. heart or lung disease; cancer; inflammatory bowel disease; nephrotic syndrome Emergency Caesarean section in labour
High risk: heparin prophylaxis and leg stockings; prophylaxis to continue for at least 5 days	A patient with three or more moderate risk factors from above Extended major pelvic or abdominal surgery, e.g. Caesarean hysterectomy Patients with a personal or family history of deep vein thrombosis; pulmonary embolism or thrombophilia; paralysis of lower limbs Patients with antiphospholipid antibody (cardiolipin antibody or lupus anticoagulant)

Key points

- Venous thromboembolism is the most common direct cause of death in pregnancy.
- If untreated, thromboembolism carries a high mortality.
- Heparin is the treatment of choice for venous thromboembolism.
- Prophylaxis against thromboembolism should be considered in all women undergoing Caesarean section.
- Low molecular weight heparin is the heparin of choice for thromboprophylaxis.

FURTHER READING

Gherman RB, Goodwin TM, Leung B, *et al.* Incidence, clinical characteristics, and timing of objectively diagnosed venous thromboembolism during pregnancy. *Obstet Gynecol* 1999; **94**: 730–4.

Bates SM, Greer IA, Hirsh J, Ginsberg JS. Use of antithrombotic agents during pregnancy: The Seventh ACCP Conference on Antithrombotic and Thrombolytic Therapy. *Chest* 2004; **126**: 627S–644S.

Royal College of Obstetricians and Gynaecologists. *Thromboprophylaxis during pregnancy, labour and after vaginal delivery.* London: RCOG, 2004.

Stone SE, Morris TA. Pulmonary embolism during and after pregnancy. *Crit Care Med* 2005; **33** (10 Suppl): S294–300.

99   THROMBOPHILIA

Thrombophilia has been defined as a familial or acquired abnormality of haemostasis likely to predispose to thrombosis. Up to 30–50% of patients with a history of venous thromboembolism may have a congenital thrombophilia and others may have a detectable phospholipid autoantibody. This is a developing area, and further congenital or acquired factors explaining a propensity to thrombosis may yet come to light.

Problems/special considerations

- Pregnancy is associated with a physiological hypercoagulable state. When a pre-existing thrombophilia is present, thrombosis may occur within the uterus, causing failure of implantation; within the placenta, causing fetal loss, abruption, pre-eclampsia, intrauterine growth retardation and fetal distress in labour; or within the systemic circulation. Patients with thrombophilia may thus present with subfertility, with a personal or family history of venous and arterial thromboses or with thromboses in pregnancy or in the puerperium.
- Diagnosis is difficult in pregnancy because of the changes in clotting factor profile associated with pregnancy.

- The usual treatment of thrombophilia complicating pregnancy is prophylactic subcutaneous heparin (usually low molecular weight) combined with low-dose aspirin. This has implications for the timing of regional analgesia and anaesthesia (see Chapter 100, Coagulopathy, p. 240).

Thrombophilias can be classified into congenital and acquired.

Congenital thrombophilias

These deficiencies are not heterogeneous; factors may be reduced quantitatively or qualitatively, underlying the importance of haematological input in their management. Subtle, subclinical deficiencies of these factors are very much more common than the figures quoted below (around 1 in 200):

- *Activated protein C resistance (APCR):* the circulating anticoagulant protein C, when activated by thrombin, inactivates factors V and VIII. APCR occurs normally in pregnancy associated with an increase in factor VIII. This makes diagnosis in pregnancy difficult. In congenital APCR, factor V is more resistant to cleavage by protein C. Factor V Leiden occurs in about 5–7% of the European population and is associated with a rate of thrombosis in pregnancy in about 1 in 400–500. Factor V Leiden is much more sinister when in the homozygous form or when combined with another thrombophilia.

  In the absence of other risk factors such patients should not need thromboprophylaxis in pregnancy.

- *Antithrombin III (ATIII) deficiency:* this is a rare defect occurring in 1 in 5000 women but may account for up to 12% of thromboembolic events in pregnancy. In untreated affected women, 55–68% of pregnancies are complicated by venous thromboembolism. Anticoagulant prophylaxis may be required throughout pregnancy and for at least 3 months postpartum. Discontinuation of heparin at the time of delivery and administration of ATIII concentrate has been advocated by some authors but is controversial.

- *Protein C or protein S deficiency:* this occurs in 1 in 15 000 pregnancies and is associated with a rate of venous thrombosis of up to 25% (protein S is a cofactor for protein C). Treatment with heparin throughout pregnancy and the puerperium is controversial. The risk of thrombosis is greatest postpartum in both protein C and S deficiencies and several authors suggest thromboprophylaxis for this period only.

- *Other causes:* these include hyperhomocystinaemia and mutations of the prothrombin gene.

Acquired thrombophilia

The antiphospholipid syndrome is the most common cause of acquired thrombophilia. Identified autoantibodies include lupus anticoagulant and anticardiolipin antibodies. However, there is some evidence that other as yet unidentified autoantibodies may cause thrombosis and fetal loss in pregnancy.

The lupus anticoagulant is so called because it causes a prolongation of the activated partial thromboplastin time even when diluted (because the autoantibody binds to phospholipid in the assay). However, it is associated with a thrombotic tendency. Anticardiolipin antibodies are detected by using an immunoassay.

Of women with recurrent miscarriage (three or more), 15% have persistently positive results for phospholipid antibodies. If untreated, 90% will have spontaneous abortions or stillbirths in subsequent pregnancies. It is possible that lupus anticoagulant (30% of cases) and anticardiolipin antibodies (70% of cases) are the same autoantibody identified in different assays. Clinical features of the antiphospholipid syndrome are recurrent fetal loss, thrombosis (arterial and venous), thrombocytopenia, haemolytic anaemia, hypertension, pulmonary hypertension and livedo reticularis. Antiphospholipid syndrome is associated with a 5% incidence of thromboembolism or cerebrovascular accident in pregnancy.

Management options

Women with a strong personal or family history of thrombosis and a poor obstetric history should be screened for known causes of thrombophilia.

Patients are at high risk of obstetric intervention in labour and may benefit from epidural analgesia and regional anaesthesia for delivery and Caesarean section. The decision to site an epidural should be based on dose and interval after heparin administration and potential benefit to the patient. Ideally, women who are likely to be receiving heparin at the time of delivery should discuss a management plan with an anaesthetist in an assessment clinic. In the majority of cases the benefits of regional analgesia and anaesthesia far outweigh the risk of epidural haematoma.

Key points

- Thrombophilias are a significant cause of fetal loss in pregnancy.
- The adverse effects on maternal and fetal health are treatable.
- The risks and benefits of regional analgesia and anaesthesia should be considered antenatally if possible.

FURTHER READING

Kujovich JL. Thrombophilia and pregnancy complications. *Am J Obstet Gynecol* 2004; **191**: 412–24.

Ralph CJ. Anaesthetic management of parturients with the antiphospholipid syndrome: a review of 27 cases. *Int J Obstet Anesth* 1999; **8**: 249–34.

Ringrose DK. Anaesthesia and the antiphospholipid syndrome: a review of 20 obstetric patients. *Int J Obstet Anesth* 1997; **6**: 107–11.

100   COAGULOPATHY

Normal coagulation is important to the obstetric anaesthetist for two reasons: firstly because of the potential risk of spinal haematoma following regional analgesia and anaesthesia and secondly because of the risk of postpartum haemorrhage.

Problems/special considerations

In general terms, increased bleeding may arise from defects in the function of:
- Blood vessels, e.g. caused by severe infections, metabolic disease (such as hepatic failure, renal failure) or congenital structural abnormalities.
- Platelets, caused by reduced numbers (e.g. thrombocytopenia, disseminated intravascular coagulation (DIC)) or impaired function (e.g. antiplatelet drugs).
- The coagulation system, caused by congenital disorders (e.g. haemophilia, von Willebrand's disease), acquired coagulation factor dysfunction (e.g. anticoagulant therapy, hepatic failure, vitamin K deficiency, DIC) or increased fibrinolysis.

Von Willebrand's disease is associated with blood vessel and platelet defects as well as coagulation factor dysfunction. Massive blood transfusion may result in dilution of both platelets and coagulation factors.

Management options

Specific disorders should be managed according to the underlying pathology and in conjunction with the appropriate specialists, usually haematologists. Coagulation studies should always be performed before considering regional analgesia and anaesthesia, although the ideal test or combination of tests and the 'safe' limits for those tests are unknown (see Chapter 81, Pre-eclampsia and eclampsia, p. 189; Chapter 103, Thrombocytopenia, p. 245). It has been suggested that regional blockade can be performed providing the activated partial thromboplastin time ratio or International Normalised Ratio is less than 1.5, although this is controversial. Symptoms of excessive bruising or bleeding should be sought since they may signify increased risk of bleeding in borderline cases.

Considerable discussion has been prompted by the problem posed by anticoagulant therapy, which is increasing as women with various medical disorders (including thrombophilia) present in pregnancy. Whereas full anticoagulation is a contraindication to regional analgesia and anaesthesia, prophylactic regimens are more controversial. Low-dose aspirin is generally felt to pose minimal risk, although the numbers of mothers who have been studied (receiving both aspirin and regional blockade) are small compared with the rarity of the outcome (spinal haematoma). Other antiplatelet drugs are less commonly used in pregnancy and experience with them is limited.

Prophylactic heparin (especially low molecular weight heparin) has been associated with spinal haematoma in non-pregnant patients who receive regional analgesia and anaesthesia, although many of these cases have been associated with relatively large doses in high-risk patients. The risk of therapeutic levels of heparin activity following a supposedly prophylactic dose in pregnancy is unknown. In addition, heparin pharmacokinetics are altered in pregnancy and larger doses are required than in non-pregnant patients, so data from series in which standard (non-pregnant) doses of heparin were used may be misleading. Most obstetric anaesthetists would follow the guidelines recommended for non-pregnant patients, in which regional analgesia and anaesthesia or removal of an epidural catheter should be avoided for 6 hours after a prophylactic dose of unfractionated heparin (12 hours after low molecular weight heparin), and heparin should not be given within 2 hours of a regional block or catheter removal. In particular cases where the risks of general anaesthesia are increased (e.g. certain forms of cardiac disease), an epidural may still represent a safer option than general anaesthesia, even within these time limits.

Key points

- Specific coagulation disorders should be managed with involvement of haematologists.
- Low-dose aspirin therapy is considered to represent minimal risk.
- Risks and benefits of regional analgesia and anaesthesia should be considered for women who are receiving prophylactic heparin therapy. In general, guidelines prohibiting regional blockade or catheter removal within certain periods of heparin administration should be followed.

FURTHER READING

Demers C, Derzko C, David M, Douglas J. Society of Obstetricians and Gynecologists of Canada. Gynaecological and obstetric management of women with inherited bleeding disorders. *J Obstet Gynaecol Can* 2005; **27**: 707–32.

Economides DL, Kadir RA, Lee CA. Inherited bleeding disorders in obstetrics and gynaecology. *Br J Obstet Gynaecol* 1999; **106**: 5–13.

Horlocker TT, Wedel DJ, Benzon H, *et al.* Regional anesthesia in the anticoagulated patient: defining the risks (the second ASRA Consensus Conference on Neuraxial Anesthesia and Anticoagulation). *Reg Anesth Pain Med* 2003; **28**: 172–97.

101 VON WILLEBRAND'S DISEASE AND HAEMOPHILIA

Von Willebrand's disease (vWD) is a heterogeneous group of mainly autosomal dominant disorders in which there is reduced or abnormal circulating von Willebrand factor (vWF). Von Willebrand factor has two functions: firstly, it combines with factor VIII in vivo to produce a pro-coagulant complex (VIIIc) that protects factor VIII from premature destruction. Hence factor VIII activity may be reduced in vWD. Secondly, vWF assists platelet adhesion to exposed subendothelium of damaged capillaries and is excreted by endothelium and activated platelets. Deficiency of vWF therefore affects platelet adherence and the clotting cascade itself. It ranges from a mild disease of little significance seen in up to 1% of the population to a very severe form in which vWF is absent.

Haemophilia A and B (factor VIII and IX deficiency respectively) are X-linked disorders and classically do not affect the female population. As many as 1 in 10 female carriers, however, may have a clinically significant clotting deficiency.

Problems/special considerations

Von Willebrand's disease

This is classified into three main variants:

- *Type I (80–90% of cases):* vWF is normal but present in diminished quantities. In pregnancy, vWF increases and may even return to normal; following delivery, VIIIc levels can fall dramatically (though this change may be delayed until late in the puerperium), and there is an increased incidence of postpartum haemorrhage. Levels of VIIIc can be increased by the administration of desmopressin (DDAVP) intravenously.

- *Type II (9–15% of cases):* there is an abnormal vWF; hence additional release of abnormal vWF with DDAVP is unlikely to improve the coagulopathy. Clotting does not improve in pregnancy. In the IIb subtype, abnormal vWF clumps inactivated platelets and causes thrombocytopenia. In this variant, DDAVP worsens the coagulopathy because increased amounts of abnormal vWF worsens the thrombocytopenia. A new variant of vWD type IIN (Normandy) has been described in which there is an isolated decrease in factor VIII concentration because of decreased affinity of the abnormal vWF for factor VIII, which results in increased factor VIII consumption. Thus it can be confused with haemophilia A.

- *Type III (autosomal recessive; < 1% of cases):* vWF is undetectable and factor VIIIc concentration is very low. The bleeding abnormality is severe and does not respond to DDAVP.

Haemophilia

A concentration of factor VIII or IX of 30% of normal is considered acceptable for vaginal delivery. For planned operative delivery, factor concentrations are usually increased to normal. Half of all fetuses will be affected and therefore fetal blood sampling and forceps or ventouse deliveries should be avoided unless chorionic villous sampling or amniocentesis has shown the fetus to be unaffected. After delivery, factor VIII level can fall abruptly, resulting in secondary haemorrhage.

Management options

Close liaison with haematologists is necessary throughout pregnancy. A management plan, which includes treatment for significant haemorrhage, is helpful. An epidural is rarely contraindicated in type I vWD, but specialist interpretation of laboratory tests (particularly VIIIc concentration) is required. Because of the sometimes precipitous drop in vWF and VIIIc following delivery, removal of the epidural catheter postpartum may be more of a problem; it is advisable either to remove epidural catheters immediately or to wait until the bleeding diathesis can be assessed.

The usual dose of DDAVP is 20 µg (0.3 µ/kg) in 50 ml of saline given over 30 minutes. DDAVP also stimulates fibrinolysis so tranexamic acid is often given simultaneously. DDAVP can cause fluid retention and therefore hyponatraemia.

Patients with type I disease may deliver vaginally. Patients with type II or III disease frequently have an elective Caesarean section, with correction of their coagulopathy. In this situation, regional anaesthesia has been used if clotting is corrected. Where DDAVP is contraindicated, fresh frozen plasma (FFP), cryoprecipitate or infusions of vWF and factor VIII may be given.

In haemophilia, close monitoring of factor VIII or IX levels as appropriate is required. Administration of FFP, cryoprecipitate, DDAVP or purified clotting factors may be necessary to bring factor levels to the 30% considered adequate for vaginal delivery or the near 100% required for operative delivery. Regional analgesia and anaesthesia is generally contraindicated unless haematological advice suggests a fully corrected coagulation profile and the possible risks are outweighed by the benefits particular to the case concerned.

Key points

- Von Willebrand's disease is a heterogeneous condition, which ranges in severity.
- The commonest form of von Willebrand's disease is improved by pregnancy.
- Coagulation may rapidly deteriorate after delivery in both von Willebrand's disease and haemophilia.
- In haemophilia, the fetus should be assumed to be affected.
- Specialist advice is necessary before, during and after delivery.

FURTHER READING

Jones BP, Bell EA, Maroof M. Epidural labor analgesia in a parturient with von Willebrand's disease type IIA and severe preeclampsia. *Anesthesiology* 1999; **90**: 1219–20.

Kadir RA, Lee CA, Sabin CA, Pollard D, Economides DL. Pregnancy in women with von Willebrand's disease or factor XI deficiency. *Br J Obstet Gynaecol* 1998; **105**: 314–21.

Kouides PA. Obstetric and gynaecological aspects of von Willebrand disease. *Bailliere's Best Prac Clin Haematol* 2001; **14**: 381–99.

102 DISSEMINATED INTRAVASCULAR COAGULATION

In disseminated intravascular coagulation (DIC) the coagulation process is activated, resulting in consumption of clotting factors and platelets, with concomitant activation of the fibrinolytic pathway. Conventional treatment of this consumptive coagulopathy is removal of the underlying trigger and support of the patient with replacement of clotting factors and platelets. In many respects, DIC can be seen as the haematological manifestation of a multiorgan disease, e.g. sepsis, pre-eclampsia.

Problems/special considerations

- Diagnosis of DIC depends on clinical features and laboratory tests. Presentation may be of rapid collapse, with shock, respiratory failure, renal impairment, acidosis, hypoxaemia and bleeding from venepuncture sites and the respiratory, gastrointestinal and urogenital tracts (the last including the uteroplacental bed). Coagulation studies show prolonged coagulation times, decreased fibrinogen concentration and platelet count and raised titres of fibrin degradation products. Some authors favour thromboelastography because it demonstrates changes in both coagulation and thrombolysis.
- In some cases there may be a more insidious progression; initially, increased circulation of activated clotting factors may even shorten coagulation times.
- The common triggers for DIC in the obstetric population are listed in Table 102.1. Many of these conditions have their own particular implications for analgesia and anaesthesia. The coagulopathy usually precludes regional anaesthesia.
- Fibrin degradation products have an anticoagulant effect and reduce the efficiency of myometrial contraction, exacerbating blood loss.

Management options

Management of DIC should be to remove the cause. This usually involves delivering the fetus if antepartum.

In fulminant DIC there may be no time to wait for laboratory results in the face of massive blood loss, haemostatic failure and multiorgan failure. Patients often

Table 102.1. Triggers of disseminated intravascular coagulation (DIC) in obstetrics

Placental abruption
Sepsis (particularly Gram-negative)
Pre-eclampsia
HELLP (haemolysis, elevated liver enzymes and low platelet count) syndrome
Acute fatty liver of pregnancy
Intrauterine death (DIC may occur after 3–4 weeks)
Amniotic fluid embolism
Massive blood transfusion (produces a dilutional coagulopathy; however, tissue factors released from the cause of blood loss may induce DIC in a compromised circulation)
Transfusion reactions
Drug reactions
Placenta accreta
Hydatidiform mole

require empirical treatment with blood and blood products and surgical treatments such as hysterectomy. The successful management of fulminant DIC requires input from senior obstetricians, obstetric anaesthetists, haematologists, laboratory staff and intensivists (see Chapter 73, Major obstetric haemorrhage, p. 173).

Conventional treatment of DIC is to fuel the consumptive coagulopathy by administering exogenous clotting factors: fresh frozen plasma to correct prolongation of the activated partial thromboplastin time or prothrombin time, cryoprecipitate to treat a low fibrinogen concentration (< 1–1.5 g/dl) and platelet concentrates.

Some authors have attempted to break the cycle of thrombosis and fibrinolysis by giving heparin, antithrombin or aprotinin. However, anticoagulating a bleeding patient or preventing fibrinolysis where deposition of fibrin is causing skin and organ necrosis is fraught with danger.

Transfer to an intensive care unit may be necessary to treat the multisystem dysfunction.

Key points

- Coagulopathy may coexist with other organ failures. Resuscitation is essential.
- Treatment includes removing the cause of the coagulopathy.
- Aggressive treatment is required to treat fulminating disseminated intravascular coagulation.
- Management of massive obstetric haemorrhage requires coordinated care with haematologists, obstetricians, obstetric anaesthetists and intensivists.

FURTHER READING

Richey ME, Gilstrap LC 3rd, Ramin SM. Management of disseminated intravascular coagulopathy. *Clin Obstet Gynecol* 1995; **38**: 514–20.

103 THROMBOCYTOPENIA

A low platelet count ($< 150 \times 10^9$/l) may occur in pregnancy for a variety of reasons ranging from the relatively benign (gestational thrombocytopenia) to the frankly sinister (HELLP [haemolysis, elevated liver enzymes and low platelet count] syndrome, thrombotic thrombocytopenic purpura (TTP)). Though the platelet count decreases in normal pregnancy possibly due to increased destruction of platelets and haemodilution a level of $\leq 115 \times 10^9$/l should be investigated. A manual count is always advisable.

Problems/special considerations

Conditions involving reduced platelet numbers or function include:
- *Gestational thrombocytopenia:* this is the most common cause of low platelet count in pregnancy, accounting for 70% of all cases. It is seen in around 5% of

parturients, is probably caused by accelerated platelet destruction and is rarely associated with a count of less than 75×10^9/l. In 75% of cases the low platelet level is clinically unimportant and it has been suggested that levels between 75×10^9/l and 115×10^9/l do not need investigation. It does not appear to increase the risk of peripartum haemorrhage and should not be regarded as a contraindication to regional analgesia, and certainly women with counts of $\geq 90 \times 10^9$/l should be regarded as normal.

- *Immune thrombocytic purpura (ITP):* this is seen in around 0.1% of pregnancies. It is characterised by the production of platelet autoantibodies that may cross the placenta, putting the fetus at risk of intracranial haemorrhage during delivery. Although the platelet count is often below 100×10^9/l, coagulation is rarely affected because the young platelets, which make up a higher than usual proportion of the platelet mass, are more aggressively haemostatic. ITP can be distinguished from gestational thrombocytopenia by the fact that the platelet count is already low in the early antenatal period. The mainstay of treatment is corticosteroid therapy and should be considered when the platelet count is $\leq 50 \times 10^9$/l, but IgG administration has proved very effective in severe cases. Platelet transfusion may stimulate autoantibody production and should therefore be avoided. A number of drugs may induce thrombocytopenia (Table 103.1).
- *Thrombotic thrombocytopenic purpura (TTP) and Haemolytic uraemic syndrome (HUS):* thrombotic thrombocytopenic purpura is a rare condition in which intra-vascular clot formation leads to platelet consumption and widespread vascular occlusion, often resulting in neurological disturbance and renal failure. A deficiency in VWF cleaving protease has been identified as a causative factor. Unlike HELLP syndrome (see below), TTP usually presents in the second trimester. The high morbidity and mortality associated with this condition warrants aggressive intervention, and exchange transfusions and plasmapheresis may be employed. Haemolyic uraemic syndrome presents clinically in a similar way to TTP but the renal problems are more severe.
- *Pre-eclampsia:* this is accompanied by a low platelet count in about 20% of cases. In its most malignant version, this manifests as HELLP syndrome. Mothers with evidence of pre-eclampsia must have their platelet count monitored frequently,

Table 103.1. Drugs that may impair platelet function or cause thrombocytopenia

Impaired platelet function	Thrombocytopenia
Aspirin	Heparin
Non-steroidal anti-inflammatory drugs	Thiazide diuretics
Colloid plasma substitutes	Hydralazine
	H_2 blockers
	Digoxin
	Cocaine

and a fall should be regarded as evidence that the condition is worsening. The thrombocytopenia of pre-eclampsia is often accompanied by clotting defects, so regular tests of the coagulation cascade should also be made. Management should be targeted at treatment of the underlying condition, ultimately by delivery, but specific therapy may be needed, including platelet transfusion and fresh frozen plasma.

- *Others:* reduced platelet concentration may also result from other causes of impaired production, e.g. bone marrow depression, vitamin B_{12}/folate deficiency, hereditary defects, paroxysmal nocturnal haemoglobinuria, alcohol toxicity; or of shortened survival of platelets, e.g. malignancy, drugs (including heparin and α-methyldopa), disseminated intravascular coagulation.

Management options

The obstetric anaesthetist is often called upon to make a decision regarding the advisability of regional analgesia and anaesthesia in these cases. Several textbooks and articles offer guidance on this subject, and the general trend in recent years has been to lower the 'cut-off point' from a platelet count of 100×10^9 / l to 75×10^9 / l. In fact, there is no evidence to support this sort of 'all-or-nothing' approach, and every case must therefore be considered on its merits, taking into account the underlying pathology, with the risk of the procedure (epidural/spinal haematoma) balanced against the benefits (pain relief, better blood pressure control, avoidance of general anaesthesia).

When monitoring platelet levels, the trend as well as the absolute value is important, and the mother with a rapidly falling count should be regarded with more suspicion than the one with a low, but stable, platelet level. In general, patients with a platelet count of greater than 75×10^9 / l in the absence of pre-eclampsia are unlikely to have significantly altered platelet function.

Tests of platelet function, such as bleeding time, are very operator-dependent and therefore of limited predictive value. Thromboelastography is a promising development in this field, but its place in clinical practice has yet to be determined. Routine coagulation studies are usually indicated in thrombocytopenia in case any other defect should be present. The mother should always be questioned about excessive bruising or bleeding since the presence of these may signify impaired platelet function in borderline cases.

Key points

- All patients with thrombocytopenia must be fully investigated.
- Trends in platelet count are more important than absolute values.
- There is no fixed 'cut-off point' for the platelet count when regional analgesia is being considered.
- Patients should be asked about excessive bruising or bleeding.

FURTHER READING

Douglas MJ. Platelets, the parturient and regional anesthesia. *Int J Obstet Anesth* 2001;
10: 113–20.

Gorton H, Lyons G. Is it time to invest in a thromboelastograph? *Int J Obstet Anesth* 1999;
8: 171–8.

Greaves M, Letsky EA. Guidelines on the investigation and management of thrombocytopenia
in pregnancy and neonatal alloimmune thrombocytopenia. *Br J Obstet Gynaecol* 1997;
104: 1108.

Kam PCA, Thompson SA, Liew ACS. Thrombocytopenia in the parturient. *Anaesthesia* 2004;
59: 225–64.

104   LYMPHOMA AND LEUKAEMIA

Haematological malignancies complicate pregnancy extremely rarely. Successful
pregnancy with chemotherapy for both acute and chronic leukaemia and
lymphoma has been described. Increasing numbers of patients are surviving childhood or adult treatment of haematological malignancies. Such treatment can leave
both physical and psychological problems associated with chemotherapeutic
treatment.

Problems/special considerations

- Treatment of haematological malignancies often involves intense periods of chemotherapy or radiotherapy followed by maintenance doses. The most aggressive
  forms of therapy result in permanent ablation of bone marrow. Bone marrow
  rescue is achieved by transplantation of stored autologous bone marrow or
  donated allogeneic bone marrow. Patients may require repeated lumbar punctures to test for disease and to administer chemotherapeutic agents
  (e.g. methotrexate).
- The limiting factor in administration of most chemotherapeutic agents is short-
  and long-term toxicity. Short-term problems include malaise, nausea and vomiting, anorexia and acute organ impairment, especially of the liver and kidneys
  (toxicity may also arise from drugs such as gentamicin and vancomycin, given
  to treat infections). Bone marrow depression may result in anaemia, neutropenia
  with increased risk of infection, and coagulopathy. Long-term toxicity of common
  chemotherapeutic agents includes neurotoxicity, neuropathies (vincristine and
  etoposide) and arachnoiditis (methotrexate). Cardiomyopathy may occur as a
  dose-dependent result of anthracycline antibiotics such as danorubicin.
  Pulmonary toxicity and fibrosis may follow busulfan and bleomycin administration. Although sterility often occurs following high-dose chemotherapeutic
  treatments, many survivors do become pregnant spontaneously or following
  infertility treatments. Central and peripheral venous access may be a persisting
  problem.

• The psychological effects of a diagnosis of cancer in a young person followed by prolonged periods of toxic therapy, infection and isolation cannot be overlooked. They may have features of a post-traumatic stress syndrome with flashbacks, nightmares and phobias of hospitals, doctors and needles. Frequently, these psychological aspects influence management far more than physical aspects.

Management options

All such patients require a detailed assessment by the antenatal team. Wherever possible, the treatment records should be obtained, preferably with a haematological summary. The patient may not (want to) remember details of their treatment, particularly if they received it as a child. In addition, repressed memories of unpleasant experiences such as general anaesthesia or lumbar puncture may induce unexpected irrational behaviour. A careful, sensitive approach is required.

Commonly performed investigations include:
• Urea and electrolytes
• Full blood count
• Liver function tests
• Pulmonary function tests
• Echocardiography
• Chest radiography.

The spectrum of such patients varies from some that can be treated as normal to those with significant hepatic, renal and cardiorespiratory disease. In the last group, regional analgesia and anaesthesia is usually recommended, depending on the pattern of disease.

Key points

• It is tempting to treat patients with active or previous haematological malignancy as normal – they are not.
• Survivors of leukaemia and lymphoma need support and sensitive, carefully planned care.

105 HAEMOGLOBINOPATHIES

Haemoglobin abnormalities result from either synthesis of abnormal haemoglobin (e.g. sickle cell anaemia) or reduced rate of synthesis of normal haemoglobin chains (the thalassaemias).

Problems/special considerations

Sickle cell disease

Patients with sickle cell disease are homozygotes for an abnormal haemoglobin (haemoglobin S). Heterozygotes have a significantly attenuated form (sickle cell trait), which is not normally of clinical significance except when combined with another abnormal haemoglobin (e.g. haemoglobin C). Haemoglobin S is poorly soluble in its deoxygenated form and therefore crystallises at a variable oxygen concentration dependent on relative concentrations of normal and abnormal haemoglobin within the red cell. Haemoglobin S in heterozygotes appears to have some protective action against malaria and is therefore more common in Africa, Asia, Arabia and southern Europe, particularly coastal Greece. Sickle cell disease is characterised by haemolysis, reticulocytosis, anaemia, recurrent sepsis, vaso-occlusive and sequestration crises and hypersplenism followed by splenic infarction. Diagnosis is based on demonstration of sickling (Sickledex test) followed by haemoglobin electrophoresis.

Sickle cell disease (homozygous SS) is a particularly aggressive disease. Affected patients may not survive into their third decade. Problems in pregnancy include vaso-occlusive and thromboembolic phenomena and infection. Placental infarction can occur and result in abortion, intrauterine growth retardation and pre-eclampsia. There is up to a 1% maternal, 20% fetal and 5% neonatal mortality rate.

Despite earlier evidence to the contrary, recent work has demonstrated that sickle cell trait is not associated with a higher incidence of pre-eclampsia.

Thalassaemias

This disease is classified according to the haemoglobin chain affected (α or β). It is common in Mediterranean countries and also occurs in a narrow band distribution crossing Africa, the Middle East, India, Burma and South-East Asia. Its distribution therefore closely follows that of sickle cell disease, and both diseases are said to give some protection against falciparum malaria.

- α-*Thalassaemia:* the α haemoglobin gene is encoded twice on each chromosome 16, giving a total of four genes controlling its production. When all four genes are deleted, α chain synthesis is completely suppressed and death occurs in utero (hydrops fetalis). Three α gene deletions lead to a moderately severe microcytic, hypochromic anaemia with splenomegaly (HbH disease). Precipitation of relatively insoluble HbH within cells induces mild haemolysis. Crises of haemolysis associated with infection may occur. Patients with two (thalassaemia trait) and one (silent carriers) α chain deletions are asymptomatic.

  Pregnancies complicated by hydrops fetalis (Bart's hydrops) are associated with pre-eclampsia, retained placenta and ante- and postpartum haemorrhage.

- β-*Thalassaemia:* in contrast to α-thalassaemia, the β haemoglobin gene is coded by a single gene; thus patients can be homozygous or heterozygous for the faulty gene. However, about 125 individual mutations of the β gene have been described, which can markedly affect the clinical picture. Hence the terms thalassaemia major, intermedia and minor have been used to describe clinical pictures of varying severity. Furthermore, the geographical distribution of thalassaemia and sickle cell trait mean that it is possible to have a mixed sickle cell–thalassaemia genotype.

In thalassaemia major either no β haemoglobin chains are produced or small amounts are produced (5–30%). Anaemia results from ineffective erythropoiesis and haemolysis and inadequate supplies of haemoglobin for formed red cells. Features include skeletal abnormalities because of bone marrow hyperactivity and failure of many organ systems, including the pancreas, liver and heart. Patients may be thrombocytopenic because of hypersplenism or thrombocythaemic following splenectomy. Thrombocythaemic patients require thromboembolic prophylaxis and may also develop arterial thrombosis, including cerebral thrombosis. Frequent cannulation may make venous access difficult (many patients have permanent indwelling intravenous catheters). There is a high incidence of blood transfusion reactions and a small incidence of transfusion-related HIV and hepatitis C. Splenectomised patients are at risk of infection.

Treatment of β-thalassaemia includes frequent transfusion. Modern haematological management means that increasing numbers of women with thalassaemia major are becoming pregnant. There is an increased incidence of intrauterine growth retardation, fetal loss and obstetric intervention because of cephalopelvic disproportion resulting from skeletal abnormalities.

In thalassaemia intermedia there are usually few symptoms. Women may have chronic anaemia and require folate therapy in pregnancy. In severe cases, however, they may develop iron overload, with a clinical syndrome that lags behind the progression seen in thalassaemia major.

Thalassaemia minor behaves as a recessive condition, with few symptoms, although there appears to be higher incidence of intrauterine growth retardation.

Management options

In sickle cell disease, the haemoglobin concentration is usually maintained at 8 g/dl (optimum haematocrit 0.26) with blood transfusion. Exchange transfusion may decrease the rate of maternal complications in pregnancy but does not change fetal or obstetric outcome. A detailed plan is essential for delivery. In general, patients should be warm, well hydrated, not acidotic or hypercarbic and venous stasis should be avoided. An epidural provides analgesia without respiratory depression, although mobility is beneficial. A combination of systemic opioids and Entonox is particularly hazardous because of the potential for respiratory depression, hypercarbia and hypoxaemia between contractions. Regional or general anaesthesia may be used for operative delivery. Oxygen administration is essential postoperatively, especially after general anaesthesia. The safety of blood patch in sickle-cell disease has not been assessed, but colloid patches have been used successfully.

α-Thalassaemia rarely results in maternal disease sufficient to cause significant problems with anaesthesia. Related problems such as haemorrhage and pre-eclampsia are covered elsewhere.

In β-thalassaemia, haemoglobin should be kept greater than 10 g/dl with transfusion. Complications such as thrombocytopenia, diabetes, hypothyroidism, cardiomyopathy and facial and vertebral abnormalities mean that choice of anaesthesia and analgesia is assessed on an individual basis.

Key points

- Patients with sickle cell disease should be kept warm, well hydrated, mobile and well oxygenated.
- Haemoglobin should be kept at 8–9 g/dl in sickle cell disease.
- Exchange transfusion reduces maternal complications of sickle cell disease.
- Thalassaemia major causes significant multisystem compromise, including cardiac, endocrine and skeletal abnormalities; it may cause intrauterine death and concomitant maternal disease.
- Non-fatal α-thalassaemias are of variable significance.

FURTHER READING

Danzer BI, Birnbach DJ, Thys DM. Anesthesia for the parturient with sickle cell disease. *J Clin Anesth* 1996; **8**: 598–602.

Howard RJ. Management of sickling conditions in pregnancy. *Br J Hosp Med* 1996; **56**: 7–10.

Serjeant GR, Loy LL, Crowther M, Hambleton IR, Thame M. Outcome of pregnancy in homozygous sickle cell disease. *Obstet Gynecol* 2004; **103**: 1278–85.

Smith JA, Espeland M, Bellevue R, *et al.* Pregnancy in sickle cell disease: experience of the Cooperative Study of Sickle Cell Disease. *Obstet Gynecol* 1996; **87**: 199–204.

Weatherall DJ. The thalassaemias. *BMJ* 1997; **314**: 1675–8.

106   RHEUMATOID ARTHRITIS

Rheumatoid arthritis (RA) is three times more common in women than in men, and although the peak time of onset is not until the mid-thirties, it is reported to complicate approximately 0.1% of pregnancies. It is a non-specific autoimmune disease. A proportion of patients are seropositive for rheumatoid factor, an anti-IgG antibody.

RA tends to run a course of remissions and relapses. Pregnancy usually has a beneficial effect on disease progress, though relapses during the puerperium are common but may be delayed by lactation.

Problems/special considerations

The pregnant woman with RA poses several concerns for the anaesthetist:
- *Effects of the disease on the joints:* RA tends to affect primarily the small joints of the hands and wrists, and although this can be disabling for the patient, it is not usually a problem for the anaesthetist. In more severe cases there may be involvement of the hips, knees and lumbar spine, which may make positioning for regional analgesia or anaesthesia difficult. In very severe cases there may be

kyphosis of the thoracic spine and fixed deformity of the ribs, causing restrictive lung disease.

RA affects the cervical spine in up to 45% of cases and it is important to remember that the cervical spine may be unstable and prone to subluxation. The temporomandibular joints may also be affected and tracheal intubation may be difficult or impossible. Cricoarytenoid arthritis may be present, causing glottic constriction.

- *Systemic effects of the disease:* these are widespread. Both pericardial and pleural effusions may occur (often asymptomatically). Systemic granulomas can form in the lungs, myocardium, heart valves, aortic root and coronary arteries. Deposits in the cardiac conducting system may occur. A vasculitic process may rarely cause coronary or pulmonary arteritis.

  Syndromes associated with RA include Felty's and Sjogren's, in both of which peripheral neuropathies may occur.

- *Long-term medication:* the general principle of drug management during pregnancy is to reduce medication to a minimum and to restrict it to those drugs with the best safety record.

Women with symptomatic RA are usually maintained on high-dose aspirin and non-steroidal anti-inflammatory drugs. Although both are relatively contraindicated during pregnancy, it may be impossible to stop them. Serial ultrasound examination of the fetal heart helps to give early warning of closure of the fetal ductus arteriosus or of developing fetal pulmonary hypertension.

Neither gold nor penicillamine therapy is indicated during pregnancy. The most frequent concern about these drugs is when conception has occurred unexpectedly, either during or shortly after treatment.

Management options

The mother with RA may have several anaesthetic risk factors and should be identified as early as possible during pregnancy and referred for anaesthetic assessment. History taking should include a drug history, and questioning about any previous anaesthetics, especially if these involved tracheal intubation. A detailed cardiorespiratory history is essential. The neck and jaw should be examined to assess potential difficulty with tracheal intubation and where appropriate cervical spine X-rays should be taken in extension and flexion. Pulmonary function tests may be considered, and electrocardiography should be performed to exclude conduction defects. If there is suspicion of a rheumatoid cardiomyopathy, echocardiography should be requested. The extent of any peripheral neuropathy must be documented.

The mother should be advised to accept early epidural analgesia. If this is precluded by coagulopathy or absolute maternal refusal, patient-controlled opioid analgesia may be offered. If Caesarean section is necessary, an epidural top-up or combined spinal–epidural (CSE) is frequently recommended in preference to a single-shot spinal anaesthesia. The careful use of a CSE reduces the risk of an unexpectedly high motor or sensory block compromising the airway, and also provides greater haemodynamic stability in the event of undiagnosed cardiac problems.

If there are known cervical spine problems and general anaesthesia is essential, the anaesthetist must have access to fibreoptic equipment and awake intubation. Even if there is severe fetal distress, general anaesthesia should not be induced without additional aids for difficult intubation (and the presence of an anaesthetist who is familiar with their use).

Key points

- Rheumatoid arthritis is a multisystem autoimmune disease.
- Pregnancy tends to be associated with remission of the disease.
- The anaesthetist should expect difficulty with tracheal intubation.
- Cardiac and respiratory manifestations of the disease may be present.
- Peripheral neuropathy may infrequently occur.
- The mainstay of drug treatment is non-steroidal anti-inflammatory drugs, which the mother may need to continue throughout pregnancy.

107   CERVICAL SPINE DISORDERS

Women may have limited cervical spine movement because of rheumatoid arthritis, ankylosing spondylitis, cervical disc disease, trauma, accessory cervical ribs and cervical spondylosis, although the last is extremely uncommon in women of child-bearing age.

A rare but important cause of cervical kyphoscoliosis is the Klippel Feil syndrome. In extreme cases the patient may present with severe webbing of the neck, marked scoliosis and virtually no neck movement, but milder cases may pass unnoticed until the woman presents to the anaesthetist in the obstetric theatre.

Problems/special considerations

The major concern of the obstetric anaesthetist is reduced flexibility of the neck and the likelihood of difficulty with tracheal intubation. In addition, there may be other features of the underlying cause of the neck problems (e.g. rheumatoid arthritis).

Management options

Whenever possible, antenatal identification and assessment should be performed. The woman with limited cervical spine movement should be advised of the potential hazards associated with general anaesthesia and advised to accept epidural analgesia for labour and regional anaesthesia for any proposed operative procedure.

If general anaesthesia is essential, the anaesthetist must fully assess the patient preoperatively (including women presenting for emergency surgery). Basic assessment must include neck movement and mouth opening. If difficulty with intubation is anticipated, senior assistance must be sought before proceeding with induction of general anaesthesia. Local protocols should be followed in the event of unexpected failed intubation.

All obstetric theatres should have a difficult intubation trolley readily available, with a variety of laryngoscopes, including McCoy and polio blades. Awake fibreoptic intubation is now thought by many to be the management of choice when general anaesthesia is required in a woman who is known to have significant cervical spine abnormality, although elective preoperative tracheostomy has also been suggested.

Key points

- The main problem posed by cervical spine disorders is potentially difficult tracheal intubation.
- Regional techniques are usually considered best.

108   KYPHOSCOLIOSIS

Kyphoscoliosis may be congenital, associated with neuromuscular disorders (muscular dystrophies, neurofibromatosis, poliomyelitis or cerebral palsy) or idiopathic. Idiopathic kyphoscoliosis is much more common in females than males (ratio of 4:1) and accounts for 80% of all cases of kyphoscoliosis.

Progressive kyphoscoliosis is almost invariably accompanied by progressive symptoms and signs of restrictive pulmonary disease and ultimately, if left uncorrected, leads to pulmonary hypertension and death.

Severe uncorrected kyphoscoliosis is extremely uncommon in the UK, and most women presenting to the antenatal clinic will either have mild deformity or will have had corrective orthopaedic surgery.

Problems/special considerations

Although kyphoscoliosis in pregnant women is likely to be idiopathic, alternative causes are important to eliminate. Neurofibromatosis is associated with other serious complications (intracranial tumours, congenital heart disease), and familial dysautonomia, characterised by massive swings in blood pressure and generalised autonomic dysfunction, is associated with kyphoscoliosis in 90% of cases.

The bony pelvis is normal in women with idiopathic scoliosis and the likelihood of vaginal delivery is not usually reduced. However, if spinal instrumentation extends near the lumbosacral junction, this may impair sacral movement and interfere with descent of the fetus within the pelvis.

Women who have had corrective surgery have two major sources of potential morbidity, firstly residual cardiorespiratory disease and secondly limited access to the thoracolumbar spine.

Management options

Antenatal assessment is important, and access to previous medical records and X-ray films should be sought as early as possible in the pregnancy. Respiratory function tests can readily be performed on an outpatient basis and may be repeated later in the pregnancy to assess any deterioration. It has been suggested that correction of scoliosis improves respiratory function, whereas in women with uncorrected scoliosis cardiorespiratory function is likely to deteriorate further as a result of pregnancy.

In women with corrected scoliosis, the major problem for the anaesthetist is provision of regional analgesia and anaesthesia. The most common means of correction of kyphoscoliosis is with Harrington rods or with the newer adaptations, Luque and Cofrel–Duousset instrumentation. Each technique involves metal instrumentation and bone grafting. Although preservation of the L5/S1 inter-space is a cardinal orthopaedic rule, instrumentation and grafting may extend down to L4/5 in up to 20% of cases. The level of skin scar is a poor guide to the level of fixation, and therefore operation notes and/or X-ray film are extremely helpful during antenatal assessment. If there are no pre-pregnancy X-ray films available and there is doubt about the extent of instrumentation of the lumbar spine, relevant radiography may be performed during the third trimester of pregnancy.

Assessment and written documentation of any existing neurological deficit and any pre-pregnancy back pain is important.

Successful insertion of both epidural and spinal needles is well described in women with Harrington rod fixation, but women should be warned that the procedure may be technically difficult. False loss of resistance has been described as a recurring problem, and the risk of inadvertent dural puncture is increased. There is an increased risk of patchy analgesia or anaesthesia with epidural tech-niques, thought to be caused by epidural adhesions and scarring following disrup-tion of the ligamentum flavum.

Because of the potential problems of epidural analgesia and anaesthesia, spinal techniques may offer significant advantages. Spinal needle insertion at the L5/S1 interspace is more likely to be successful, even in very low fusions. There is a definite endpoint, which overcomes the problem of false loss of resis-tance, and deliberate dural puncture with an appropriate needle avoids the risks of inadvertent dural puncture with an epidural needle. Spread of local anaesthetic within the cerebrospinal fluid is unlikely to be affected by previous surgery, and therefore anaesthesia for operative delivery is more reliable with spinal than with epidural techniques. There are theoretical reasons to recommend continuous spinal catheter analgesia for labour as an alternative to epidural analgesia.

It is important to discuss in advance alternative methods of analgesia and the potential need for general anaesthesia in case regional techniques fail.

Key points

- Although at least 80% of kyphoscoliosis is idiopathic, association with other diseases such as neurofibromatosis and familial dysautonomia should not be forgotten.
- Uncorrected progressive kyphoscoliosis leads to severe restrictive pulmonary disease and pulmonary hypertension.
- The major anaesthetic problem in pregnant women with corrected kyphoscoliosis is provision of regional anaesthesia and analgesia. Spinal techniques offer several advantages over epidural.
- When no previous X-ray films or records are available, it is helpful to know that lumbar fusions should not involve the L5/S1 interspace.
- Radiography of the lumbar spine may be performed during the third trimester to aid management of regional analgesia.

FURTHER READING

Smith PS, Wilson RC, Robinson AP, Lyons GR. Regional blockade for delivery in women with scoliosis or previous spinal surgery. *Int J Obstet Anesth* 2003; **12**: 17–22.

109 LOW BACK PAIN

Low back pain, sacroiliac pain and sciatic pain are common during pregnancy, affecting between 50% and 90% of women. Symptoms vary from mild 'normal' backache to severe pain that may render the woman bed bound and necessitate early delivery.

The prevalence of low back pain during pregnancy increases with increasing maternal age. Numerous other risk factors have been investigated, but reports are contradictory about the relevance of maternal weight, socioeconomic class, number of pregnancies and previous history of back pain, although it is thought that women with a previous history of spinal surgery are not necessarily at increased risk of back pain during pregnancy.

Retrospective studies significantly under-report low back pain, usually quoting an incidence of 20–25%. This accounts for the conflicting data concerning any putative relationship between epidural analgesia and backache. Several prospective studies have now confirmed the absence of any relationship between epidural analgesia and the development of new long-term backache.

Problems/special considerations

- *Non-specific back pain:* the majority of back pain in pregnancy is directly attributable to the physiological changes that occur. The influence of relaxin, which is produced by the corpus luteum, leads to generalised ligamentous laxity. Serum levels of relaxin are highest during the first trimester of pregnancy. The pelvis widens, which may lead to sacroiliac joint instability. This may in turn allow anterior displacement of the sacrum, causing stretching of the lumbosacral plexus and subsequent pain. The expanding uterus alters the woman's centre of gravity and causes an increased lumbar lordosis and pelvic tilt, and this, combined with the additional weight carried as pregnancy progresses, contributes to development of back pain. Some women complain of night-time back pain, for which a vascular mechanism has been proposed. It is suggested that inferior vena caval compression and increased intravascular volume occurring during recumbency may lead to distension in the vertebral venous plexus and subsequent stagnant hypoxia in the nerve roots and vertebral bodies, producing radicular and low back pain.
- *Pelvic girdle pain:* some women have symptoms relating specifically to the sacroiliac joints or the symphysis pubis. These women complain of pain localised to the pelvis and pubic symphysis, with radiation to the buttocks and thighs but not to the calf or foot, and commonly complain of pain when turning over in bed at night. In extreme cases there may be separation of the pubic symphysis, in which case the woman may become unable to walk or weight bear at all. Abduction of the legs and external rotation of the hips may be difficult, and women may have anxieties about their ability to cope with labour and vaginal delivery.
- *Acute disc prolapse:* central disc herniation occurs in about 1 in 10 000 pregnancies and may require surgical decompression. Large central disc herniations can occur during pregnancy and at the time of delivery, and if there is an associated significant neurological deficit, surgical decompression is indicated. If magnetic resonance imaging is used, disc bulges and herniations can be demonstrated in approximately half of all pregnant women, which is the same incidence as in asymptomatic non-pregnant women. Low back pain with sciatic radiation is common in pregnancy, and careful history taking and examination are needed to ensure that the availability of magnetic resonance imaging does not lead to unnecessary surgical intervention.
- *Other causes:* less common causes of back pain should not be overlooked. Spinal cord tumours are extremely rare and most reported during pregnancy are angiomas, presumed to be present before pregnancy. The increased vascularity of pregnancy is assumed to cause the tumours to become symptomatic. Secondary metastasis to the spine of primary malignancies such as breast can occur during pregnancy.

Management options

General management

Back care advice early in pregnancy has been reported to reduce the incidence and severity of low back pain during pregnancy. This may be particularly important for women with a history of prepregnancy back pain, who may be at increased risk of worsening pain during pregnancy. Simple physiotherapy, exercise programmes and the use of lumbosacral corsets have all been reported to provide symptomatic pain relief during pregnancy.

Use of simple analgesics such as paracetamol and codeine-based preparations is acceptable during pregnancy but non-steroidal anti-inflammatory drugs should be avoided whenever possible. If their use is considered essential, treatment should be agreed with the obstetrician and fetal cardiac ultrasound monitoring arranged because of the risk of premature closure of the ductus arteriosus. Amitriptyline may be prescribed as a co-analgesic, especially if pain is disrupting normal sleep patterns. In cases of severe back pain, strong opioid analgesia may be required.

Transcutaneous electrical nerve stimulation for back pain during the second half of pregnancy is not recommended by the manufacturers of the machines but is used in clinical practice, frequently with good effect. Injection of local anaesthetic and steroid into the epidural space, the sacroiliac joints or the symphysis pubis may be considered necessary if symptomatic control of pain cannot be achieved by other methods. The safety of such procedures during pregnancy is unknown, and a risk–benefit analysis must be undertaken for each woman.

Delivery before term may be considered when pain control is difficult to achieve.

Anaesthetic management

Women with pre-existing musculoskeletal pathology should be fully assessed during the antenatal period. Previous spinal surgery is not a contraindication to regional analgesia and anaesthesia, although many women may have been told by their midwife, general practitioner or orthopaedic surgeon that they will be unable to have epidural analgesia. There may be respiratory impairment following significant corrective surgery, and some postoperative neurological deficit, and if so these must be documented antenatally. Women should be told that epidural analgesia for labour does not increase the likelihood of experiencing postnatal backache.

There is no contraindication to vaginal delivery nor to the use of regional anal-gesia in women with pregnancy-related back pain, although many women request (and some obstetricians suggest) delivery by elective Caesarean section to avoid any risk of exacerbating existing back symptoms.

Previous hospital records are helpful, since the position of the scar on the woman's back is not a reliable guide to the level of surgery. Most women will know whether they have had metal instrumentation of the spine or merely bony fusion. Those who have had instrumentation should be warned about possible technical difficulties in correctly positioning an epidural needle; it may be easier to perform spinal anaesthesia or analgesia. If successful epidural catheterisation is achieved, it may be difficult to obtain reliable spread of local anaesthetic, and this should be explained before starting the procedure.

Regional anaesthesia and analgesia in women who have had discectomy or laminectomy is not usually technically difficult, but there may be a slightly increased risk of inadvertent dural puncture, and patients should be warned about this.

Key points

- Low back pain is common in pregnancy; it is usually mechanical and should be treated symptomatically.
- Acute disc prolapse with neurological deficit is rare but may occur and should be treated surgically.
- There is no contraindication to epidural or spinal analgesia or anaesthesia in women with low back pain.
- Serious spinal and neurological pathology may, rarely, present during pregnancy and should always be considered in the differential diagnosis of new back pain.

FURTHER READING

MacEvilly M, Buggy D. Back pain and pregnancy: a review. *Pain* 1996; **64**: 405–14.

Rathmell JP, Viscomi CM, Ashburn MA. Management of nonobstetric pain during pregnancy and lactation. *Anesth Analg* 1997; **85**: 1074–87.

Young G, Jewell D. Interventions for preventing and treating pelvic and back pain in pregnancy. *Cochrane Database Syst Rev* 2002: CD001139.

---

110   NEUROLOGICAL DISEASE

The pregnant woman may develop neurological disease while pregnant or she may have an established neurological disease before she becomes pregnant (Table 110.1).

Problems/special considerations

- Acute neurological conditions may put both the mother and fetus at risk. Anaesthetic input may be required for peripartum analgesia or anaesthesia, acute medical management of critically ill patients or surgery indicated by the neurological condition.
- Traditionally, regional analgesia and anaesthesia have been avoided in most chronic neurological disease because of the fear of making the woman's condition worse or being blamed should a worsening occur. Since randomised

Table 110.1. Neurological conditions that may be seen in pregnancy

Arising during pregnancy		
	Trauma	Acute head injury
		Acute spinal cord injury
	Infection	Meningitis
		Acute post-infective neuropathy
	Tumour	
	Cerebrovascular accident	
Pre-existing		
Past history of:	Trauma	Head injury
		Spinal cord injury
	Infection	Meningitis
		Acute post-infective neuropathy
	Tumour	
	Cerebrovascular accident	
Established neurological disease	Migraine	
	Myasthenia gravis	
	Spina bifida	
	Epilepsy	
	Multiple sclerosis	
	Benign intracranial hypertension	

controlled trials are lacking for most of these conditions, traditional prejudices persist, although such evidence that there is supports regional techniques in many cases.

Management options

The management of both groups of women depends on the nature of the disease, its effects on pregnancy and delivery and the implications of the physiological changes of pregnancy.

Ideally, women who have a diagnosed neurological disease should be counselled before conception, so that they are aware of the possible problems that may be associated with their disease during pregnancy and delivery. In practice, the majority of women are seen after conception, and the aim should be early antenatal assessment. The effect of maintenance therapy and the necessity to change treatment to avoid teratogenic effects must also be considered. Good communication between the clinicians involved is essential in the management of these women. Clear guidelines for care should be written in the medical record and should be revised and updated as necessary.

Key points

- Neurological conditions may arise acutely during pregnancy or may already be present before pregnancy.
- Management depends on the condition, the effects on pregnancy and the effects of pregnancy on the condition.
- Early assessment and drawing up of management plans should take place whenever possible.

FURTHER READING

Karnad DR, Guntupalli KK. Neurologic disorders in pregnancy. *Crit Care Med* 2005; **33** (10 Suppl): S362–S371.

111   MENINGITIS

Acute infections of the nervous system may occur at any time during pregnancy or the peripartum period. The most important infection for the anaesthetist to consider is meningitis, as this can (rarely) occur as a sequel to spinal anaesthesia and confuse the differential diagnosis of a postdural puncture headache.

Women may also present having previously had meningitis.

Problems/special considerations

- Meningitis may be:
  - (i) Infective caused by bacteria, viruses and, rarely, others, e.g. tuberculosis, fungal infections.
  - (ii) Aseptic caused by chemical agents (e.g. disinfectants) and drugs, e.g. H_2-blockers or non-steroidal anti-inflammatory drugs.
- Meningitis that occurs as a complication of regional anaesthesia may be either of the above, and in each case prevention is better than cure. Meticulous attention to technique (this includes the use of a facemask to prevent droplet spread) is an essential part of minimising the risk of introducing infection or chemical contamination at the time of performing the regional block.
- The classic signs of meningitis are:
  - (i) Headache
  - (ii) Neck stiffness
  - (iii) Photophobia
  - (iv) Vomiting
  - (v) Fever
  - (vi) Raised white cell count.

    Many of the above symptoms are also produced by an accidental dural puncture, and so the exclusion of meningitis is essential in the differential diagnosis of any headache that develops after a regional anaesthetic.

- Almost all women with a history of previous meningitis have had a diagnostic lumbar puncture and that may have been a frightening experience, leading to apprehension of any further similar procedures. Some may have residual neurological impairment, although this is uncommon with modern management.

Management options

Meningitis should be considered as a possible diagnosis in any patient who has a raised temperature or white cell count associated with a headache. Differentiation between meningitis and accidental dural puncture as the cause of the headache may be difficult.

When there is any doubt, a neurological consultation is essential, and where appropriate a diagnostic lumbar puncture should be performed (Table 111.1). Antibiotics are usually prescribed empirically whilst awaiting the results of microbiological investigation.

Ideally, women with a previous history of meningitis should be seen antenatally by the obstetric anaesthetist for assessment and reassurance. It is important to ascertain whether the meningitis was bacterial or viral as there is some evidence that those women who have had a bacterial meningitis have increased risk of accidental dural puncture (unpublished personal series), especially if the meningitis was caused by tuberculosis, and they can be advised of this risk. In general, most women can be reassured that they are not at extra risk from regional analgesia and anaesthesia.

Key points

- Meningitis is the most important acute neurological infection in obstetrics.
- Meningitis should always be considered in a woman with severe postpartum headache.
- Analysis of cerebrospinal fluid may aid the diagnosis.

Table 111.1. Typical cerebrospinal fluid (CSF) findings in meningitis

	Postdural puncture headache	Viral meningitis	Bacterial meningitis	Aseptic meningitis
CSF	Clear, normal	Clear, normal	May be cloudy	May be cloudy
CSF protein	_	↑	↑	↑
WBC in CSF	_	↑Lymphocytes	↑	↑*
Glucose	Normal	↓	↓	Normal
Culture	Negative	Negative	May be positive	Negative

*Variable, usually leucocytes. WBC; white blood cells.

FURTHER READING

Loo CC, Dahlgren G, Irestedt L. Neurologiacl complications in obstetric regional anaesthesia. *Int J Obstet Anesth* 2000; **9**: 99–124.

Wong CA. Neurological deficits and labor analgesia. *Reg Anesth Pain Med* 2004; **29**: 341–51.

112   ACUTE POST-INFECTIVE PERIPHERAL NEUROPATHY (GUILLAIN–BARRÉ SYNDROME)

Acute post-infective peripheral neuropathy (Guillain–Barré syndrome) is a rare condition that usually follows an acute respiratory infection, although it may follow clostridial diarrhoea or surgery. Recent evidence suggests a slight increase in incidence in the early postpartum period. The symptoms usually commence some days after the infection, which triggers an autoimmune acute demyelinating neuropathy. The first symptoms are peripheral sensory paraesthesiae followed by a loss of motor power. The neuropathy ascends and may affect respiratory muscles. Generally, the disease is short lived, and full recovery is usual over a period of weeks or months.

Problems/special considerations

- Rarely, an acute episode of Guillain–Barré syndrome may occur during pregnancy, when the course may be very rapid. Because of the physiological changes of pregnancy, the respiratory reserve is less than normal, making patients especially prone to respiratory impairment.
- Women with a past history of Guillain–Barré syndrome may present for obstetric analgesia and anaesthesia. The most common clinical problems are:
  - (i) There may be concerns that whether regional analgesia or anaesthesia will cause a recurrence of the disease.
  - (ii) Women are often very frightened about having a needle in their back as they may have had a bad experience with a lumbar puncture during investigation of the acute episode.
  - (iii) Regional anaesthesia or analgesia causing a significant motor block (e.g. when a Caesarean section is performed) may provoke a panic reaction.

Residual neurological impairment is rare after an acute episode.

Management options

Management of the acute illness should take into account the physiological changes of pregnancy and the wellbeing of the growing fetus. Careful monitoring of respiratory function is required, with ventilatory support when necessary. If the mother becomes immobilised it is important to avoid aortocaval compression and to give thromboprophylaxis.

There is no contraindication to regional analgesia or anaesthesia when there is a past history of Guillain–Barré syndrome, and the woman can be reassured that it will not cause a recurrence of the acute episode. The risks and benefits of regional blocks should be discussed before the woman is in pain and preferably at an antenatal consultation. The woman's fears of a motor block need to be considered by the anaesthetist, particularly if she has required ventilation for her acute illness. If there is any neurological deficit this should be assessed and documented before a regional anaesthetic is performed.

Considerable reassurance by the anaesthetist may be required.

Key points

- Acute Guillain–Barré syndrome is rare in pregnancy.
- Antenatal assessment of women with a previous history of Guillain–Barré syndrome is advisable since they may be very worried about regional analgesia and anaesthesia.
- Regional analgesia and anaesthesia is not contraindicated.

FURTHER READING

Brooks H, Christian AS, May AE. Pregnancy, anaesthesia and Guillane–Barré syndrome. Case Report. *Anaesthesia* 2000; **55**: 894–8.

Chan LY, Tsui MH, Leung TN. Guillain–Barré syndrome in pregnancy. *Acta Obstet Gynecol Scand* 2004; **83**: 319–25.

113   PAST HISTORY OF NEUROLOGICAL TRAUMA

It is not uncommon for patients with previous head or spinal cord injury to become pregnant. Many of these women will seek preconceptual advice, but others will present in the antenatal period.

Problems/special considerations

The extent of the problems depends on the neurological deficit. For head-injured patients, the main concerns are related to:

- The presence of upper motor neurone lesions (causing difficulties with positioning and mobility; possible hyperkalaemic response to suxamethonium)
- Immobility (increasing the risk of thromboembolism, pressure sores and atelectasis following general anaesthesia)
- Any associated injuries, especially neck (affecting the airway) and pelvis or vertebral column (affecting mode of delivery and regional analgesia/anaesthesia)
- Difficulties in communication.

For spinal cord injured patients, the above concerns may also exist. The level of the neurological deficit is the most important issue; the major considerations are:

- *Pulmonary function and the effect of pregnancy and delivery:* if the level is above T4, there is likely to be some reduction in respiratory reserve. The phrenic nerve supply to the diaphragm arises from cervical roots 3–5 so this is usually spared in paraplegics; however, the intercostal nerves which contribute to ventilation and which may be particularly important in pregnancy will be affected.
- *Risk of autonomic hyperreflexia:* this is associated with injuries above T4–6 and results in increased sensitivity of sympathetic reflexes in response to cutaneous or visceral stimulation below the level of the lesion. There is resultant labile blood pressure, typically causing massive vasoconstriction and hypertension associated with high levels of circulating catecholamines; there may be a compensatory bradycardia. Susceptibility usually develops within a few weeks of injury.
- *Mode of delivery:* a sensory level above T10 is usually associated with a painless labour and these women are also more likely to deliver prematurely. This may result in a painless precipitate delivery. Some of these women will suffer from muscle spasms and many will need an assisted delivery.

Management options

These women should be seen antenatally and any neurological deficit carefully assessed. When the delivery is planned, the above points should be taken into consideration, with epidural analgesia part of the management in most cases.

Epidural analgesia has been shown to be effective in prophylaxis and treatment of autonomic hyperreflexia. The epidural should be carefully managed to minimise any cardiovascular changes, and a low concentration of local anaesthetic combined with an opioid is usually considered the method of choice, although the need for more concentrated local anaesthetic has been suggested in order to block the powerful afferent triggers of autonomic hyperreflexia. Autonomic hyperreflexia is difficult to treat pharmacologically, and the use of α- and β-blocking drugs and nifedipine are of limited value. The use of magnesium sulphate has been described, although experience is limited.

Regional anaesthesia is the anaesthetic of choice for operative delivery in most cases. If general anaesthesia is used, alternatives to suxamethonium should be considered if within the period of risk of hyperkalaemia (10 days to 6–7 months). Care must be taken to avoid autonomic hyperreflexia, and deep anaesthesia is needed.

Key points

- Each patient requires individual assessments of her neurological deficit and associated injuries in order to estimate her risk factors.
- Regional analgesia and anaesthesia is indicated in most cases.
- Autonomic hyperreflexia is best prevented or controlled by epidural block.

FURTHER READING

Crosby E, St-Jean B, Reid D, Elliott RD. Obstetrical anesthesia and analgesia in chronic spinal cord injured women. *Can J Anaesth* 1992; **39**: 487–94.

Greenspoon S, Paul RH. Paraplegia and quadriplegia: special considerations during pregnancy and labour and delivery. *Am J Obstet Gynecol* 1986; **155**: 738–41.

114   BENIGN INTRACRANIAL HYPERTENSION

Benign intracranial hypertension (pseudotumour cerebri) is defined as raised intracranial pressure that is not associated with intracranial pathology. It is a rare but well-recognised syndrome that generally affects young to middle-aged overweight females, causing headache and visual disturbances. The aetiology is unclear and there are no focal neurological signs.

Problems/special considerations

- There may be fear of puncturing the dura in someone with raised cerebrospinal fluid (CSF) pressure. However, dural puncture (deliberate or accidental) will not lead to coning in this group of patients and it may even be temporarily beneficial in relieving CSF pressure.
- The epidural space may be compressed by the increased pressure of CSF within the dural sac. Theoretically, spinal anaesthetic solutions may not spread in the normal way in the presence of benign intracranial hypertension. If epidural analgesia or anaesthesia is performed, the increased pressure in the epidural space often leads to an increased spread so that a block may extend much higher than would be expected. This is particularly relevant if the block is to be extended for a Caesarean section. Spinal anaesthesia may be potentially difficult as the CSF is under pressure, and drainage of some CSF may be needed before injection of the local anaesthetic.
- Headache and visual disturbances may also occur in pre-eclampsia and postdural puncture headache, possibly causing confusion.

Management options

General treatment is to advise weight loss and if necessary to prescribe diuretics. In more severe cases, lumbar puncture and the removal of CSF may be recommended. Insertion of lumboperitoneal shunts and optic nerve sheath decompression have been performed in very severe cases.

There is no reason that these women should not be given appropriate regional analgesia or anaesthesia. There need be no anxiety about accidental dural puncture. Because of the relatively benign nature of the disease, general anaesthesia is not contraindicated, although peaks of raised intracranial pressure are to be avoided.

> **Key points**
>
> • Benign intracranial hypertension may present with severe headache and visual disturbances.
> • Regional analgesia and anaesthesia (including spinal block) are not contraindicated.

FURTHER READING

Bedard JM, Richardson MG, Wissler RN. Epidural anesthesia in a parturient with a lumboperitoneal shunt. *Anesthesiology* 1999; **90**: 621–3.

Bedson CR, Plaat F. Benign intracranial hypertension and anaesthesia for caesarean section. *Int J Obstet Anesth* 1999; **8**: 288–90.

115   INTRACRANIAL TUMOUR

A tumour may present during pregnancy or labour; the obstetric anaesthetist may be involved in looking after a woman with acutely raised intracranial pressure (ICP) or in the diagnosis of the tumour in the peripartum period. Women may also present with a previous history of intracranial tumour.

Problems/special considerations

Tumour diagnosed during pregnancy

Particular problems may be related to:

• The nature of the tumour
• The treatment the patient is receiving, e.g. steroids
• Whether there is raised ICP, how severe it is and whether there is an associated risk of coning
• The effect of pushing in the second stage of labour on ICP and the tumour
• The presence of any other medical problems
• The risks of regional analgesia or anaesthesia and general anaesthesia.

Tumour manifesting itself in the peripartum period

The woman may present with neurological signs or symptoms that may be related to the position of the tumour or to the development of raised ICP. The obstetric anaesthetist may be asked to see the woman, particularly if she had a regional anaesthetic and the symptoms arose in the postpartum period.

The patient may present with altered consciousness, focal signs, a fit or a headache. The differential diagnosis will include eclampsia, epilepsy, meningitis and postdural puncture headache. The headache associated with raised ICP is usually present when the patient is supine and does not have the same postural changes as a postdural puncture headache. The headache will be made worse by stooping, coughing or straining. The associated symptoms and signs of photophobia, vomiting and neck stiffness may be present both in raised ICP and following dural puncture.

Previous history of tumour

There may be residual neurological impairment, as for a past history of neurological trauma. A small number of women have residual tumour left and this may be affected by the pregnancy. There may be a shunt to maintain normal cerebrospinal fluid (CSF) pressures. Generally, these shunts drain from the brain into the peritoneal cavity; however, some drain CSF around the spinal cord into the peritoneum. The latter may be placed in the lumbar region and thus cause a problem if regional block is to be considered. The risk of introducing infection at the time of a regional block is very small but may be a deterrent to regional block in these women. Many patients will be particularly anxious about the effects of both regional and general anaesthesia on their neurological function.

Management options

If a tumour has been diagnosed during pregnancy, the obstetric anaesthetist should be consulted about the management of the labour. It is generally accepted that the delivery should be as stress free as possible, and normally regional analgesia would be part of the management. The benefits of regional anaesthesia for these patients must be balanced against an accidental dural puncture causing coning. If epidural analgesia is considered to be the best management, a senior anaesthetist should be involved. Pushing in the second stage should be minimised to reduce the possibility of bleeding into the tumour. If the patient is suffering from a significant increase in ICP and the obstetrician advises urgent delivery, Caesarean section under general anaesthesia may be the technique of choice. General anaesthesia may need to be modified to give a 'neuro' anaesthetic that would minimise raised ICP at the time of induction of anaesthesia. It is important to remember that decreased arterial partial pressure of carbon dioxide from the normal value in pregnancy (approximately 4 kPa) in the mother will reduce placental perfusion and this may compromise the fetus.

When new headaches, convulsions or other neurological symptoms and signs present in the peripartum period, it is easy to assume more common conditions such as postdural puncture headache and eclampsia rather than think of intracranial tumour. A careful history and examination (where appropriate by a neurologist) is important in reaching the correct diagnosis. Magnetic resonance imaging and/or computerised tomography should be considered. Once diagnosed, treatment is as for any non-pregnant patient.

The majority of women who have had previous intracranial tumours are entirely normal and have no residual problems. Neurological advice will be necessary to know if the pregnancy will affect any residual tumour. Examination of the medical records and discussion with the neurosurgeon is wise.

Key points

- Regional analgesia is usually indicated during labour, but an accidental dural puncture may be catastrophic; thus the decision should depend on the individual features of each case.
- Underlying intracerebral pathology should always be considered when new symptoms or signs present postpartum.
- A neurologist should be consulted if in doubt.

FURTHER READING

Chang L, Looi Lyons L, Bartosik L, Tindal S. Anaesthesia for cesarean section in two patients with brain tumours. *Can J Anaesth* 1999; **46**: 61–5.

Dutton DA. A 'postspinal headache' associated with incidental intracranial pathology. *Anaesthesia* 1991; **46**: 1044–6.

Finfer SR. Management of labour and delivery in patients with intracranial neoplasms. *Br J Anaesth* 1991; **67**: 784–7.

116   CEREBROVASCULAR ACCIDENT

Cerebrovascular accidents (CVAs) may occur during pregnancy and delivery and may be due to intracranial haemorrhage or thrombosis. The Confidential Enquiry into Child and Maternal Health 2000–02 describes 21 deaths caused by intracranial haemorrhage, 17 due to subarachnoid haemorrhage and 4 due to intracerebral haemorrhage. Four deaths were caused by cerebral thrombosis.

Problems/special considerations

CVA presenting during pregnancy or peripartum

Pregnancy and labour in themselves increase the risk of CVAs. This risk will be further increased if there is associated obesity, smoking or hypertensive disease of pregnancy.

- *Intracerebral haemorrhage:* this may occur at any stage during the pregnancy, including the peripartum period. The most common problem is subarachnoid haemorrhage (SAH), which presents as an acute onset of severe headache, often with associated neck stiffness, photophobia and vomiting. There may be loss of consciousness. SAH is often associated with an underlying berry aneurysm or arteriovenous malformation and is also a cause of death associated with pre-eclampsia.
- *Cerebral thrombosis:* pregnancy predisposes to cerebral thrombosis, including cortical vein thrombosis. Other predisposing factors include dehydration and other hypercoagulable states (e.g. thrombophilias). Although cortical vein thrombosis is rare, it is important to the obstetric anaesthetist in the differential diagnosis of postdural puncture headache. The patient may present with focal neurological signs or signs of raised intracranial pressure.

Sudden collapse carries the risk of airway obstruction and hypoxaemia, aspiration of gastric contents, aortocaval compression and fetal compromise. As for many acute medical emergencies in the maternity suite, staff may be unfamiliar with basic resuscitative measures unless these are regularly practised.

Previous history of CVA

The most common presentation in the child-bearing age group is a previous history of SAH. Some of these women will have made a complete recovery and others will have a neurological deficit of which the anaesthetist should be aware. They may be very frightened by the thought of a needle in their back after a bad experience with lumbar puncture. There may be an exaggerated hyperkalaemic response to suxamethonium 10 days to 6–7 months after CVA. Women with a previous cerebral thrombosis may be taking heparin or aspirin.

Management options

If there is loss of consciousness, basic resuscitation must be performed, with particular attention to uterine displacement and avoidance of aspiration of vomit. There is a significant risk of rebleeding following SAH; therefore assessment by neurosurgeons with a view to surgical treatment is essential. The indication for surgical intervention should not be altered by the fact that the woman is pregnant. The risk of SAH is one reason for ensuring adequate blood pressure control in pre-eclampsia, particularly in the peripartum period.

Management of delivery depends on the clinical condition of the patient, who may still have a significant neurological deficit. If the patient is well recovered, a stress-free vaginal delivery with epidural analgesia is the management of choice, taking care to avoid significant fluctuations in blood pressure. The indications for Caesarean section should only be obstetric. However, if the patient is confused or has a problem with cognitive function, the wisest course of action may be delivery by Caesarean section under general anaesthesia. General anaesthesia should be carefully managed to minimise the hypertensive response to tracheal intubation. Each patient will need to be considered individually in consultation with the obstetrician and neurosurgeons and other disciplines where appropriate. Combined Caesarean section and neurosurgery has been performed.

Diagnosis of CVA is by computerised tomography or magnetic resonance imaging of the brain; if the diagnosis is suspected, it is wise to involve the neurologists early. Although the use of lumbar puncture has largely been superseded by imaging techniques for the diagnosis of SAH, partly because of the risk of coning if intracranial pressure is increased, lumbar puncture may still have a place in selected cases.

The management of women with previous SAH depends on whether the underlying pathology has been surgically treated. If so, the woman can be regarded as relatively normal. The risk of a further bleed is increased if there is hypertension and in particular if there are sudden surges in blood pressure. The control of blood pressure and the avoidance of stress during labour or delivery are therefore important. Generally, regional analgesia should be recommended for labour. If a Caesarean section is required, regional anaesthesia is appropriate. No regional technique should be performed without a detailed discussion with the woman, and this ideally should take place in the antenatal period, when a plan for the management of analgesia and anaesthesia should be written in her notes. If general anaesthesia is necessary, the hypertensive response to intubation should be modified and alternatives to suxamethonium used if within the period of risk.

Rarely, CVA (usually subdural or subarachnoid haemorrhage) has followed spinal anaesthesia or accidental dural puncture.

Key points

- Control of blood pressure in hypertension is important in pregnancy, whether or not it is pregnancy related.
- Headaches are not always due to dural puncture.
- Pregnancy is not a contraindication to neurosurgery.
- Regional analgesia or anaesthesia is usually indicated unless there is significant neurological impairment.

FURTHER READING

Eggert SM, Eggers, KA. Subarachnoid haemorrhage following spinal anaesthesia in an obstetric patient. *Br J Anaesth* 2001; **86**: 442–4.

James AH, Bushnell CD, Jamison MG, Myers ER. Incidence and risk factors for stroke in pregnancy and the puerperium. *Obstet Gynecol* 2005; **106**: 509–16.

Levy DM, Jaspan T. Anaesthesia for Caesarean section in a patient with recent subarachnoid haemorrhage and severe pre-eclampsia. *Anaesthesia* 1999; **54**: 994–9.

Witlin AG, Mattar F, Sibai BM. Postpartum stroke: a twenty-year experience. *Am J Obstet Gynecol* 2000; **183**: 83–8.

117   EPILEPSY

Epilepsy is the most common neurological disease: it is estimated that 2–5% of the population have suffered a fit in the past and around 0.5–1% of the population suffer from epilepsy. Therefore pregnancy and epilepsy may commonly coexist. However, fits may develop for the first time in pregnancy and cause a problem in differential diagnosis.

Problems/special considerations

- *Pre-existing epilepsy:* it is generally accepted that epilepsy is affected by the hormonal changes of pregnancy and that the frequency of fits may increase during pregnancy. If the woman has not sought advice before conception, it is possible that she may stop her medication as she may be worried about teratogentic effects on the fetus. In addition, the pharmacodynamics and pharmacokinetics of antiepileptic drugs may be affected by the physiological changes of pregnancy. Both hyperventilation and the pain and stress of labour may trigger a fit.

In recent Reports on Confidential Enquiries into Maternal Deaths/Maternal and Child Health, epilepsy (especially poorly controlled) has been a major factor in deaths from neurological disease, frequently associated with drowning in the bath.

- *Convulsions occurring in pregnancy:* these may present immediate problems, including aortocaval compression, hypoxaemia, cerebrovascular accident and aspiration of gastric contents. In addition, differential diagnosis may include a number of conditions both related and unrelated to pregnancy.

Management options

Ideally, the woman with diagnosed epilepsy should have had counselling before pregnancy to discuss the management of her epilepsy during pregnancy. Preconception planning aims to simplify the drug regimen, and medication may be stopped in a woman who has been fit free for a long time.

During pregnancy, normal medication should be maintained. This may necessitate alternative routes of administration when gastric absorption is affected. The risks and benefits of changing the treatment requires specialist advice for each individual. It is important to remember the effects of pregnancy on the pharmacodynamics and pharmacokinetics of the antiepileptic drugs and the regular monitoring of drug levels during pregnancy is useful.

When carefully managed, the woman with epilepsy does not usually experience problems during pregnancy and most can be offered any form of pain relief that they wish. The poorly controlled epileptic will benefit from epidural analgesia to reduce the stress of labour and hyperventilation. General anaesthesia is not a greater problem in these women, and thiopental remains a good anticonvulsant.

Convulsions are managed in the normal way, taking into account the risk of aortocaval compression and aspiration of gastric contents (see Chapter 122, Convulsions, p. 280).

Key points

- Epilepsy is the commonest neurological disease.
- Eclampsia is not the only cause of convulsions in pregnancy.
- Epilepsy may become poorly controlled in pregnancy.
- Management of the well-controlled epileptic is as for normal women.

FURTHER READING

Morrell MJ. Guidelines for the care of women with epilepsy. *Neurology* 1998; **51** (suppl. 4): S21–S27.

Sabers A, a'Rogvi-Hansen B, Dam M, *et al.* Pregnancy and epilepsy: a retrospective study of 151 pregnancies. *Acta Neurol Scand* 1998; **97**: 164–70.

Zahn CA, Morrell MJ, Collins SD, Labiner DM, Yerby MS. Management issues for women with epilepsy: a review of the literature. *Neurology* 1998; **51**: 949–56.

118   MIGRAINE

The classic presentation of migraine is with a paroxysmal unilateral headache preceded by visual and sensory phenomena, accompanied by or followed by nausea and vomiting. Migraine may present for the first time in or shortly after pregnancy.

Problems/special considerations

- Migraine often improves in pregnancy. However, many women are anxious about how labour and the pain-relieving drugs given in labour will affect them and seek advice as to whether regional analgesia is a problem.
- Many drugs used for migraine cross the placenta, and therapy may need altering during pregnancy.
- Stress, including pain and starvation, can precipitate an attack of migraine.
- An acute migraine attack presenting with severe headache and visual disturbances may be confused with pre-eclampsia. Rarely, migraine may be associated with other neurological symptoms.
- In the postpartum period, migraine may be confused with postdural puncture headache (PDPH); indeed, the cerebral vasodilation, which is thought to cause the headache of migraine, may in part be responsible for the headache that follows dural puncture.

Management options

There is no contraindication to epidural or spinal analgesia or anaesthesia.

Migraine can usually be easily distinguished from PDPH. In migraine, the headache is usually unilateral and frontal whereas in PDPH the headache is usually bilateral, occipital and frontal. The dramatic improvement in PDPH on lying down is not present with migraine. New onset severe headache should always alert medical staff to the possibility of other underlying conditions (see Chapter 44, Postdural puncture headache, p. 114).

Key points

- Migraine is common but often improves during pregnancy.
- Migraine may resemble pre-eclampsia and postdural puncture headache.
- Anaesthetic management is routine.

119   MULTIPLE SCLEROSIS

Multiple sclerosis is a disease of unknown aetiology in which the clinical symptoms are caused by patches of damage to the myelin sheath of the central, but not peripheral, neurones. The onset of the disease is generally between the ages of 20 and 40 years and it is usually a disease of relapse and remission.

The incidence of the disease is around 110 per 100 000 in the UK and it is more common in females (two out of three patients will be female). Therefore it is not uncommon in women who present for obstetric care. The rate of relapse may decrease during pregnancy and the latter is usually well tolerated, although the rate of relapse may increase in the first three months postpartum before returning to the basal rate.

Problems/special considerations

- Many anaesthetists feel reluctant to perform regional analgesia in these women since a relapse may occur after a stressful event such as delivery of a baby. The regional anaesthetic may then erroneously be blamed. Previous studies have suggested an increased incidence of relapse if higher concentrations of bupivacaine are used, although more recent evidence has not confirmed this.
- Women who are very disabled may have impairment of laryngeal reflexes and ventilation. They also may be unable to position themselves for regional blockade and may be physically unable to achieve a vaginal delivery without assistance.
- Women will be concerned about any possible effect of regional analgesia and anaesthesia on their disease.

Management options

Antenatal counselling is advised if possible, to enable a plan for analgesia and anaesthesia to be drawn up and documented in the mother's notes. Time should be taken to discuss the risks and benefits of regional techniques so that the woman may give informed consent where appropriate. It is difficult to discuss such problems effectively when she is in pain and in labour.

There is no logical reason why these women should not have regional analgesia and there may be benefits in reducing the stress of labour that is caused by pain. Where practical, it is good practice to assess the neurological deficit before performing a regional block and to maintain as much motor power as possible. Similarly, both spinal and epidural anaesthesia are suitable if Caesarean section is necessary. If general anaesthesia is used, standard techniques are used.

Key points

- Antenatal consultation is the gold standard to ensure informed consent.
- Epidural analgesia should not be denied in labour.
- Relapse is not more common with than without regional anaesthesia.
- Routine techniques are used, taking into account any pre-existing neurological deficit.

FURTHER READING

Confavreux C, Hutchinson M, Hours MM, *et al.* Rate of pregnancy-related relapse in multiple sclerosis. *NEJM* 1998; **339**: 285–91.

Lorenzi AR, Ford HL. Multiple sclerosis and pregnancy. *Postgrad Med J* 2002; **78**: 460–4.

Whitaker JN. Effects of pregnancy and delivery on disease activity in multiple sclerosis. *N Engl J Med* 1998; **339**: 339–40.

---

120   MYASTHENIA GRAVIS

Myasthenia gravis is an autoimmune disease affecting the neuromuscular junction, at which circulating antibodies compete with acetylcholine. It has an incidence of around 1 per 100 000. It is more common in females, with an onset at any age. The muscles that are most commonly involved are the oculomotor, facial, pharyngeal and respiratory. The weakness of the muscles is improved by rest. The effect of pregnancy on the disease is variable.

The disease is treated with acetylcholinesterase inhibitor therapy. The treatment of choice is pyridostigmine in a dose range of 30–120 mg orally at regular intervals through the day. The side effects of treatment may include bradycardia, sweating and increased salivary secretion.

Problems/special considerations

- As with many neurological diseases, women with myasthenia gravis may be very worried about regional analgesia and anaesthesia and any adverse effect on their disease.
- Myasthenia gravis is generally made worse by stress, physical exertion, minor infections and fatigue. During labour an increase in weakness can be expected. In severe disease there is a risk of respiratory insufficiency and aspiration of gastric contents, which may thus increase as labour progresses.

- Maternal expulsive efforts may be markedly reduced at the end of labour, increasing the need for instrumental delivery.
- Requirements for acetylcholinesterase inhibitors may be difficult to estimate during labour because of worsening weakness and possibly reduced gastric absorption of oral pyridostigmine (especially if opioids have been administered). Inadequate dosage may lead to severe weakness (myasthenic crisis), whereas overdosage with acetylcholinesterase inhibitors may lead to a cholinergic crisis (muscle weakness and fasciculation, sweating, miosis, lacrimation, abdominal colic, etc.).
- There is increased sensitivity to non-depolarising neuromuscular blocking drugs, with the risk of prolonged neuromuscular blockade during and after general anaesthesia. Resistance to suxamethonium has been reported, although most authorities recommend a normal dose. Magnesium sulphate worsens muscle weakness.
- Placental transfer of maternal antibodies may cause neonatal myasthenia.

Management options

There should be a team approach to the management of women with myasthenia gravis during the antenatal period. The extent of her muscle weakness and whether this affects the bulbar and respiratory muscles should be carefully assessed. The variable effect of pregnancy on the disease means that the mother will need constant monitoring of her disease. Treatment will need to be adjusted to maintain muscle strength, and pulmonary function tests may be useful in assessing the strength of the respiratory muscles.

The mode of delivery should be decided on obstetric grounds, taking into account the severity of the illness and the ability of the woman to tolerate the work of labour.

Regional analgesia is advisable, to minimise the stress of labour and to avoid the sedative effects of pethidine or Entonox. If opioids have not been given, gastric function can be considered to be near-normal and oral medication continued. If in doubt in severe cases, equivalent doses of parenteral acetylcholinesterase inhibitors can be given (Table 120.1). Atropine should also be given to reduce unwanted cholinergic effects. If in doubt over whether worsening weakness

Table 120.1. Oral and parenteral acetylcholinesterase inhibitors (all the following dosages are equivalent in clinical effect)

Neostigmine:	15 mg orally
	0.7–1.0 mg i.m.
	0.5 mg i.v.
Pyridostigmine:	60 mg
	3–4 mg i.m.
	2 mg i.v.

represents a myasthenic or cholinergic crisis, edrophonium 2 mg intravenously will improve the former but worsen or have no effect on the latter.

In well-controlled myasthenia gravis, Caesarean section may be performed under regional anaesthesia. If the disease is not well controlled, the risk of aspiration and respiratory impairment with a high regional block must be weighed against the risks of respiratory impairment following general anaesthesia. Non-depolarising neuromuscular blocking drugs are usually not necessary. Following general anaesthesia, mothers may require postoperative ventilation until their medication is reintroduced and their muscle power has returned to normal.

Key points

- Team management is essential.
- Regular monitoring of muscle strength throughout pregnancy is essential.
- Oral medication can be continued throughout labour unless the disease is very severe and gastric function is in doubt, when parenteral medication may be substituted.
- Both myasthenic and cholinergic crises may occur.
- Regional analgesia and anaesthesia is indicated in most cases.

FURTHER READING

Batocchi AP, Majolini L, Evoli A, *et al.* Course and treatment of myasthenia gravis during pregnancy. *Neurology* 1999; **52**: 447–52.

D'Angelo R, Gerancher JC. Combined spinal and epidural analgesia in a parturient with severe myasthenia gravis. *Reg Anesth Pain Med* 1998; **23**: 201–3.

121   SPINA BIFIDA

Spina bifida is a congenital neural tube defect with a spectrum of severity. Neural tube defects in survivable form are estimated to occur in 3 in 1000 live births, of whom 60% will survive the first year of life. Many of these will have a significant neurological deficit, in spite of which they will strive to achieve as normal a lifestyle as possible; for women this includes pregnancy and childbirth. Spina bifida is generally categorised as occulta and cystica:

- *Spina bifida occulta:* its reported incidence is between 5% and 20% of the population and it is not associated with a neurological deficit. It may only be discovered incidentally on radiography or when a woman presents for regional analgesia. It is a vertebral defect and occurs when the two halves of the vertebral arch fail to fuse.
- *Spina bifida cystica:* this is a collective term for the more severe forms of spina bifida. Common to all these malformations is a sac-like protrusion through the defect in the vertebral arch. The neurological deficit depends on the severity and level of the defect and, to an extent, on the effect of subsequent surgery.

Problems/special considerations

Pregnancy in women with spina bifida can prove to be a serious challenge to both obstetric and anaesthetic staff, depending on both the severity of the neurological deficit and any associated skeletal abnormality:

- Kyphoscoliosis and pelvic distortion may make vaginal delivery difficult.
- There may be an intraventricular shunt to maintain normal cerebrospinal fluid pressure.
- There is an increased risk of accidental dural puncture, particularly when the needle is inserted at the level of the defect.
- The spinal cord may be tethered, with risk of neurological injury.
- There is a risk of abnormal spread of local anaesthetic resulting in either excessive cranial spread or inadequate sacral spread.
- There is often anxiety regarding the conduct of regional anaesthesia, particularly in patients with an established neural deficit.
- If Caesarean section is required, surgery may be difficult because of previous urological surgery, such as ileal conduit.
- Latex allergy is more common in patients with spina bifida cystica.

Management options

Women who have spina bifida occulta usually have no neurological deficit and may be offered regional analgesia or anaesthesia when appropriate. Ideally, they should be seen by the anaesthetist in the antenatal period when the risks of regional anaesthesia can be assessed and explained. Cord tethering is unlikely in the absence of any neurological symptoms, in which case imaging is of little value. Occasionally, spina bifida occulta may only be discovered incidentally during siting the epidural/spinal, but this is not a reason to deny appropriate analgesia or anaesthesia. The above considerations should be taken into account.

In spina bifida cystica, there may be significant neurological deficit, including skeletal abnormalities and impairment of bladder and bowel function. Some women may be wheelchair bound. The aim is to achieve as normal a pregnancy and labour as possible for the individual; for this, effective antenatal consultation and team planning is essential in order that all the options for delivery are discussed and documented. Before regional analgesia is contemplated, baseline clinical findings should be documented in the records, including neurological assessment and where possible pre-existing spinal and pelvic X-ray films (pelvic radiography in pregnancy may not be advisable). The neurological examination is helpful in assessing whether the pain pathways of labour are intact and how regional analgesia can be used to help in labour and delivery. Many women may have been told that they will not feel the pain of labour because of their pre-existing sensory deficit. However, this ignores the fact that most are neurologically intact above the lower lumber segments and therefore they will experience the normal pain of the first stage of labour, although it is true that the pain of the second stage may be modified.

For analgesia in labour, epidural analgesia is generally not contraindicated. However, siting the epidural may be difficult and it is advisable to insert it above the defect and/or the scar from previous surgery. The woman should be warned of the increased risk of dural tap and inadequate block. Because of the latter, a combined epidural–spinal may be indicated.

For Caesarean section, regional anaesthesia is acceptable. Spinal anaesthesia may be more predictable than epidural anaesthesia, particularly for spread of the block to the sacral roots. Normal volumes of subarachnoid injectate may be used. However, depending on the complexity of the previous surgery and the wishes of the women, some may opt for general anaesthesia. This usually poses no particular problems, although tracheal intubation may be difficult in some patients with kyphoscoliosis. These patients have a normal response to suxamethonium.

Key points

- Antenatal assessment is important.
- Regional analgesia or anaesthesia may be difficult but should not be denied.
- Women should be warned of the risks of accidental dural tap and inadequate block.
- Spinal anaesthesia may be preferable to epidural anaesthesia for Caesarean section.

FURTHER READING

Anderson KJ, Quinlan MJ, Popat M, Russell R. Failed intubation in a parturient with spina bifida. *Int J Obstet Anesth* 2000; **9**: 64–8.

Tidmarsh MD, May AE. Epidural anaesthesia and neural tube defects. *Int J Obstet Anesth* 1998; **7**: 111–14.

122   CONVULSIONS

Convulsions occurring ante-, peri- or postpartum are uncommon but important causes of collapse on the labour ward; they may herald significant maternal disease or reflect a transient disturbance, but in either case management must be prompt and appropriate. Although petit mal (absence seizures) and focal seizures may occur, they are less common in the maternity suite than grand mal (tonic–clonic seizures).

Problems/special considerations

- Diagnosis may be uncertain if not witnessed by an experienced observer; e.g. a simple faint may be labelled as a 'fit'. A history of a tonic–clonic seizure may not always be obtained. Furthermore, collapse from non-neurological causes may themselves lead to convulsions if severe hypotension or hypoxaemia occurs.

Table 122.1. Causes of convulsions on the labour ward

Neurological disease	Pre-existing epilepsy
	Stroke
	Cerebral vein thrombosis
	Infection
	Migraine
	Incidental disease, e.g. tumours
Hypoxaemia	Cardiovascular collapse, e.g. haemorrhage
	Pulmonary embolus
Obstetric	Eclampsia
	Amniotic fluid embolism
Metabolic	Hypoglycaemia
	Hypocalcaemia
	Hyponatraemia*
	Uraemia
Drugs	Anaesthetic, e.g. local anaesthetics, possibly propofol
	Others, e.g. cocaine intoxication, overdoses, acute withdrawal (including alcohol)

*Hyponatraemia is especially important in the delivery suite, where it may follow prolonged infusion of oxytocin diluted in dextrose solutions.

- Physiological effects include increased cerebral and whole body oxygen requirement, with increased carbon dioxide production. Together with hypoventilation arising from airway obstruction and chest wall rigidity, this may result in hypoxaemia, acidosis, hypercapnia and increased sympathetic activity. These effects may be exacerbated by the increased cardiac output and metabolic requirements of the pregnant woman compared with the non-pregnant one. Convulsions in pregnancy may be more likely to lead to stroke than in the non-pregnant state. Aortocaval compression further exacerbates the situation before delivery. If inadequately treated, convulsions may merge into each other without breaks in between (status epilepticus).
- As for collapse generally, the labour ward staff may be less familiar with emergency equipment and drugs than staff elsewhere. Although most of the possible causes of convulsions are the same as outside of the maternity suite (Table 122.1), the emphasis is different in this setting.

Management options

Initial management includes avoidance of aortocaval compression, protection of the airway (remembering the risk of aspiration) and support of the ventilation and circulation.

The differential diagnosis (Table 122.1) is usually one of exclusion; the initial task is to distinguish between a primary convulsion and one resulting from hypoxaemia and/or cardiovascular collapse, hence the importance of a careful history from the patient and observer(s). Since eclampsia is such an important and relatively common cause in the peripartum period, it should be assumed until proven otherwise. Although 'pre-eclampsia screening' investigations are commonly performed, eclampsia may precede other evidence of pre-eclampsia. Baseline laboratory investigations should be done and computerised tomography/magnetic resonance imaging scan of the head is generally advised unless a clear history of epilepsy is obtained. Blood gas analysis may be useful in guiding management but not in the differential diagnosis; it may reveal marked metabolic and respiratory acidosis resulting from the seizure itself, although this may also represent cardiorespiratory collapse preceding the convulsion. Hypoxaemia may be apparent if aspiration has occurred. Further investigations are guided by the results of preliminary testing and the clinical course.

Drug treatment is with standard anticonvulsant drugs (e.g. diazepam 5–10 mg boluses intravenously; phenytoin 10–15 mg/kg slowly intravenously, preferably with electrocardiographic monitoring), although magnesium sulphate has been shown to be more effective in preventing recurrent eclamptic fits and should be the first choice unless eclampsia can be excluded. Thiopental, tracheal intubation and controlled ventilation may be required if convulsions are severe and continuous; however, this does prevent further neurological assessment.

Fetal monitoring should not be forgotten. Once control of the fits has been achieved, delivery should be considered, depending on the aetiology of the convulsions, the gestation and the state of the mother and fetus. In eclampsia, delivery is usually indicated as soon as the stability of the mother allows.

Key points

- Convulsions on the labour ward should be considered as eclampsia until proven otherwise, although other causes should not be forgotten.
- Immediate management is with support of the airway, breathing and circulation and avoidance of aortocaval compression; magnesium sulphate is the treatment of choice in eclampsia to prevent further convulsions.

---

123   RESPIRATORY DISEASE

An increasing number of women with respiratory disease are becoming pregnant; the incidence of asthma is increasing, and more women with chronic conditions such as cystic fibrosis are surviving into reproductive life.

Problems/special considerations

Both primarily obstructive and primarily restrictive disease may be exacerbated by the increased respiratory demands of pregnancy (although asthma often improves in pregnancy), with further worsening in labour. In addition, the physiological changes of pregnancy may further hinder respiratory function, in particular airway oedema, upward displacement of the diaphragm and reduced functional residual capacity. It is also important to remember the increased risk factors associated with obesity, smoking and kyphoscoliosis, any of which may complicate the underlying respiratory condition.

Management options

The clinician must be familiar with the physiological changes of pregnancy in the respiratory system in order to understand the relevant pathophysiology. Early antenatal assessment of the woman, including pulmonary function tests, is essential. Ideally, this should be in the first trimester. If the condition is severe, preconception counselling may be advisable. The effect of the pregnancy and delivery may then be assessed in light of the physiological changes of pregnancy and the respiratory stresses of delivery. Specifically, pulmonary function tests will give an idea of how the mother might cope with labour.

Women with mild disease can be treated as normal. In more severe disease, regional analgesia and anaesthesia is usually indicated to reduce the stress and demands of labour. Continuous pulse oximetry is advisable throughout labour. If operative delivery is required, regional techniques avoid the depressant effects of general anaesthetic drugs but care must be taken in the case of high regional blocks.

Key points

- Respiratory disease may be exacerbated by the physiological changes of pregnancy and the increased demands of the fetus.
- Careful antenatal assessment is important.
- Regional analgesia and anaesthesia is usually indicated.

124 ASTHMA

Asthma is defined as reversible airways obstruction characterised by the narrowing of the small and large airways. This is caused by spasm in the smooth muscle, oedema of the bronchial wall, inflammation in the mucosa and mucous plugging. Patients with asthma have hyperreactive bronchi and are sensitive to a variety of external and internal stimuli.

Asthma is one of the most common diseases in the UK, with a prevalence of 15% in children and 10% in adults. Its incidence is increasing. Asthma is thus the most common respiratory condition seen in pregnancy, occurring in approximately 1% of pregnant women. Of these, around 10% will need hospital admission for an acute exacerbation.

Anaesthetists may be involved in looking after women who have an exacerbation of their asthma during pregnancy or when in the delivery suite.

Problems/special considerations

- In pregnancy, asthma usually improves from the first trimester, an effect thought to be caused by progesterone and cortisol. However, in the first trimester the respiratory centres are reset and this causes hyperventilation, which may cause anxiety in the asthmatic patient, who is more aware of a change in her breathing pattern.
- In severe cases, patients may be taking a number of bronchodilator and anti-inflammatory drugs, including steroids.
- Stress, especially pain and anxiety, may precipitate an acute exacerbation.
- The increased demands of pregnancy make mothers more vulnerable to acute exacerbations of asthma. During an acute attack, physicians not accustomed to the assessment of pregnant patients may misinterpret blood gas results, e.g. by not appreciating that an arterial partial pressure of carbon dioxide of 5.5–6.0 is grossly abnormal.
- Both maternal and neonatal complications are more common in mothers with asthma, especially if poorly controlled.
- Pethidine has been implicated in worsening asthma because of its histamine-releasing action, though it is thought to be better than other opioids as it has a smooth muscle relaxant effect.
- General anaesthesia in an asthmatic pregnant patient may provoke severe bronchospasm, especially when the airway is instrumented. Thiopental has been implicated in causing bronchospasm, although this is disputed. Non-steroidal anti-inflammatory drugs are well known to induce bronchospasm in susceptible patients.

Management options

Ideally, moderate and severe asthmatics should be counselled in the antenatal period and a plan set out for their management in labour. The prime aim of treatment is the maintenance of oxygenation. As asthmatics often play down their symptoms, direct questioning about their exercise tolerance and their current treatment, including steroids, is required for the antenatal record.

Basic techniques for analgesia and anaesthesia are as for non-asthmatic mothers, bearing the above points in mind. Bronchospasm in labour may interfere with effective self-administration of Entonox. The woman should be fully alert and in control during her labour as much as possible, and therefore able to manage her asthma treatment with her inhalers. Epidural analgesia should be generally recommended.

Regional anaesthesia is indicated for operative deliveries, although a high block may reduce the ability to cough.

There is no contraindication to the standard treatments for an asthmatic attack in pregnancy or labour, including the use of inhaled or systemic steroids. It is important to remember that peak flow measurements are useful for monitoring the condition and that respiratory reserve is less during pregnancy, particularly if the mother's attack is precipitated by a respiratory tract infection.

Key points

- Both maternal and neonatal complications are more common in mothers with asthma, especially if poorly controlled.
- Epidural analgesia should be encouraged in labour.
- Regional anaesthesia is indicated for operative delivery.
- Acute exacerbations should be treated as for non-pregnant patients.

FURTHER READING

Hanania NA, Belfort MA. Acute asthma in pregnancy. *Crit Care Med* 2005; **33** (10 Suppl): S319–24.

Kwon HL, Belanger K, Bracken MB. Effect of pregnancy and stage of pregnancy on asthma severity: A systematic review. *Am J Obstet Gynecol* 2004; **190**: 1201–10.

Liu S, Wen SW, Demissie K, Marcoux S, Kramer MS. Maternal asthma and pregnancy outcomes: A retrospective cohort study. *Am J Obstet Gynecol* 2001; **184**: 90–6.

Nelson-Piercy C. Asthma in pregnancy. *Thorax* 2001; **56**: 325–8.

Schatz M. Asthma and pregnancy. *Lancet* 1999; **353**: 1202–4.

125   CYSTIC FIBROSIS

Cystic fibrosis is an autosomal recessive genetic disorder with a frequency of approximately 1 in 2000 births. It is primarily a disease of exocrine gland function. Because of improved medical care, women with cystic fibrosis are increasingly reaching childbearing age and presenting in pregnancy. Pregnancy itself is not thought to increase mortality in women unless pre-pregnancy forced expiratory volume in one second (FEV_1) is less than 50–60% of predicted, there is respiratory colonisation with *Burkholderia cepacia,* or she has pancreatic insufficiency. Overall mortality has been reported as 5% within two years of pregnancy and 10–20% within 5–10 years.

Problems/special considerations

- The main anaesthetic consideration is limited pulmonary reserve. These patients have tenacious secretions and they suffer multiple respiratory infections. They may also develop bronchiectasis for which regular postural drainage is required. Regional blockade may further impair respiratory function, especially if extensive.

- Pulmonary hypertension with right heart failure may also occur; it carries with it a poor outcome for both mother and baby.
- Diabetes, renal impairment and obstructive jaundice may occur.

Management options

The outcome of the pregnancy will depend on the degree of pulmonary insufficiency and this is best assessed by performing pulmonary function tests in the first and third trimesters. Careful cardiac assessment is also required to exclude the coexistence of right heart failure.

Vaginal delivery

Oxygenation should be optimal at all times. Stress and pain during labour will increase the respiratory demands and it is thus important to reduce these. The respiratory depressant effect of drugs and in particular opioids should be considered. Mobility is important to facilitate postural drainage. Low-dose epidural analgesia is the management of choice in most cases in order to satisfy these conditions.

Caesarean section

Regional anaesthesia is to be recommended, although many women with severe respiratory impairment are unable to lie flat. Care should be taken to avoid a high block and an incremental technique may be best if impairment is already severe. If general anaesthesia is undertaken, bronchial secretions will need regular suction, particularly before extubation. Postoperative analgesia is particularly important and is best provided by neuraxial opioids. During the recovery period, high-dependency care is essential and should include regular physiotherapy.

Key points

- Antenatal planning is essential.
- Maintenance of oxygenation should be given high priority at all times.
- Regional analgesia and anaesthesia is usually indicated but high blocks should be avoided if possible.

FURTHER READING

Cameron AJ, Skinner TA. Management of a parturient with respiratory failure secondary to cystic fibrosis. *Anaesthesia* 2005; **60**: 77–80.

Gillet D, de Braekeleer M, Bellis G, Durieu I and the participating centres to the French Cystic Fibrosis Registry. Cystic fibrosis and pregnancy. Report from French data (1980–1999). *Br J Obstet Gynaecol* 2002; **109**: 912–18.

McMullen AH, Pasta DJ, Frederick PD, *et al.* Impact of pregnancy on women with cystic fibrosis. *Chest* 2006; **129**: 706–11.

Muammar M, Marshall P, Wyatt H, Skelton V. Caesarean section in a patient with cystic fibrosis. *Int J Obstet Anesth* 2005; **14**: 70–3.

126   PULMONARY FIBROSIS

The most common fibrotic pulmonary lesion in young women is pulmonary fibrosis secondary to radiotherapy and will be discussed here. The progressive alveolar and pulmonary fibrotic conditions tend to occur in later life; the general principles are the same, although these conditions are potentially life threatening.

Problems/special considerations

Many women who have had a successfully treated malignancy expect to have children. Many of them are unaware that their pulmonary function is not normal as they have no symptoms during ordinary activities, nor are all of them told that there has been any pulmonary damage as a result of treatment of their malignancy. Pulmonary function tests show a reduction in the vital capacity and forced expiratory volume. They show no evidence of restrictive lung disease unless they have other pathology. Most of these women tolerate the pregnancy with little or no problem, although they need a plan for their delivery. Patients who have had a treated malignancy have usually had chemotherapy and may have had drugs that cause myocardial damage, e.g. bleomycin. It is therefore important that these women have echocardiography to assess their cardiac function.

Management options

It is important to assess these women antenatally so that they may understand their restrictions and how these may affect the management of labour and delivery. The delivery plan will depend on the degree of pulmonary damage. Some women may be treated as entirely normal whereas others require a clear plan comprising avoidance of general anaesthesia and sedative drugs, epidural analgesia during labour and regional anaesthesia for operative delivery.

Key points

- Antenatal assessment is essential, including pulmonary function tests and echocardiography when appropriate.
- Intrapartum management is as for respiratory disease in general.

127   SARCOIDOSIS

Sarcoidosis is a systemic granulomatous reaction affecting many organs. The main effects of the disease are seen in the peripheral and central nervous systems and the pulmonary and cardiac systems. An important aspect of the disease for the anaesthetist is the pulmonary infiltration, which occurs in up to 80% of cases and produces a restrictive type of lung disease; therefore it is considered with the respiratory diseases.

The disease is treated with steroids and is not made worse by pregnancy.

Problems/special considerations

- Sarcoidosis produces a restriction of the lungs; therefore the vital capacity and functional residual capacity will be reduced. These changes, compounded by the physiological changes of pregnancy, mean that many of these patients have no significant pulmonary reserve and may tolerate pregnancy (and especially labour) poorly.
- Cardiac impairment may be related to the primary disease (e.g. causing heart block or heart failure) or secondary to pulmonary involvement (causing pulmonary hypertension and right sided failure).
- There may also be renal impairment and central nervous system involvement, including isolated cranial nerve lesions.

Management options

The main consideration is to assess the pulmonary and cardiac functions of the woman and to assess the effect of pregnancy and delivery on function. All these women should have pulmonary function tests performed in the first and third trimester of their pregnancy unless mildly affected, and the management of the labour should be guided by the results. Electrocardiography should also be performed, with echocardiography in selected cases.

In labour, the respiratory challenge of the work of labour and the ventilatory response to pain may be poorly tolerated; therefore epidural analgesia is recommended as part of the management of labour.

For Caesarean section, general anaesthesia is best avoided, regional anaesthesia being the technique of choice.

Key points

- It is important to be aware of the generalised nature of the disease.
- Pulmonary involvement occurs in up to 80% of cases.
- Pulmonary and cardiac function should be assessed carefully in the antenatal period.
- Regional analgesia and anaesthesia is usually indicated in severe cases.

FURTHER READING

Euliano TY, White SE, Aleixo L. Sarcoidosis in a pregnant woman. *J Clin Anesth* 1997; **9**: 78–86.

128   ACUTE LUNG INJURY (ACUTE RESPIRATORY DISTRESS SYNDROME)

The syndrome of lung inflammation and increased permeability that is not explained by left atrial or pulmonary capillary hypertension (although they may coexist) is now called acute lung injury (ALI). The previous term, adult (now acute) respiratory distress syndrome (ARDS), is now reserved for the most severe form of ALI. Both conditions are characterised by their acute onset; bilateral diffuse infiltrates on chest radiography; pulmonary artery wedge pressure < 18 mmHg or absence of clinical evidence of left atrial hypertension; and arterial hypoxaemia resistant to oxygen therapy alone (ratio of arterial partial pressure: inspired fractional concentration of oxygen < 39.9 kPa [300 mmHg] for ALI; < 26.6 kPa [200 mmHg] for ARDS). Other features include reduced respiratory compliance and lung volumes, increased work of breathing, ventilation/perfusion mismatch and increased shunt. ALI or ARDS associated with pulmonary oedema is a common feature of deaths associated with pregnancy, and has received special attention in past Reports on Confidential Enquiries into Maternal Deaths. It has been suggested that ALI may be more likely in the pregnant state, possibly as result of the physiological changes of pregnancy, especially the increased cardiac output, lower colloid osmotic pressure and leaky capillaries. It is also suspected that aggressive fluid therapy, especially in obstetric haemorrhage and pre-eclampsia, has led to many cases of ALI. In the case of haemorrhage, this may be related to rapid transfusion in the presence of high circulating levels of catecholamines and a relatively constricted pulmonary circulation; in pre-eclampsia, over-emphasis on treating oliguria by 'pushing fluids' may lead to pulmonary oedema and ALI.

Problems/special considerations

The causes of ALI in pregnancy are generally the same as those in the non-pregnant state, although particularly important causes include pre-eclampsia, haemorrhage, sepsis, aspiration of gastric contents, presence of a dead fetus and amniotic fluid embolism. Use of β_2-agonists in premature labour may also contribute by causing pulmonary oedema (although whether this in itself leads to ALI and ARDS is uncertain).

The increased demands on the maternal cardiovascular and respiratory systems make the obstetric patient with ALI less able to cope with hypoxaemia, especially in the third trimester. The decreased functional residual capacity increases the likelihood of airway closure and ventilation/perfusion mismatch. However, established ALI has a similar mortality in both pregnant and non-pregnant women. The fetus is particularly at risk from hypoxaemia and this is compounded by any associated cardiovascular instability and the risk of aortocaval compression.

Management options

Management requires early referral to the intensive care unit and involves increasing levels of respiratory support as ALI increases in severity. Management of the predisposing condition should continue as for any acutely ill patient. The physiological changes of pregnancy pose particular problems for the critically ill obstetric patient (see Chapter 143, Intensive care in pregnancy, p. 321).

Key points

- Obstetric patients may be especially prone to acute lung injury.
- Acute lung injury is a common feature in deaths caused by pre-eclampsia, sepsis and massive obstetric haemorrhage.
- The increased physiological demands of pregnancy make obstetric patients especially susceptible to hypoxaemia.

FURTHER READING

Bandi VD, Munnur U, Matthay MA. Acute lung injury and acute respiratory distress syndrome in pregnancy. *Crit Care Clin* 2004; **20**: 577–607.

Catanzarite V, Willms D, Wong D, *et al.* Acute respiratory distress syndrome in pregnancy and the puerperium: causes, courses, and outcomes. *Obstet Gynecol* 2001; **97**: 760–4.

Cole DE, Taylor T, McCullough DM, Shoff CT, Derdak S. Acute respiratory distress syndrome in pregnancy. *Crit Care Med* 2005; **33** (10 Suppl): S269–78.

Karetzky M, Ramirez M. Acute respiratory failure in pregnancy. *Medicine* 1998; **77**: 41–9.

Tomlinson MW, Caruthers TJ, Whitty JE, Gonik B. Does delivery improve maternal condition in the respiratory-compromised gravida? *Obstet Gynecol* 1998; **91**: 108–11.

129   PSYCHIATRIC DISEASE

Suicide ± psychiatric disease is now the most common cause of death in recent Reports on Confidential Enquiries into Maternal Deaths in the United Kingdom (now Confidential Enquiry into Maternal and Child Health; CEMACH). The most recent increase results partly from the improved ascertainment of cases. As well as women with pre-existing psychiatric disease, it is estimated that 10–15% of women suffer from postnatal depression, and as many as 60% experience postnatal 'blues'. The risk of admission to hospital with psychosis in the first three months after childbirth is more than 300 times greater than at other times.

Much of the challenge in providing effective care to women with psychiatric disease relates to the organisation and funding of services, and the identification of women at risk. Anaesthetists' involvement is usually restricted to care for women who present peripartum or who have attempted suicide.

Problems/special considerations

- *Pre-existing disease:* patients may be taking drugs that are affected by pregnancy, that have important maternal or fetal effects, or that affect anaesthesia. Women with manic-depressive illness may be maintained on lithium or, less commonly, carbamazepine. Serial monitoring of plasma drug levels is particularly important for these drugs. Lithium may potentiate neuromuscular blockade (with both suxamethonium and non-depolarising neuromuscular blocking drugs). Women with schizophrenia are likely to be taking a variety of antipsychotic drugs, high doses of which can cause sedation, and postural hypotension due to α blockade. The latter is likely to be exacerbated by the physiological changes of pregnancy. Monoamine oxidase inhibitors (MAOIs) have a number of potential interactions, the most important of which concern pethidine and vasopressors.

  Women who have been psychiatrically well and taking maintenance drugs may stop their medication when they become pregnant and present with recurrence of symptoms. Many of the psychotropic drugs are relatively contraindicated during pregnancy, but a risk–benefit analysis must be made before changing or stopping such medication.

  Women with psychiatric disease may lack capacity to give consent to treatment (see below). In acute mental states, they may also refuse treatments, disrupt the care of other patients and not follow feeding policies.
- *Postnatal psychiatric disease:* women who develop postnatal depression may not have had any warning symptoms or signs. Women with a past history of psychiatric disease or drug dependence may conceal this from obstetricians and midwives because of the perceived stigma of these conditions. Those with a previous history of postnatal depressive psychosis run a 50% risk of recurrence, classically at the same time postnatally as before. It is important for all healthcare professionals to maintain a high level of awareness of such disorders, and ask all women at booking about previous psychiatric illness.
- *Substance abuse:* drug abuse is more common in North America than in the UK but nevertheless is an important cause of morbidity and mortality in the UK (see Chapter 139, Substance abuse, p. 312).

Management options

Antenatal care

Women with poorly controlled psychiatric disease may default from antenatal care and may thus be at increased risk from undetected complications of pregnancy. They may exhibit hospital phobia and may lack insight into the need for medical care if pregnancy-related problems occur. Continuity of care, which enables a trusting relationship to be developed with one or two healthcare professionals, is vital. Antenatal discussion about options for analgesia in labour and the possibility of needing anaesthesia for operative delivery are particularly important, and such discussions should be documented and witnessed by the woman's partner, and a third party if possible. There must be discussion between the psychiatrist, obstetrician, general practitioner and the woman herself about continuing drug therapy throughout pregnancy.

Women who are maintained on drug therapy should be monitored regularly to ensure that the pregnancy-related increase in blood and plasma volume does not result in sub-therapeutic drug levels.

Labour and delivery

Regional analgesia and anaesthesia are not contraindicated for women with psychiatric disease.

Women taking a MAOI can receive ephedrine or phenylephrine to correct hypotension caused by regional anaesthesia, but the anaesthetist should use smaller doses than usual and be aware that pressor responses may be exaggerated. Pethidine should be avoided, but fentanyl and morphine have both been used uneventfully. Use of patient-controlled intravenous analgesia is preferable to intramuscular analgesia postoperatively.

There is a need for a high level of awareness amongst all healthcare professionals involved in intrapartum and postnatal care. Symptoms and signs suggestive of depressive illness must be treated promptly. Tri- and tetracyclic antidepressants, the selective serotonin reuptake inhibitor group of antidepressants and MAOIs may all be necessary in the treatment of both non-pregnancy-related and postnatal depression. Electroconvulsive therapy may also be indicated.

Women known to abuse illegal drugs should be treated with caution. There are numerous interactions with medical drugs, and women frequently abuse multiple drugs.

Consent

A psychiatrist's input may be invaluable in characterising a psychiatric patient's illness and advising on her state of mind, though the decision on whether she has capacity should be made by the treating doctor, after considering such advice. The doctrine of necessity allows treatment to be administered without consent if this is in the patient's best interests, but it cannot be assumed that what the obstetric team would wish to do always reflects the mother's 'best interests', and a psychiatrist's advice may be useful here too. In the UK, the unborn fetus has no legal status or rights (though it may have moral ones). If the mother is held in hospital under the Mental Health Act (1983), this only covers treatment of the primary mental condition and does not allow other treatments to be enforced unless they are considered to affect it directly.

Patients in whom consent may be problematic require multidisciplinary discussion antenatally in order to formulate a management plan. Often there is extensive discussion but the obstetric anaesthetist is not invited, so that the first contact he/she has may be when analgesia or anaesthesia is required.

Key points

- Psychiatric disease is common in pregnancy.
- A patient's drug therapy requires careful monitoring during and after pregnancy.
- The possibility of substance abuse should always be considered.
- Difficulties with consent should be anticipated and plans made in good time.

FURTHER READING

Brockington I. Postpartum psychiatric disorders. *Lancet* 2004; **363**: 303–10.

Hofberg K, Ward MR. Fear of pregnancy and childbirth. *Postgrad Med J* 2003; **79**: 505–10.

Jablensky AV, Morgan V, Zubrick SR, Bower C, Yellachich LA. Pregnancy, delivery, and neonatal complications in a population cohort of women with schizophrenia and major affective disorders. *Am J Psychiatry* 2005; **162**: 79–91.

130 OBESITY

Obesity is so prevalent in North America and the UK that the associated risks are often underestimated. However, the obese mother presents significant challenges to the obstetric anaesthetist, and obesity has been highlighted as an important contributory factor in maternal mortality.

Problems/special considerations

- The risks of diabetes, hypertension and coronary artery disease are all increased. Airway closure may occur within tidal volume, especially in supine and semi-supine positions. A small number of morbidly obese women may develop secondary pulmonary hypertension and chronic right ventricular failure.
- Antenatal assessment, including accurate estimation of gestation, may be difficult. The obese mother has an increased likelihood of developing pre-eclampsia, of requiring operative delivery and of developing thromboembolic disease and infective postoperative complications.
- Symptomatic reflux occurs in nearly all obese pregnant women.
- Aortocaval compression will occur in all but the full upright and full lateral positions.
- Fetal growth retardation is possible, as well as the more commonly occurring macrosomic fetus.
- The massively obese woman may not fit on a standard operating table and she may exceed the weight limit of a standard hospital lift.
- Intravenous access and non-invasive monitoring of both mother and fetus may be difficult.

Management options

Thromboprophylaxis should be used, preferably with low-dose heparin (in increased doses), and graduated compression stockings should be worn for the entire hospital admission. H_2-antagonists and antacids should be used throughout labour.

Difficulty in securing intravenous access should be anticipated, as should difficult tracheal intubation. Early use of epidural analgesia should be recommended for labour; the benefits usually outweigh the risks of epidural haematoma resulting from heparin prophylaxis. The initial failure rate of epidural analgesia is higher in obese women, who should therefore be persuaded to accept regional analgesia early in labour. Although identification of landmarks is difficult, standard length needles can be used for the majority of women. The lowest effective concentrations of local anaesthetic combined with an opioid should be used; combined spinal–epidural analgesia offers a suitable alternative. The aim should be to minimise any motor blockade whilst providing effective analgesia. There is some circumstantial evidence suggesting that the incidence and severity of postdural puncture headache is reduced in obesity, perhaps because of increased intra-abdominal pressure.

Regional anaesthesia is usually recommended in preference to general, and an existing epidural can be readily extended for emergency Caesarean delivery. Combined spinal–epidural anaesthesia is recommended for elective Caesarean section or for emergency section when there is no pre-existing epidural analgesia. Single-shot spinal anaesthesia is less suitable for the obese woman, because control over the final height of the block is difficult and surgical difficulty may lead to prolonged operating time. It is important to pay meticulous attention to avoidance of aortocaval compression.

If general anaesthesia is necessary, the risks of hypoxia and regurgitation of gastric contents should be assumed to be higher than in the non-obese pregnant woman. Adequate preoxygenation is essential. Difficulty with tracheal intubation should be anticipated and suitable aids to intubation should be readily available. Often, extra pillows are required under the patient's shoulders and neck to position the mother optimally. Trained and experienced anaesthetic assistance is essential, and the presence of a second anaesthetist is desirable.

Residual neuromuscular blockade has been implicated in maternal death and is a particular hazard in the obese woman. A peripheral nerve stimulator should be used to confirm reversal of neuromuscular blockade, and recovery from general anaesthesia should take place in a well-lit recovery area under the supervision of trained recovery staff.

Good postoperative analgesia, e.g. with epidural or spinal opioids, is important to allow early mobilisation. Intravenous patient-controlled opioid analgesia is recommended for women in whom the central neuraxial route is unavailable. Postoperative physiotherapy should be provided, and high-dependency midwifery care should also be available.

Key points

- The obese mother has an increased risk of obstetric and anaesthetic complications.
- Early regional analgesia for labour should be encouraged.
- Difficulty with tracheal intubation should be anticipated.
- Thromboprophylaxis should be used.

FURTHER READING

Andreasen KR, Andersen ML, Schantz AL. Obesity and pregnancy. *Acta Obstet Gynecol Scand* 2004; **83**: 1022–9.

Saravanakumar K, Rao SG, Cooper GM. Obesity and obstetric anaesthesia. *Anaesthesia* 2006; **61**: 36–48.

Yu CKH, Teoh TG, Robinson S. Obesity in pregnancy. *BJOG* 2006; **113**: 1117–25.

131 PYREXIA DURING LABOUR

Variously defined as core temperature exceeding 37.5 °C or 38 °C, pyrexia in labour has traditionally been taken to be a marker of infection requiring investigation and antibiotic therapy. However, there are many other medical causes of pyrexia (e.g. inflammatory disease, thyrotoxicosis, pulmonary embolism, malignancy, malignant hyperthermia) which should not be forgotten. In addition, it has recently been recognised that epidural analgesia itself may be associated with a gradual increase in maternal (and thus fetal) temperature after about 5–6 hours, of up to 1 °C or thereabouts, although most studies are poorly controlled and the phenomenon is controversial (for example, women with predisposing factors for infection are often those who request epidural analgesia). Fetal heart rate may increase as a direct consequence of maternal pyrexia. Suggested mechanisms include alteration of afferent temperature-related neural input to the hypothalamus, impaired thermoregulatory mechanisms in the lower body (such as absent shivering in the legs) and a resetting of the central 'thermostat'.

The fetal temperature is ~1 °C higher than the maternal core, and follows maternal oral readings more closely than tympanic.

Problems/special considerations

Pyrexia itself has been implicated in causing premature labour and may stress an at-risk fetus. Neonatal encephalopathy is more common if mothers are pyrexial during labour, although whether this is related to the increased temperature itself or to any underlying cause (particularly infection) is uncertain.

Infection causing pyrexia is a potentially serious problem since severe sepsis may affect both the mother and the fetus. Thus most protocols call for screening tests and possibly antibiotic therapy if infection is suspected.

It has been claimed that huge amounts of money are spent each year investigating neonates born of pyrexial mothers in whom the only cause of pyrexia was epidural analgesia, although the epidural's role in causing the pyrexia is disputed. Nevertheless, it is thus important that all anaesthetists, obstetricians, midwives and paediatricians are aware that the phenomenon may exist. In protocols and guidelines for the management of pyrexia during labour, provision should be made for the effect of epidurals; separate instructions may be required for mothers with epidurals and those without.

Management options

In most cases, mild pyrexia is not in itself troublesome. Fanning, sponging or treatment with paracetamol may be used, although the possibility of masking underlying sepsis should not be forgotten. Pyrexia above 38.5 °C is unlikely to be related to epidural analgesia, especially if it occurs within 6 hours of the epidural. If infection is suspected, screening should include blood cultures, high vaginal swabs and mid-stream urine sampling. Infection may not be accompanied by localising signs, at least initially; in addition, white cell count may increase during normal labour to as high as $40 \times 10^9/l$.

Mothers who are pyrexial and who request epidural analgesia present a separate dilemma since regional blockade may be complicated by severe cardiovascular compromise or epidural/meningeal infection in the presence of systemic infection, which is therefore usually a contraindication to regional anaesthesia. For mild localised infection such as chorioamnionitis (which may be associated with subclinical bacteraemia), regional analgesia is generally felt to be safe if covered with antibiotic therapy.

Set procedures should exist for monitoring of maternal temperature and management of pyrexia, including provision of regional blockade in pyrexial mothers and neonatal screening. A high level of general awareness and education is important since staff of all disciplines are often unaware of the relationship between epidural analgesia and pyrexia.

Key points

- There are many causes of fever, including infection.
- Epidural analgesia exceeding 5–6 hours has been associated with pyrexia.
- Protocols should exist for monitoring of temperature during labour and screening ± treatment of pyrexial mothers.

FURTHER READING

Banerjee S, Cashman P, Yentis SM, Steer PJ. Maternal temperature monitoring during labor: concordance and variability among monitoring sites. *Obstet Gynecol* 2004; **103**: 287–93.

Camann W. Intrapartum epidural analgesia and neonatal sepsis evaluations: a casual or causal association? *Anesthesiology* 1999; **90**: 1250–2.

Kuczkowski KM, Reisner LS. Anesthetic management of the parturient with fever and infection. *J Clin Anesth* 2003; **15**: 478–488.

Mercier FJ, Benhamou D. Hyperthermia related to epidural analgesia during labour. *Int J Obstet Anesth* 1997; **6**: 19–24.

132   CONNECTIVE TISSUE DISORDERS

The connective tissue disorders are a diffuse group of diseases, which include the rheumatoid diseases (rheumatoid arthritis, ankylosing spondylitis), the collagen vascular diseases (systemic lupus erythematosus [SLE], scleroderma, the vasculitides), granulomatous diseases and inherited connective tissue disease (e.g. Ehlers–Danlos syndrome).

The factors of importance to the anaesthetist are firstly the widespread systemic nature of the diseases and secondly the drug treatment that is used.

Problems/special considerations

With the exception of the rheumatoid diseases, connective tissue disorders are rare in the antenatal population. The onset of significantly symptomatic disease is frequently towards the end of reproductive life. Both spontaneous abortion and late pregnancy loss are increased in women who do become pregnant.

Drug treatment

Drug treatment frequently includes long-term oral corticosteroids and may also include immunosuppressive agents such as azathioprine, chlorambucil, cyclophosphamide or methotrexate. Low-dose aspirin and subcutaneous heparin are often used in SLE. In arthritic conditions, non-steroidal anti-inflammatory drugs (NSAIDs) are invariably used.

Cardiac involvement

Pericardial effusions are common, especially in rheumatoid and collagen disorders. A restrictive pericarditis may ensue. Valvular dysfunction can occur. A miscellany of electrocardiographic changes may be seen, and echocardiography is useful in assessing both valvular and ventricular function.

Pulmonary involvement

Pleural effusions are common. Impaired pulmonary function of both restrictive and obstructive patterns may occur, and pulmonary vasculitis can occur in both collagen and vasculitic disorders, rarely leading to spontaneous pulmonary haemorrhage.

Women with scleroderma may be at increased risk of chronic aspiration because of impaired gastrointestinal motility. These women may also have significant airway problems.

Multiple antibody formation

This is a significant problem in women with SLE and can also occur in other auto-immune connective tissue disorders. Maternal antibodies cause difficulty and delay in obtaining adequately cross-matched blood for transfusion. In severe cases there may be coagulation disorders in the mother that may be thrombotic or may increase risk of bleeding.

Anti-cardiolipin antibodies are associated with increased pregnancy loss and increased maternal morbidity. Anti-Ro antibodies may cross the placenta and cause fetal cardiac conduction defects, rendering the fetus bradycardic and unable to mount a tachycardic response to stress.

Musculoskeletal problems

Musculoskeletal involvement is a feature of a number of the connective tissue disorders. Women with scleroderma classically have very tight perioral skin and may also have involvement of the temporomandibular joints; both may limit mouth opening.

Cervical arthritis and consequent reduction of neck mobility is a feature of several connective tissue disorders.

Bullous diseases such as pemphigus and epidermolysis bullosa are characterised by formation of large bullae on the skin and mucous membranes in response to minor trauma. Although extremely rare, cases have been reported in pregnancy, and there are significant implications for the anaesthetist. Any airway instrumentation (including pressure from a facemask) can provoke bullous formation, and bullae may also form in the trachea. Regional anaesthesia has been recommended.

Tissue fragility

Several conditions (e.g. certain forms of Ehlers–Danlos syndrome) may be associated with increased fragility of tissues including blood vessels, leading to an increased susceptibility to trauma and bleeding.

Management options

Early antenatal assessment is vital, and preconception counselling may be desirable. If pregnancy has occurred unexpectedly, expert advice should be sought about the relative risks of teratogenicity of immunosuppressive drugs, and the patient counselled appropriately.

Many women with connective tissue disorder have multisystem involvement. Detailed history and examination are necessary, with particular reference to drug treatment and symptoms or signs suggestive of cardiac or pulmonary disease.

The possibility of difficulty with airway management and cardiopulmonary involvement should be remembered if anaesthesia is required for termination of pregnancy. The skin should be examined for fragility and ease of intravenous access. Investigations should include electro- and echocardiography, pulmonary function tests, chest radiography and full biochemical and haematological investigation.

Women who are continuing with a pregnancy should be regarded as high risk and receive consultant obstetric care. Serial monitoring of the mother should include assessment of cardiac, pulmonary and renal reserve. Mothers needing maintenance NSAIDs throughout pregnancy will require fetal cardiac monitoring during the third trimester because of the risk of premature closure of the ductus arteriosus and potential fetal renal compromise.

Individual plans will be required depending on the particular disorder with which a woman is presenting. Some general principles apply:

- It is usually beneficial to admit women with significant disease for a short time at about 28–30 weeks' gestation for assessment and formulation of plans for delivery.
- There should be provision for high-dependency level of care during and after delivery.
- The obstetrician, anaesthetist and patient should discuss the relative risks and benefits of spontaneous labour, induction of labour, or delivery by elective Caesarean section.
- In the absence of coagulation disorder, regional analgesia is not contraindicated. Regional anaesthesia is considered unwise by some authorities because of the risk of major haemorrhage during surgery, but a risk–benefit analysis must be made for each patient.

If difficulty with the airway is considered to be a major potential risk, relative contraindications to regional anaesthesia are usually outweighed by the benefits. There are no absolute contraindications to regional anaesthesia in these circumstances. Published case reports indicate successful management of individual cases with both general and regional techniques.

Key points

- Connective tissue disorders encompass a wide variety of clinical conditions. Each woman must be assessed on an individual basis.
- Many connective tissue disorders are associated with cardiac, pulmonary and renal dysfunction.
- Drug treatment frequently includes corticosteroids.
- Early and detailed antenatal assessment and serial monitoring during pregnancy are essential.
- Regional analgesia and anaesthesia are not contraindicated, but careful assessment of the balance of risks and benefits is necessary.

FURTHER READING

Mok CC, Wong RWS. Pregnancy in systemic lupus erythematosus. *Postgrad Med J* 2001; **77**: 157–65.

Rayburn WF. Connective tissue disorders and pregnancy. Recommendations for prescribing. *J Reprod Med* 1998; **43**: 341–9.

133   RENAL FAILURE

Renal failure may be present before the patient becomes pregnant or it may develop during (or following) pregnancy, perhaps as a complication of a pregnancy-related problem. Either way, it has implications for the obstetric anaesthetist.

Although pregnancy was uncommon in patients with renal failure in the past, improvements in the care of patients requiring renal replacement means that women on dialysis programmes or having received renal transplants are increasingly likely to present to the maternity department. Conversely, acute renal failure (ARF) related to an obstetric complication should be becoming less common as care of the sick mother (in both the maternity suite and the intensive care unit) improves, although there are no data relating to this.

It should be remembered that the normal physiological changes of pregnancy result in an increased glomerular filtration rate and a lowering of the 'normal' blood indices of renal function. Thus the usual blood urea concentration in pregnancy is 3.0–4.0 mmol/l and the creatinine concentration 55–65 μmol/l. An increase in blood urea concentration from, say, 4.0 mmol/l to 9.0 mmol/l thus may represent significant renal impairment, which may not be the case in non-pregnant subjects.

Problems/special considerations

Pre-existing disease

In terms of general anaesthetic management, the problems of pre-existing renal disease are the same as in the non-pregnant population. These include the underlying cause of renal impairment, systemic manifestations of renal failure (in particular, hypertension and ischaemic heart disease, thrombocytopenia and anaemia), the patient's medication, altered handling of drugs and fluid management, including the nature and timing of dialysis.

Obstetric management may be influenced by the above factors and any history of previous abdominal surgery, including the presence of a transplanted kidney. There is an increased risk of pre-eclampsia in mothers with renal impairment. The fetus may be at risk from the underlying disease that caused renal impairment or from the above complications.

Acute renal failure related to pregnancy

Typically, pregnancy-related ARF is especially associated with pre-eclampsia, HELLP (haemolysis, elevated liver enzymes and low platelet count) syndrome, septic abortion and massive haemorrhage (traditionally caused by placental abruption, although any cause of hypovolaemia may be followed by renal failure). Other important causes include pyelonephritis, drug reactions (especially non-steroid anti-inflammatory drugs [NSAIDs]), acute fatty liver and incompatible blood transfusion. In most cases, ARF is caused by acute tubular necrosis, although cortical necrosis has been seen after abruption and pre-eclampsia. Problems are those of ARF generally, especially related to fluid balance and the apparently increased susceptibility of pregnant women to developing pulmonary oedema.

Management options

Pre-existing disease

Standard anaesthetic and analgesic techniques are suitable, given the above considerations. Renal function and blood pressure should be closely monitored during pregnancy. Discussion with the renal physicians and obstetricians is required regarding the timing of dialysis and method of delivery. Any arteriovenous shunt should be noted and steps taken to protect it during labour and/or delivery. Drugs excreted renally should be used with caution, and those known to impair renal blood flow or function (especially NSAIDs) should be avoided.

Acute renal failure related to pregnancy

Management of renal failure is along standard lines. Careful fluid balance is especially important given the propensity of obstetric patients to pulmonary oedema. Individual predisposing conditions are considered under their own headings. Most mothers regain normal renal function, depending on the underlying cause, although a degree of renal impairment may persist.

Key points

- Mothers with pre-existing renal failure require careful monitoring and an interdisciplinary approach.
- Obstetric anaesthetic management uses standard techniques, taking into account the underlying cause and systemic effects of renal failure, use of drugs and problems relating to fluid management.
- Renal failure may develop during or after obstetric catastrophes; management is along standard lines, and recovery of function is usual.

FURTHER READING

Gammill HS. Jeyabalan A. Acute renal failure in pregnancy. *Crit Care Med* 2005; **33** (10 Suppl): S372–84.

Tighe KE, Smith ID, Bogod DG. Caesarean section in chronic renal failure. *Eur J Anaesthesiol* 1995; **12**: 185–7.

Williams DJ. The implications of pre-existing renal disease in pregnancy. *Curr Obstet Gynaecol* 1999; **9**: 75–81.

134   HEPATITIS

Hepatitis may predate pregnancy or may occur coincidentally during pregnancy. The diagnosis of acute viral hepatitis is made from the history and from blood tests of liver function (increased conjugated bilirubin, markedly increased transaminases, and slightly increased alkaline phosphatase). Chronic hepatitis (active, persistent, drug- or alcohol-induced) also causes abnormality of liver function tests, but definitive diagnosis is made by liver biopsy.

Problems/special considerations

Viral hepatitis

Viral hepatitis accounts for 40% of all liver disease associated with pregnancy. It is thought that pregnant women might be more susceptible to viral hepatitis because of their relatively immunosuppressed state.

- Hepatitis A is highly contagious and spread by the faecal–oral route. The incidence in pregnancy is unknown since many infections are mild, but is thought to be low in the UK.
- Hepatitis B is thought to infect up to 1:50 pregnant women in UK inner cities, in which there is a large immigrant population. It is readily spread by contact with blood and body fluids. Women who are known to have been exposed to intravenous drug use or to have had multiple sexual partners should be assumed to be at high risk of having hepatitis B, and appropriate precautions should be taken. Prostitutes are at particularly high risk, since many are using illegal drugs and working as prostitutes to fund their drug habit. Pregnant women have been screened for hepatitis B in the UK since 2000. There is a ~10% risk of developing chronic liver disease; this may be increased by co-infection with hepatitis D.
- Hepatitis C is unusual in pregnancy in the UK; it is thought to be prevalent in 0.5–1% of parturients in inner cities. It is spread mainly by contact with blood, although sexual transmission may also occur. There is a ~5% risk of transmission to the baby during pregnancy/delivery and a 50–80% risk of developing chronic liver disease.
- Hepatitis E is similar to hepatitis A. It may cause serious infection during the last trimester and may also cause miscarriage. It is unusual in the UK.

Symptoms are non-specific, and include fatigue, general malaise, loss of appetite, nausea, vomiting, headache and pyrexia. There may be some abdominal discomfort. Overt jaundice only occurs in about a quarter of cases. Treatment is symptomatic, and in the majority of cases there is complete resolution of all signs and symptoms over the course of a few weeks. Women with significantly impaired liver function may be thrombocytopenic or have abnormal clotting studies. Renal function may also be impaired. In end-stage hepatitis, alteration in mental state may occur as a result of hepatic encephalopathy. There is no evidence that pregnancy affects the course of the disease nor that hepatitis has any significant effect on pregnancy in the majority of cases. For the small number of pregnant women who develop hepatitis C it has been suggested that maternal morbidity and mortality is higher than in the non-pregnant woman. However, this increased risk may be apparent, due to misdiagnosis of conditions such as fatty liver of pregnancy, rather than a genuine risk.

Chronic hepatitis

Chronic persistent hepatitis is usually unaffected by pregnancy. Chronic active hepatitis is associated with impaired fertility; if pregnancy does occur it may be associated with accelerated deterioration in liver function. Treatment includes corticosteroids and antiviral drugs, including interferon. Lupus antibodies may occur in up to 20% of women with chronic active hepatitis. Chronic active hepatitis may be complicated by arthritis, impaired renal function, myocarditis and neuropathies. Diabetes, hypertension and osteoporosis may also occur as a result of long-term steroid therapy.

Management options

Regional analgesia and anaesthesia is not contraindicated if coagulation studies are normal. If there is chronic impairment of liver function, invasive venous pressure monitoring may assist fluid management, especially if regional anaesthesia is performed. Although fluid overload must be avoided, hypotension will aggravate any reduction in liver blood flow.

There may be impaired clearance of lidocaine; dose reduction is advisable.

Patients with severe liver disease may have oesophageal varices and often have severely impaired liver function and coagulopathy. Avoidance of pushing during vaginal delivery is recommended, but frequently superimposed obstetric complications (pre-eclampsia, intrauterine growth retardation) will necessitate operative delivery. Rapid sequence induction of general anaesthesia for Caesarean section should be used. Suxamethonium can be used safely, despite the greater than normal reduction in plasma cholinesterase levels that is likely to be present. Use of a peripheral nerve stimulator is mandatory, since the action of non-depolarising muscle relaxants is variable though usually prolonged.

Standard infection control precautions should be used if women with viral hepatitis are hospitalised.

Key points

- Viral hepatitis is highly contagious.
- Regional analgesia and anaesthesia are not contraindicated, but impaired liver function is frequently associated with disorders of coagulation.

FURTHER READING

Guntupalli SR, Steingrub J. Hepatic disease and pregnancy: an overview of diagnosis and management. *Crit Care Med* 2005; **33** (10 Suppl): S332–39.

Liddle C. Hepatitis C. *Anaesth Intens Care* 1996; **24**: 180–3.

Rahman TM, Wendon J. Severe hepatic dysfunction in pregnancy. *QJM* 2002; **95**: 343–57.

135   HERPES SIMPLEX INFECTION

The herpes simplex virus (HSV) is a common infective agent during both childhood and adult life. Although HSV-1 is traditionally considered to be responsible for orolabial herpes and HSV-2 for genital herpes, there is considerable overlap. HSV is important in pregnancy because of the adverse effects of primary infection on maternal health and premature labour and also because of the risks of primary neonatal infection, which may be severe.

Problems/special considerations

Primary infection may result in local lesions and viraemia with systemic effects, e.g. malaise, myalgia, meningitis, encephalitis and hepatitis. Local lesions may reappear weeks to years later, often following emotional or physical stress. Primary infection is associated with a ~40% incidence of neonatal transmission. Secondary infection is not associated with viraemia and the risk of neonatal transmission is <3%.

Women with severe primary infection may present in premature labour or with acute systemic manifestations, whereas those with active genital lesions may present for Caesarean section, performed to reduce neonatal transmission.

It is not known whether epidural or spinal anaesthesia increases the likelihood of central nervous system involvement if there is a history of secondary HSV infection, although there are published series of successful obstetric regional anaesthesia performed without problems. Epidural morphine is associated with up to 11 times the risk of recurrence of oral lesions compared with parenteral morphine; the mechanism is unclear but may be related to direct activation of the dormant virus in cranial nerve nuclei. There is little information available about reactivation of HSV by other opioids.

Avoidance of regional anaesthesia in primary infection is often advised but less is known about the risks since primary infection at the time of delivery is rare. There are series of successful regional blocks in the presence of primary infection but numbers are very small.

Management options

Aciclovir is generally avoided during pregnancy because of fears of interfering with fetal thymidine metabolism. However, aciclovir is indicated in cases of severe disseminated infection (e.g. 200 mg orally five times a day or 5 mg/kg i.v. 8-hourly). In recurrent HSV infection, routine genital culturing is no longer recommended as an indicator of the need for Caesarean section, since the presence of visible genital lesions has been shown to be more reliable and easier to ascertain. Thus vaginal delivery is generally advised unless genital lesions are present, in which case Caesarean section is performed (unless the membranes have been ruptured for more than 4 hours, in which case Caesarean section makes no difference to neonatal transmission).

Mothers should be fully informed of the theoretical risks and benefits of regional anaesthesia, especially before Caesarean section when the alternative (i.e. general anaesthetic) is generally perceived as being more hazardous. The neonate born of a mother with HSV should be carefully evaluated for evidence of infection.

Key points

- Primary herpes simplex virus (HSV) infection may cause severe systemic illness and premature labour.
- Neonatal infection may occur if there are active genital lesions.
- The risk of central neural infection following regional anaesthesia in secondary HSV infection is thought to be theoretical only.
- Epidural morphine may cause recurrence of orolabial HSV lesions.

FURTHER READING

Bader AM, Camann WR, Datta S. Anesthesia for cesarean delivery in patients with herpes simplex virus type-2 infections. *Reg Anesth* 1990; **15**: 261–3.

Boyle RK. A review of anatomical and immunological links between epidural morphine and herpes simplex labialis in obstetric patients. *Anaesth Intens Care* 1995; **23**: 425–32.

Boyle RK. Herpes simplex labialis after epidural or parenteral morphine: a randomized prospective trial in an Australian obstetric population. *Anaesth Intens Care* 1995; **23**: 433–7.

Smith JR, Cowan FM, Munday P. The management of herpes simplex infection in pregnancy. *Br J Obstet Gynaecol* 1998; **105**: 255–60.

136   HIV INFECTION

The prevalence of human immunodeficiency virus (HIV) has been found on population screening to be present in about 0.22% of women giving birth in England (0.04% in those born in the UK and 2.4% in those born in sub-Saharan Africa), and 0.07% of those in Scotland in 2005. In inner London the prevalence is ~0.5%, a figure similar to that in New York. In parts of central and east Africa, the incidence may reach 20–30% in the larger cities. The natural course of infection is an acute viral-type illness, followed on average 3 months later by seroconversion when the patient becomes 'HIV-positive'; progression to the acquired immunodeficiency syndrome (AIDS; characterised by lymphadenopathy and conditions indicating reduced cell-mediated immunity, e.g. chronic opportunistic/invasive infections, chronic diarrhoea, malignancies, neurological involvement) occurs in about two-thirds of cases over the next 10 years, although up to 20% of cases survive for 20 years without progression to AIDS. Median survival once AIDS is diagnosed is currently about 30–50 months; in Africa, survival is shorter, with about one-third of cases progressing to death without developing AIDS itself.

HIV infection has altered the way in which contaminated materials are handled in the labour ward and the way in which blood and blood products are administered. In addition, it has sparked debates over the testing of expectant mothers, e.g. whether routine screening should be offered only if the mother chooses (opt-in) or whether it should be performed unless the mother specifically chooses not to be tested (opt-out). The argument favouring testing is that neonatal transmission occurs in 25–30% of cases, with a further 14% increase if the mother breastfeeds; with appropriate medical management of known cases (see below) this can be reduced to under 3%. The Department of Health recommended in 1999 that testing should be offered and recommended to all pregnant women; since this recommendation the proportion of HIV-infected women diagnosed before delivery has risen to ~95%. Human T cell leukaemia/lymphoma virus (HTLV) types I and II have been found to have a similar prevalence to that of HIV in pregnancy, and screening of blood donations and/or pregnant women is performed in some countries.

Since the target of infection is primarily the lymphocyte, plasma counts of the CD4 positive cells (mainly helper T-lymphocytes) have been used to monitor the course of infection and guide treatment. The CD4:CD8 ratio and plasma viral load (amount of viral RNA measurable in the plasma, representing degree of viral replication) are also used.

Problems/special considerations

Problems may be related to:
- The acute viral illness of initial HIV infection
- Impaired organ function and immunodepression of AIDS
- The risk of transmission of HIV to the neonate
- The risk of transmission of HIV to medical and midwifery staff and to other patients.

Management options

All units should offer counselling and testing for at-risk women prenatally or even pre-pregnancy, and this should continue during pregnancy. Many units have protocols in place for joint management of HIV-positive women by obstetricians and HIV specialists.

Acute HIV infection is rarely a known problem on the labour ward and in general is managed as for any acute viral illness. For those with acute organ dysfunction, supportive management is directed at the organ system affected.

Patients with chronic HIV infection are managed according to their degree of organ impairment, which in most cases presenting to the labour ward will not be severe. All systems may be affected, either by primary HIV infection or secondary infection, e.g. with fungi or other atypical organisms. Neurological manifestations are especially important to anaesthetists and include neuropathy, encephalopathy, meningitis, focal brain lesions, dementia, myelopathy and myopathy. In addition, HIV-positive subjects' life expectancy is increased by taking prophylactic highly active antiretroviral therapy (HAART). These drugs may cause blood dyscrasias, gastrointestinal disturbances, neurological and hepatic impairment and increased drug metabolism via hepatic enzyme indication. Prior to any anaesthetic intervention all patients must therefore be assessed carefully for evidence of organ system impairment.

In general, patients with HIV infection are managed as for any obstetric patient, unless specific contraindications exist. Particular care with invasive techniques has been suggested, to reduce the risk of introducing infection, but standard aseptic methods should be adequate if they are followed. The use of epidural or spinal anaesthesia has been questioned for fear of seeding the virus into the cerebrospinal fluid (CSF) and thus accelerating the central nervous system (CNS) progression of the infection; seeding opportunistic infective organisms into the CNS; and complications related to underlying and undiagnosed CNS pathology. Since CSF involvement occurs very early in HIV infection, no further risk is generally felt to exist, and this is supported by clinical experience, albeit limited. Epidural blood patch has also been performed in HIV-positive patients without apparent adverse consequences. There has been no report of secondary CNS infection introduced during administration of regional anaesthesia in the HIV-infected mother and this risk is generally felt to be theoretical only. Further, if no evidence of CNS involvement exists then most authorities recommend regional anaesthesia as routine. If CNS abnormalities do exist then management is dependent on their severity and other considerations such as the presence of other complications.

Most units now treat HIV-positive mothers with antiviral drugs, e.g. zidovudine, which has been shown to reduce transmission to the neonate by up to two-thirds. Combination with elective Caesarean section reduces the risk further, to about 1%, although some authorities have suggested that vaginal delivery is an acceptable option in the UK since the risk of vertical transmission has fallen to ~1% if the mother is well controlled on HAART. There is wide consensus that breastfeeding should be discouraged.

Because of the implications of testing for HIV, most health authorities advocate the approach of 'universal precautions' to potentially at-risk patients; thus routine management of all women on the labour ward should involve the use of protective clothing where appropriate (gloves, goggles etc., according to individual choice), use of disposable equipment or proper sterilisation techniques and careful handling and disposal of contaminated sharps. If these practices are routinely followed, the known HIV-positive patient should need no extra measures. Many units have policies such as this and have accepted the cost implications of such all-inclusive guidelines, especially given the high cost and high profile of legal proceedings against establishments where cross-infection has occurred. If an accidental needle-stick injury or similar event occurs, local protocols and specialists should be consulted for guidance about prophylactic zidovudine therapy, since this is a controversial area. The risk of seroconversion after needlestick is about 0.3%.

Key points

- HIV infection affects 0.03–2.4% of UK obstetric patients.
- HIV-positive mothers may have many systems affected and may be taking several drugs.
- General anaesthetic management is according to standard criteria for indications and contraindications.
- Universal precautions should apply to all patients to reduce contamination of staff.

FURTHER READING

Avidan MS, Groves P, Blott M, *et al.* Low complication rate associated with cesarean section under spinal anesthesia for HIV-1-infected women on antiretroviral therapy. *Anesthesiology* 2002; **97**: 320–4.

Evron S, Glezerman M, Harow E, Sadan O, Ezri T. Human Immunodeficiency Virus: anesthetic and obstetric considerations. *Anesth Analg* 2004; **98**: 503–11.

Gershon RY, Manning-Williams D. Anesthesia and the HIV-infected parturient: a retrospective study. *Int J Obstet Anesth* 1997; **6**: 76–81.

Royal College of Obstetricians and Gynaecologists. *Management of HIV in pregnancy.* London: RCOG, 2004.

137 SEPSIS

A number of infections, especially those affecting the genitourinary tract, are more common during pregnancy, possibly related to maternal immunosuppression. Many have the potential to cause systemic involvement if untreated. Genital tract sepsis (particularly puerperal) was the leading cause of maternal death in the UK from the 1700s to the early/mid 1900s; the incidence fell in subsequent years but the number of deaths increased from the mid 1980s. Sepsis is therefore still an important cause of maternal mortality.

Problems/special considerations

Severe sepsis in obstetrics is usually associated with bacterial infection. It is thought that endogenous inflammatory mediators (including cytokines, histamine and complement products) are produced from peripheral mononuclear cells, mast cells and vascular endothelium in response to endotoxin from the cell walls of Gram-negative bacteria or to polysaccharide from Gram-positive bacteria. This results in widespread organ dysfunction, with renal impairment and acute respiratory distress syndrome (ARDS) common manifestations. Whether these target organs are more at risk in the parturient because of the physiological changes that occur during pregnancy is uncertain.

Bacteria commonly involved include *Escherichia coli* (Gram-negative) and Group B haemolytic streptococci (Gram-positive), the latter of great historical importance as the major cause of puerperal deaths.

Clinically, patients become hypermetabolic, with pyrexia, tachycardia, tachypnoea and classically warm and well-perfused peripheries. White cell count is typically increased but may be normal early on (or decreased if infection is overwhelming); it must be remembered also that white cell count may increase during normal labour to up to 40×10^9/l, and may also increase after steroid therapy given for prematurity. A left shift in peripheral blood white cell profile may be an early marker of infection. As organ impairment develops, hypotension, circulatory shutdown, oliguria, dyspnoea and impaired consciousness occur. Severe sepsis associated with (especially Gram-positive) bacteraemia may present with non-specific signs such as abdominal pain and diarrhoea, with or without pyrexia. It is typically rapid and overwhelming; when death occurs it often does so within 36 hours of presentation.

Unusual organisms may be responsible occasionally, especially in immunocompromised patients such as those with HIV infection or a history of drug abuse.

Institution of an epidural or spinal block in the presence of systemic infection is potentially very hazardous since cardiovascular compensation, which may be just adequate to maintain blood pressure etc. within normal limits, may be abolished, with catastrophic results as sympathetic blockade develops. In addition, there is a risk of epidural/meningeal infection arising from blood-borne organisms.

The fetus is at increased risk from many infections during pregnancy, whether manifested by increased incidence of congenital malformations, premature delivery, the consequences of general maternal illness or neonatal infection. Chorioamnionitis itself has been implicated in causing premature labour; thus prophylactic antibiotics have been studied as a means of delaying onset of labour in premature rupture of membranes.

Management

Prophylactic intraoperative antibiotic therapy has been shown to reduce the incidence of sepsis following Caesarean section and should be routine. Usually this is given by the anaesthetist; administration is often delayed until after delivery to avoid drugs passing into the fetus. Also, should an allergic reaction occur, the baby will already have been delivered.

As with sepsis generally, management is primarily supportive with intravenous fluids, anti-infective agents and oxygen therapy. Minor bacterial infections must be taken seriously and treated promptly, especially on the labour ward where antibiotics may easily be forgotten amongst other things going on. Antibiotic therapy should be with broad-spectrum drugs initially, guided by the most likely responsible organisms, e.g. cefuroxime/metronidazole $\pm$ gentamicin for chorioamnionitis.

Swabs and blood cultures should always be taken and therapy adjusted according to any organisms grown. If severe Gram-positive sepsis is suspected, high-dose intravenous penicillin should precede microbiological confirmation because of the rapid course of the disease.

The decision whether to use regional anaesthesia for labour or operative delivery depends on cardiovascular (in)stability, severity of infection and the individual circumstances of the case, given the risks outlined above. It has been suggested that epidural block is preferable to spinal in the presence of infection since the dura acts as a barrier to infection, but evidence for this is lacking. Regional anaesthesia is commonly administered in the presence of mild localised infection (e.g. chorioamnionitis) so long as there is antibiotic cover in case of subclinical bacteraemia; this is supported by experimental animal work and also by clinical experience.

Infection should always be borne in mind when cardiovascular collapse or other adverse events occur in the maternity suite. Prompt management is crucial in preventing an otherwise relatively minor problem becoming life threatening. Many units have protocols and guidelines for management of the more common or serious infections in pregnancy.

Key points

- Infections are common in pregnancy.
- Minor infections may have serious implications for the mother and baby unless treated.
- Sepsis should always be considered if adverse events occur.

FURTHER READING

Bader AM, Gilbertson L, Kirz L, Datta S. Regional anesthesia in women with chorioamnionitis. *Reg Anesth* 1992; **17**: 84–6.

Fernandez-Perez, Evans R, Salman, S, Pendem S, Farmer JC. Sepsis during pregnancy. *Crit Care Med* 2005; **33** (10 Suppl): S286–93.

Goodman EJ, DeHorta E, Taguiam JM. Safety of spinal and epidural anesthesia in parturients with chorioamnionitis. *Reg Anesth* 1996; **21**: 436–41.

Morgan PJ. Maternal death following epidural anaesthesia for caesarean section delivery in a patient with unsuspected sepsis. *Can J Anaesth* 1995; **42**: 330–4.

138   STEROID THERAPY

In pregnancy, steroids are used for the same conditions as in the non-pregnant state, i.e. inflammatory conditions such as sarcoidosis, rheumatoid arthritis, etc. They may also be used for obstetric medical conditions, e.g. antiphospholipid syndrome. Finally, maternal administration of glucocorticoids (usually dexamethasone or betamethasone) has been shown to reduce the incidence of respiratory distress syndrome and related complications in premature babies; the drugs are usually given as two doses 12–24 hours apart, with delivery 24 hours after the second dose if possible. The benefit is greatest at 30–32 weeks' gestation.

Problems/special considerations

Anaesthetic concerns are related to the underlying reason for steroid therapy, the presence of side effects of steroids and the requirement for supplementary steroids to cover the stress of delivery.

Reason for steroid therapy

This may be related to maternal disease or premature delivery, as described above.

Side effects

These are well known and no different in the pregnant state to those in the non-pregnant state, and they may be of relevance to the anaesthetist (e.g. electrolyte disturbance, osteoporosis). In general, hydrocortisone and prednisolone are about 90% metabolised by the placenta and therefore little reaches the fetus. However, maternal dosage above 10 mg prednisolone per day has been associated with neonatal adrenal suppression, and similar effects are theoretically possible in breastfed neonates, although reported measured concentrations of steroids in breast milk have been extremely low. There are unlikely to be adverse maternal effects of short-term administration of steroids given for premature delivery, although transient reductions in fetal heart rate variability have been reported.

Steroid supplementation

Severe hypotension characterises the acute adrenocortical insufficiency of Addison's disease, and hypotension may also occur following surgery or trauma in chronic takers of steroids who do not receive supplementation, presumably as a result of suppression of the adrenals' ability to mount a stress response. This has led to the recommendation that all patients on steroid therapy should receive supplementation perioperatively; however, the population at risk is uncertain, although most authorities would include all those with more than a week's steroid therapy within the last 3–6 months. The dosage prescribed is often chosen in a heavy-handed and non-scientific manner. If too much steroid is given, there is at least a theoretical risk of increased susceptibility to infection; in addition, many patients dislike taking increased doses because depression and other mood changes may be apparent even after a short time, although other side effects typically take longer to occur. Finally, the amount of steroid reaching the neonate through breast milk should be kept to a minimum, even though small.

Management options

For general surgery, a more logical approach than the traditional '200 mg hydrocortisone 6-hourly' is to consider the normal endogenous response to surgery and to ensure that the equivalent amount of steroid is provided, e.g. 25–50 mg hydrocortisone for minor surgery, 75–100 mg for intermediate surgery and 100–150 mg for major surgery (N.B. 1 mg prednisolone is equivalent to 4 mg hydrocortisone). This daily amount is required for 1–3 days depending on the extent of surgery and should include any therapy the patient is already taking, e.g. maintenance dose.

The situation concerning labour and delivery is less clear; although Caesarean section could be considered intermediate/major surgery, the stress of a prolonged and difficult labour is likely to be greater than that of a simple and rapid one. In general, the above plan may be adapted according to the particular circumstances of the case. If the patient is already taking adequate steroid to cover the daily requirement, no extra steroid should be required so long as the usual dose can be taken orally. If supplementation is necessary, it can be given as hydrocortisone intravenously divided into 2–4 doses per day or oral prednisolone, each tailing off after the required period.

Key points

- Steroids may be given for medical or obstetric purposes.
- Side effects may be important to the anaesthetist just as in the general population, although they are usually not a problem after administration for premature delivery.
- Steroid cover should be given according to the particular circumstances of the case but most patients require less than is traditionally given.

FURTHER READING

Nicholson G, Burrin JM, Hall GM. Peri-operative steroid supplementation. *Anaesthesia* 1998; **53**: 1091–104.

139   SUBSTANCE ABUSE

The definition of this term is difficult, since use of non-medically indicated substances ranges from socially acceptable activities such as smoking and moderate alcohol intake to abuse of intravenous drugs. Many types of abuse coexist.

Drug abuse is an increasing problem in inner city units. Most experience is from the USA, where up to 20% of pregnant women are thought to have abused illicit substances (usually marijuana or cannabis) at some point during their pregnancy.

Problems/special considerations

Problems may be related to the maternal effects of drug use, including acute intoxication, chronic organ impairment and the risk of HIV infection and endocarditis for intravenous drug users; the control of drug use and withdrawal during pregnancy and labour; and the effects of drug abuse on the fetus and neonate. Because delivery is seen as a 'normal' process and the mothers may not consider themselves as unwell, they may continue taking the drug up to and through the peripartum period, thus presenting with the acute effects of intoxication, including altered mental state. This may make communication, and especially consent, difficult or impossible. Many addicts present for the first time in labour, with poor antenatal care. There is a greater incidence of sexually transmitted disease in addicts.

Alcohol

Alcohol abuse is a more widespread problem than abuse of many recreational drugs, with well-known manifestations including malnutrition, hepatic and cardiac impairment, etc. Acutely intoxicated mothers may be aggressive and may have taken other drugs as well. If the stomach is full there may be increased risk of aspiration. Acute withdrawal typically reaches its worst about 24–36 hours after cessation of intake. A particular feature of alcohol abuse in pregnancy is the fetal alcohol syndrome, which comprises craniofacial, neurological, cardiac, urological and musculoskeletal abnormalities. The upper safe limit of alcohol consumption in pregnancy has not been determined, but recent evidence suggests that even minimal intake may be associated with behavioural difficulties.

Tobacco

Smoking is a common problem worldwide; in the UK there has been a recent upward trend in smoking in women and especially young people, despite its overall decline in popularity as socially acceptable behaviour. Maternal effects are well known; in the neonate it has been long associated with low birth-weight, although the precise mechanism is unclear.

Cocaine

Cocaine, or its water-insoluble derivative crack, causes central and peripheral dopaminergic and adrenergic stimulation resulting in euphoria, increased alertness, vasoconstriction and hypertension. Myocardial ischaemia and arrhythmias may occur, and convulsions, intracranial haemorrhages and renal, hepatic and haematological impairment (including thrombocytopenia) have been reported. Cocaine abuse has been associated with increased incidence of spontaneous abortion, placental abruption, premature labour and fetal morbidity and mortality. Prolonged action of suxamethonium has also been reported. Diagnosis may be difficult since its use is often denied and the presentation may resemble that of pre-eclampsia and phaeochromocytoma. Urine remains positive for cocaine metabolites up to 3 days after use, and testing has been suggested in all at-risk groups (e.g. known users of other drugs, unbooked pregnancies, etc.).

Opioids

Opioid abuse is associated with hepatic, renal, pulmonary and cardiovascular impairment. Gastric emptying is impaired. The incidence of pre-eclampsia is reportedly increased. Addicts may require central venous cannulation because of their poor peripheral veins. Apart from these considerations, opioid withdrawal may complicate labour and delivery, and postoperative analgesia may be dificult to provide. Withdrawal typically occurs 8–16 hours after cessation of intake, with features increasing over 1–3 days. Opioid antagonists may precipitate acute withdrawal (including neonatal). Neonatal withdrawal may occur several days postpartum. Other neonatal effects of opioid addiction include increased fetal loss and growth retardation.

Cannabis

Cannabis has been associated with increased incidence of peripartum complications, including arrest of labour and fetal morbidity. Cardiac arrhythmias, especially tachycardia, and myocardial depression have also been reported.

Amphetamines

Although less commonly abused than the above drugs, amphetamines acutely cause similar effects to cocaine, including hypertension, arrhythmias, agitation, fever and confusion. Fetal effects include growth retardation, premature labour and abruption. Acute ingestion may increase the requirement for anaesthetic drugs, whereas chronic abuse may result in central depression and depletion of catecholamine stores. Both regional and general anaesthesia may be accompanied by severe hypotension in chronically abusing patients.

Others

Experience with methylenedioxymethylamphetamine (MDMA; 'Ecstasy') and solvent abuse in obstetrics is limited but the same maternal manifestations may occur as is seen in non-pregnant subjects. Barbiturate abuse is less common now; its main problems are acute intoxication and chronic addiction/withdrawal.

Management options

General management is directed at any specific organ impairment (including central nervous system depression) and providing appropriate nutrition and psychological support and counselling. Substance abuse should always be considered in the differential diagnosis of any atypical case, e.g. unexplained collapse or acute confusion.

Management of acute alcohol withdrawal includes oral clomethiazole or benzodiazepines. Alcohol infusion may also be used (10–150 ml/h of a 5–10% solution), although it may suppress uterine contractions.

If abusers of cocaine require general anaesthesia, pretreatment with antihypertensive drugs should be considered, since severe hypertension and arrhythmias may follow tracheal intubation. Labetalol has been suggested as the drug of choice since pure β-blockade may precipitate severe hypertension via unopposed α stimulation. Glyceryl trinitrate has also been used. Benzodiazepines have been recommended to reduce sympathetic activity. Drugs causing sympathetic stimulation or arrhythmias (e.g. ketamine or halothane respectively) should be avoided. During regional anaesthesia, haemodynamic instability may be greater than normal and resistance to ephedrine has been reported, possibly related to noradrenaline depletion (directly acting vasopressors such as phenylephrine may be preferable). Increased requirement for analgesic supplementation during Caesarean section has also been described.

Many anaesthetists avoid opiods altogether and use local anaesthetic alone for regional analgesia/anaesthesia, though this is controversial.

Key points

- Problems of substance abuse in pregnancy/labour include the maternal effects of chronic abuse, acute effects on presentation and fetal/neonatal effects.
- A high index of suspicion is required in all atypical cases on the labour ward.

FURTHER READING

Cassidy B, Cyna AM. Challenges that opioid-dependent women present to the obstetric anaesthetist. *Anaesth Intens Care* 2004; **32**: 494–501.

Kuczkowski KM. Anesthetic implications of drug abuse in pregnancy. *J Clin Anesth* 2003; **15**: 382–94.

Kuczkowski KM. The cocaine abusing parturient: a review of anesthetic considerations. *Can J Anesth* 2004; **51**: 145–54.

Ludlow JP, Evans SF, Hulse G. Obstetric and perinatal outcomes in pregnancies associated with illicit substance abuse. *Aust N Z J Obstet Gynaecol* 2004; **44**: 302–6.

140   TRAUMA IN PREGNANCY

Trauma during pregnancy may be coincidental or related to instability and difficulty moving, especially in the third trimester. It is a consistent cause of maternal death, usually associated with road traffic accidents but also including other forms such as violence, suicide and falls. Although the general principles are the same as in non-pregnant women, the physiological effects of pregnancy and the presence of the fetus impose particular conditions upon the presentation, assessment and management of injured mothers.

Problems/special considerations

- The increased metabolic demands of pregnancy make the mother less tolerant of hypotension, poor organ perfusion and hypoxaemia. Assessment of circulating volume status may be complicated by the increased cardiac output, pulse rate and blood volume of pregnancy and the potential for aortocaval compression. Injury to the abdomen and/or pelvis may result in fetal injury, maternal urinary tract injury or severe haemorrhage from the increased vascularity.

- Obstetric complications include premature rupture of membranes, premature labour and placental abruption, the last an especially common cause of fetal death. Fetomaternal haemorrhage may occur, with maternal sensitisation to fetal blood antigens if susceptible.
- The fetus is susceptible to the effects of drugs given to the mother.

Management options

General resuscitation is as for any injured patient, with the risk of aortocaval compression and regurgitation borne in mind. The choice of drugs administered to the mother will be influenced by the stage of the pregnancy. In the early stages of pregnancy teratogenicity should be considered, and in the second and third trimesters the effect of the drugs on fetal growth and uterine function must be considered.

In the management of acute head injury, the normal blood gas values for pregnancy (arterial partial pressure of carbon dioxide approximately 4 kPa) must be remembered, especially when artificial ventilation is required. The risk of acid aspiration should be considered when airway reflexes are obtunded, and early intubation and ventilation may need to be considered.

Many of these women will require diagnostic radiological investigations, especially for head or spinal cord injury. Computerised tomography requires that the fetus is screened from the ionising radiation. Magnetic resonance imaging (MRI) requires an immobile patient, which may necessitate general anaesthesia with all its attendant risks. Aortocaval compression must be avoided at all times. Access to the MRI scanner may not be possible in an advanced state of pregnancy.

If indicated by the clinical condition, neurosurgical procedures can be performed in pregnancy.

The fetus should be monitored for at least several hours since abruption or fetomaternal haemorrhage may be delayed. In addition, the fetus may have suffered direct injury itself or be stressed by any concomitant hypotension, hypoxaemia or maternal therapeutic drugs or maneouvres (e.g. inotropes, mannitol, furosemide, hyperventilation for control of intracranial pressure).

Caesarean delivery should be for obstetric reasons; epidural analgesia can be an integral part of the management of labour or operative delivery.

Key points

- General principles are as for non-pregnant patients.
- Pregnant women are more susceptible to the effects of hypotension and hypoxaemia.
- Aortocaval compression must be avoided at all times.
- Assessment may be complicated by the physiological changes of pregnancy.
- Placental abruption and fetomaternal haemorrhage are particular risks.

FURTHER READING

Coleman MT, Trianfo VA, Rund DA. Nonobstetric emergencies in pregnancy: trauma and surgical conditions. *Am J Obstet Gynecol* 1997; **177**: 497–502.

Connolly AM, Katz VL, Bash KL, McMahon MJ, Hansen WF. Trauma and pregnancy. *Am J Perinatol* 1997; **14**: 331–6.

Mattox KL, Goetzl L. Trauma in pregnancy. *Crit Care Med* 2005; **33** (10 Suppl): S385–89.

Polko LE, McMahon MJ. Burns in pregnancy. *Obstet Gynecol Surv* 1998; **53**: 50–6.

Weinberg L, Steele RG, Pugh R, *et al.* The pregnant trauma patient. *Anaesth Intens Care* 2005; **33**: 167–80.

141 MALIGNANT DISEASE

There have been continuing improvements in the treatment of malignancies affecting children and young adults and in the management of reduced fertility that commonly follows such treatment. There are thus increasing numbers of women with treated (but not necessarily cured) malignant disease becoming pregnant. In addition, malignant disease may occasionally present for the first time during pregnancy and may also be related to the pregnancy itself.

Problems/special considerations

General problems of malignancy

These may be local (compression effects, local invasion, scarring, etc.), metastatic (e.g. liver involvement etc.) or general (malaise, anaemia, endocrine effects, weight loss and cachexia). There may also be problems relating to treatment, e.g. cytotoxic drugs, steroids, fibrotic effects of radiotherapy. There may be coagulation abnormalities or increased risk of deep-vein thrombosis necessitating anticoagulant therapy. Electrolyte disturbances may be a feature of the malignancy (e.g. hypercalcaemia) or its treatment.

Problems during pregnancy

Malignancies may be affected by the different hormonal profile of pregnancy and its effects on the tissues; this may make certain tumours more aggressive (e.g. breast cancer, melanoma). Some maternal malignancies may metastasise to the fetus or placenta (e.g. melanoma), although in general this is rare.

The patient's medication may need altering, especially in early pregnancy, since many cytotoxic drugs are harmful to the fetus. Similarly, there may be concerns about the use of radiotherapy or even surgery to treat malignancy during pregnancy, and the risks and benefits to both the mother and the fetus of administering or withholding treatment need careful consideration. In addition, the normal psychological stresses of pregnancy and delivery are especially intense if the mother has (or has had) cancer. The physiological demands of normal pregnancy may stress the more susceptible systems in the mother with malignant disease, e.g. anaemia may become more pronounced; mild cytotoxic-induced cardiomyopathy may become more severe. Finally, there may be direct effects of the malignancy or its treatment on the uterus and birth canal, e.g. cervical surgery and scarring, perineal scarring and abdominal adhesions.

A particular form of malignant disease affecting pregnancy is that arising from the placenta itself (gestational trophoblastic neoplasia), comprising hydatiform mole, invasive mole, choriocarcinoma and placental site trophopbastic tumour. It is more common at the extremes of reproductive age, in the Far East and Asia and if previous pregnancies have been affected. The pregnancy itself is non-viable and concerns about the fetus do not apply. These tumours generally respond well to chemotherapy, even if metastatic spread has occurred, with a mortality of < 1%. Molar pregnancy may be associated with hyperemesis, hypertensive disease, anaemia, ovarian cysts and rarely hyperthyroidism. Surgical evacuation may be followed by pulmonary oedema or acute lung injury, possibly related to trophoblastic pulmonary embolism.

Management options

General care is directed towards the particular organs or systems affected by the malignancy itself and its treatment. Thus all mothers require careful antenatal assessment with particular attention to haematological, cardiac, renal and hepatic function etc., with decisions concerning anaesthetic management made accordingly. Some mothers may knowingly have put their lives at risk in order to give the fetus the best chance of survival, and this must be respected when managing their analgesia and anaesthesia.

In trophoblastic neoplastic disease, uterine evacuation may be adequate surgical management but hysterectomy may be required in more invasive disease, especially in older women. Surgery may also be required for torsion of, or haemorrhage into, ovarian cysts. Chemotherapy may be required if human chorionic gonadotrophin levels remain elevated or in metastatic disease. In terms of anaesthetic management, the above considerations should be taken into account and appropriate measures taken regarding investigation (including liver and thyroid function blood tests and chest radiography), monitoring and management. General anaesthesia is usually recommended since uterine bleeding may be rapid and severe, and blood should be cross-matched and ready before surgery.

Key points

- Malignancies may be present before pregnancy, may develop or be diagnosed during pregnancy or may arise from the pregnancy itself.
- Problems may be related to general effects of malignancies or those related to the interaction between malignancy, its treatment and pregnancy.
- Gestational trophoblastic neoplasia represents a particular form of malignancy.

FURTHER READING

Maxwell C, Barzilay B, Shah V, *et al.* Maternal and neonatal outcomes in pregnancies complicated by bone and soft-tissue tumors. *Obstet Gynecol* 2004; **104**: 344–8.

Ward RM, Bristow RE. Cancer and pregnancy: recent developments. *Curr Opin Obstet Gynecol* 2002; **14**: 613–17.

142 TRANSPLANTATION

Advances in transplant surgery and in immunosuppressive drug treatment have led to increasing numbers of women with transplanted organs choosing to embark on pregnancy. Pregnancy following renal transplantation is now almost commonplace, and successful pregnancy following liver, heart and heart–lung transplantation has been reported. The major considerations for the medical staff caring for the pregnant transplant recipient are the effects of immunosuppressive therapy, the alteration in physiological function of the transplanted organ and the impact of the physiological changes of pregnancy.

Problems/special considerations

Immunosuppressive therapy

All transplant patients are at risk of organ rejection and therefore require long-term immunosuppressive therapy. There is no evidence that pregnancy itself increases the risk of rejection, which, in the case of renal transplants, is about 10% in the first year and up to 40% after 5 years.

Infections, both bacterial and viral, are more common because of the immunosuppressed state, with urinary tract infections (already more common during pregnancy) being the most frequent infectious complication. The immunosuppressed patient is at risk of infection with uncommon pathogens, and it is therefore important to take appropriate cultures before beginning treatment.

Cyclosporin, azathioprine and corticosteroids are the most frequently used immunosuppressive drugs, although newer agents that may reduce the rate of organ rejection are being introduced. Frequent monitoring of drug levels is required because of the changing blood volume during pregnancy, although in some cases the dose requirement may be reduced rather than increased.

Cyclosporin is associated with systemic hypertension (caused by activation of the sympathetic nervous system), and women with transplanted organs also have an increased risk of developing pre-eclampsia – an incidence of 30% has been reported. Pre-eclampsia may be difficult to diagnose because of the pre-existing hypertension and proteinuria. There have also been reports of thrombotic complications occurring in patients receiving cyclosporin, leading to recommendations that prophylactic heparin should be considered during pregnancy.

Azathioprine is associated with abnormal liver function tests and thrombocytopenia.

The problems associated with long-term corticosteroid therapy are well known; of specific concern during pregnancy are hypertension and glucose intolerance.

Immunosuppressive drugs are associated with a relatively low rate of fetal abnormality (cyclosporin is less teratogenic than azathioprine) but an increased rate of pre-term delivery and intrauterine growth retardation.

Renal function

The background rate of deterioration in renal function following transplantation is about 10% per year, and this is not affected by pregnancy. It is important to monitor renal function closely throughout pregnancy; as with hypertension, there may be difficulty with differential diagnosis if pre-eclampsia develops.

Heart and heart–lung transplant

The transplanted heart is denervated, and thus there are no vagal influences acting upon it. Adequate cardiac output is dependent on maintenance of adequate preload. Heart rate can increase in response to hypovolaemia or vasodilatation, but this response is delayed compared with that of the normal pregnant woman. There is considerable controversy regarding the response of the denervated heart to adrenergic agonists, with reports of both extreme hypersensitivity and blunted response. Likewise there have been reports of bradycardia and even sinus arrest following administration of neostigmine, despite theoretical grounds for believing that the drug should not alter the rate of the denervated heart.

Afferent denervation of the heart prevents the patient experiencing angina; the anaesthetist and obstetrician should be aware that the woman with a cardiac transplant is at increased risk of coronary artery disease (20% by one year post-transplant and up to 50% by 5 years), which can only be reliably detected by cardiac catheterisation.

Obstetric outcomes

Apart from the increased incidence of pre-eclampsia with cyclosporin, parturients who are recipients of transplanted organs have an increased risk of premature delivery, intrauterine growth retardation and the need for operative delivery. Surgery may be complicated by the previous transplant and the risk of postoperative infection is increased.

Management options

Most women are advised not to become pregnant for 18–24 months after tranplantation, in order to allow organ function and immunosuppressive therapy to stabilise.

There are reports of successful vaginal delivery following renal, heart, heart–lung and hepatic transplants. As a general rule Caesarean section is only indicated for obstetric complications, although each case must be considered individually. The woman with a renal transplant can be treated as normal and may receive epidural analgesia and either regional or general anaesthesia. Particular attention should be paid to venous access, keeping cannulae as peripheral as possible and preserving any sites for shunts and fistulae.

Epidural analgesia has been used for heart transplant recipients in labour, and regional anaesthesia (both epidural and spinal) has been used successfully for operative delivery. It is important to avoid dehydration and to use adequate preloading, but the risks of catheter-related sepsis probably outweigh the benefits of central venous pressure monitoring in these patients. Ephedrine has been used in normal doses, but it is wise to use small increments because of the risk of exaggerated response to the drug.

Infectious complications remain one of the major risks for all transplant recipients, and scrupulous attention to aseptic technique is therefore vital.

Key points

- Immunosuppressive drugs are used by all transplant recipients.
- Cyclosporin is associated with systemic hypertension and proteinuria.
- Transplanted hearts are denervated and cardiac output is primarily dependent on preload.
- Successful vaginal delivery with epidural analgesia has been reported following organ transplantation.

FURTHER READING

Cardonick E, Moritz M, Armenti V. Pregnancy in patients with organ transplantation: a review. *Obstet Gynecol Surv* 2004; **59**: 214–22.

Kallen B, Westgren M, Aberg A, Olausson PO. Pregnancy outcome after maternal organ transplantation in Sweden. *Br J Obstet Gynaecol* 2005; **112**: 904–9.

McKay DB, Josephson MA. Pregnancy in recipients of solid organs – effects on mother and child. *New Eng J Med* 2006; **354**: 1281–93.

Rigg CD, Bythell VE, Bryson MR, Halshaw J, Davidson JM. Caesarean section in patients with heart-lung transplants: a report of three cases and review. *Int J Obstet Anesth* 2000; **9**: 125–32.

143 INTENSIVE CARE IN PREGNANCY

Information about intensive care in pregnancy is hampered by the lack of detail provided in published reports, differing admission criteria used by different units and the absence of systematic data collection schemes. The Report on Confidential Enquiries into Maternal Deaths/Maternal and Child Health recognises the importance of adequate intensive care unit (ICU) provision and care, but since it focuses solely on deaths it does not give a complete picture of critical illness and pregnancy, although recent enquiries have included questions about ICU management. The need for adequate provision of ICU or high-dependency beds, especially in smaller delivery units, is repeatedly stressed. More recently, emphasis has been on providing 'intensive care' to the sick mother within the maternity unit – i.e. before she is actually admitted to the ICU.

Most series give an overall ICU admission rate of 0.2–9 per 1000 deliveries, although there is much variation between countries and even units as a result of differences in patient population and selection. The most common reasons for admission are haemorrhage and hypertensive disorders (including HELLP [haemolysis, elevated liver enzymes and low platelet count] syndrome). Most patients stay in the ICU for less than 3–4 days. Mortality rates are difficult to estimate for the above reasons but are generally low overall (in the order of 3–4% in reported UK series), although they range from 0–20% in published series worldwide. Objective prediction of mortality is hampered by the relative inability of standard scoring systems (e.g. APACHE) to allow for obstetric factors; e.g. platelet count has greater importance in obstetric patients than in the non-pregnant population.

Problems/special considerations

General ICU care is as for non-obstetric patients. Particular points to note are the risks to the fetus and the need for fetal monitoring (if antepartum), the requirements of the patient's partner and family, the midwifery care required in the puerperium (if postpartum) and the physiological changes of pregnancy. Of particular importance amongst the latter are the increased risk of aspiration; the increased oxygen demands and changes in respiratory function; the apparently increased propensity of critically ill obstetric patients to develop acute lung injury, susceptibility to aortocaval compression, increased cardiac output and other cardiovascular changes; and haematological changes including anaemia, increased risk of deep-vein thrombosis (DVT) and the readiness towards disseminated intravascular coagulation. These effects of pregnancy may be overlooked by intensivists unfamiliar with managing pregnant women. Finally, there may be psychological problems in the mother who is, or has been, critically ill, both before and after delivery. The fetus is likely to have been affected by her illness, increasing the stress upon her. The ICU environment is a far from ideal place to deliver or care for a baby.

Management options

Routine ICU support includes DVT and stress ulcer prophylaxis. Management of any associated organ failure is along standard lines. Premature labour is always a risk of severe maternal illness; however, the use of tocolytic drugs may be considered too risky for the mother. Aortocaval compression must be avoided at all times.

Caesarean section may be required in order to improve the mother's condition, e.g. in severe cardiac or respiratory disease or hypertensive disorders. Postpartum haemorrhage may be severe if a coagulopathy is present. Breast milk may be collected postpartum but may be unsuitable for use because of maternally administered drugs. If breast milk is not collected for neonatal feeding or to maintain lactation until the mother is well enough to nurse, lactation can be suppressed with bromocriptine, although this is not recommended routinely (especially in pre-eclampsia) since hypertension, stroke and myocardial infarction have followed its use.

Good communication between all the involved clinicians (obstetricians, intensivists, etc.) and midwife/ICU nursing staff is vital to ensure that continuity of care is achieved with regard to treatment decisions and information given to relatives.

Key points

- About 0.2–9 per 1000 obstetric patients require intensive care.
- Hypertensive disorders and haemorrhage are the most common causes of admission.
- Basic principles apply but the special needs of the fetus/neonate, mother and family, and the physiological effects of pregnancy, must be remembered.
- Overall mortality of intensive care unit admission in UK series is 3–4%.

FURTHER READING

Gernaina S, Wyncolb D, Nelson-Piercyc C. Management of the critically ill obstetric patient. *Curr Obstet Gynacol* 2006; **16**: 125–33.

Gopalan PD, Muckart DJJ. The critically ill obstetric patient:what's the score? *Int J Obstet Anesth* 2004; **13**: 144–5.

Hazelgrove JF, Price C, Pappachan VJ, Smith GB. Multicenter study of obstetric admissions to 14 intensive care units in southern England. *Crit Care Med* 2001; **29**: 770–5.

Martin SR, Foley MR. Intensive care in obstetrics: an evidence based review. *Am J Obstet Gynecol* 2006; **195**: 673–89.

Soubra SH, Guntupalli KK. Critical illness in pregnancy: An overview. *Crit Care Med.* 2005; **33** (10 Suppl): S248–55.

Waterstone M, Bewley S, Wolfe C. Incidence and predictors of severe obstetric morbidity: case-control study. *BMJ* 2001; **322**: 1089–93.

144   INVASIVE MONITORING

The increase in the number of pregnant women with significant coexisting medical disease has led to a need for high-dependency facilities during labour, delivery and the puerperium. In addition, women with complications of pregnancy such as pre-eclampsia may require high-dependency care. In these situations, an understanding of the pathophysiological changes that are taking place may be improved by the use of invasive monitoring.

Recent Reports on Confidential Enquiries into Maternal Deaths/Maternal and Child Health in the United Kingdom (CEMD/CEMACH) have recommended the more frequent and earlier use of invasive monitoring in the management of obstetric haemorrhage.

Problems/special considerations

Midwives are not intensive care nurses, and invasive monitoring can only aid management if the data obtained are reliable and correctly interpreted. All invasive cardiovascular monitoring has significant morbidity associated with its use, such as line sepsis, inadvertent arterial puncture, pneumothorax and even death. Insertion of pulmonary artery catheters is associated with a particularly high morbidity, and their use is becoming increasingly controversial.

The relative risks and benefits of invasive monitoring need to be assessed carefully – the difficulties of conducting labour and delivery on an intensive care unit may, in some circumstances, outweigh the potential benefits of such monitoring. However, major obstetric haemorrhage can occur in any maternity unit at any time. The implications of the CEMD/CEMACH recommendations are that all obstetric units should be able to care for women with central venous pressure (CVP) monitoring, and that if they cannot do so these women should be transferred to an intensive care unit.

Management options

Central venous pressure monitoring

Insertion of a central venous catheter to measure right atrial pressure may give valuable information in women with coexisting cardiac disease (see relevant chapters for further details). Most protocols for managing women with severe pre-eclampsia also suggest insertion of a CVP line to aid in fluid management, although it is important to realise that the information obtained (right atrial pressure) may not accurately reflect left atrial pressure.

The least invasive technique is recommended for women who are undelivered; that is, use of a long line inserted from a peripheral vein (usually in the antecubital fossa). It may be technically difficult to cannulate the subclavian or internal jugular vein in the neck of a pregnant woman. She will be intolerant of the head-down position, and the need to adopt lateral tilt or the supine wedged position may distort the usual anatomical landmarks. The apprehension caused by attempting insertion of a neck line may provoke hypertension or arrhythmias caused by increased circulating catecholamines. In addition, the pre-eclamptic woman may have considerable soft tissue oedema of the face and neck and may also be thrombocytopenic.

A directly transduced trace is preferable to use of a manometer set. A clear right atrial pressure waveform may provide confirmation of correct placement of the line without the need for radiological confirmation, although the decision about whether to perform radiography should follow consideration of the relative risks and benefits. Chest radiography should be performed regardless of whether the woman is delivered if there is any anxiety about correct placement or complications of insertion.

Midwives should be able to look after women with CVP lines, and there should be an ongoing programme of in-service training to ensure that new staff are familiar with this aspect of care of high-risk patients.

Pulmonary artery catheterisation

The place of pulmonary arter catheterisation is becoming increasingly disputed, since its use has been linked to increased mortality in some studies (although patient selection may be a confounding factor). In obstetrics, many authorities would reserve its use for extreme cases of impaired global cardiac function such as cardiomyopathy, or for severe pre-eclampsia with impaired left ventricular function. The risks are those of CVP monitoring plus the potential for pulmonary artery rupture and infarction, as well as technical problems such as knotting of the catheter.

Direct arterial pressure monitoring

Intra-arterial monitoring provides valuable information in conditions where even brief periods of hypotension may cause significant morbidity or mortality. Women with cardiac disease resulting in relatively fixed cardiac output require continuous blood pressure monitoring if epidural analgesia is used in labour and before induction of either general or regional anaesthesia for operative delivery.

Direct arterial pressure monitoring is desirable in women with severe pre-eclampsia.

On rare occasions an intra-arterial cannula may be inserted to facilitate frequent arterial blood gas analysis in women with severe respiratory pathology.

Most midwives are not used to managing arterial lines, and it is therefore vital to ensure that the line is clearly labelled to minimise the risk of it being confused with an intravenous line. The insertion site must be readily accessible and kept visible at all times. It is sensible to explain the purpose of the line to the mother and to involve her in responsibility for its care.

Key points

- High-dependency care of women with coexisting medical disease or obstetric complications of pregnancy may require invasive monitoring.
- If appropriate monitoring cannot be provided in the maternity unit in which the woman is intending to deliver, arrangements should be made to transfer her care to another unit.

FURTHER READING

Nolan TE, Wakefield ML, Devoe LD. Invasive hemodynamic monitoring in obstetrics. *Chest* 1992; **101**: 1429–33.

VII The neonate

145 NEONATAL ASSESSMENT

Formal assessment of the newborn baby is important to allow documentation of the neonate's general state of wellbeing; as a prognostic exercise, to identify neonates at risk and focus medical attention on them; possibly as a means of following progress over time; and as a research tool for determining the effects of various interventions or conditions on neonatal outcome (e.g. drug therapy, anaesthetic techniques, epidemiological factors). Various methods have been described; as far as obstetric anaesthesia is concerned the important ones are those that focus on the neonate's gross physiological status at or shortly after birth and those that assess its neurobehaviour.

Problems/special considerations

The easier the system for assessment (and therefore the more attractive it is to busy clinicians), the less its ability to discern subtle differences and thus the less useful it is as a tool, especially when the effects being studied are likely to be small (e.g. a possible difference in effects of two similar drugs in labour). Conversely, tiny differences revealed by very sensitive measurements may be of uncertain significance clinically. In addition, factors that might ordinarily be prognostic may be susceptible to the actions of anaesthetic agents, e.g. ketamine may be associated with falsely high scores when using systems that rely heavily on muscle tone.

Methods of assessment

Measures of overall physiological status

- *Time to sustained respiration (TSR):* the time between delivery and sustained spontaneous ventilation is a very crude indicator of neonatal wellbeing but does indicate babies that need special attention and attempts to quantify the degree of impairment. It does not distinguish between babies who are slow to breathe unsupported for different reasons (e.g. drugs, congenital defects)

Analgesia, Anaesthesia and Pregnancy: A Practical Guide Second Edition, ed. Steve Yentis, Anne May and Surbhi Malhotra. Published by Cambridge University Press. © Cambridge University Press 2007.

Table 145.1. Apgar scoring system

	0	1	2
Heart rate	Absent	<100	>100
Respiratory effort	Nil	Weak cry	Strong cry
Muscle tone	Limp	Poor tone	Good tone
Reflex irritability	Nil	Some movement	Strong withdrawal
Colour	Blue/pale	Pink body/blue extremities	Pink

and is best suited to birth asphyxia. It is rarely performed routinely.

- *Apgar system:* described by the American anaesthetist Apgar in 1953, the system comprises five variables, each scoring 0–2 (Table 145.1). The Apgar score is now a standard tool and is recorded routinely after virtually all deliveries. It is usually performed at 1 and 5 minutes after birth, although it may be repeated thereafter. A modified system, 'Apgar minus colour' (maximum of 8), has been suggested but is rarely used.

Tests of neurobehavioural status (sometimes referred to eponymously)

- *Neurobehavioural assessment score (NBAS):* developed in 1973 by the British paediatrician Brazelton, the NBAS is the most commonly used of the detailed neurobehavioural assessment systems. It takes 45–60 minutes and requires trained staff to perform it.
- *Early neonatal neurobehavioural scale (ENNS):* developed in 1974 by the American anaesthetist Scanlon, the ENNS is less complicated than the NBAS and therefore quicker to perform (about 5–10 minutes). It examines wakefulness, tone and the response to various stimuli, including the presence or absence of neonatal reflexes.
- *Neurological and adaptive capacity score (NACS):* developed in 1982 by the paediatrician Amiel-Tison and anaesthetic colleagues in San Francisco, the NACS takes about 5 minutes to perform and is a relatively crude measure, mainly examining neonatal tone. It has been claimed that the NACS can distinguish between the effects of asphyxia and those of drugs, although this has been challenged. It has, however, been widely used in obstetric anaesthetic studies because of its ease of use.

Effects of anaesthetic drugs

In general, the more gross an effect, the easier it is to show it; thus, for example, maternal pethidine can readily be demonstrated to suppress neonatal condition at birth and affect neurobehaviour and feeding for 1–2 days postpartum, by using relatively crude scoring systems. However, more subtle tools such as the NBAS are required to investigate smaller effects, and their significance may be disputed. Finally, the difficulty in conducting randomised studies and the inadequate size of most studies that have looked at measures of neonatal assessment in depth mean that no clear conclusions can be drawn in many cases. However, overall effects of anaesthetic and analgesic drugs are summarised in Table 145.2.

Table 145.2. Effects of maternal anaesthetic and analgesic drugs on the neonate

Systemic drugs:	Impairment is seen depending on the dosage and the test used: the more sensitive the assessment system, the greater the effect. Thus effects on alertness and responsiveness may be detected by using NBAS and ENNS before respiratory depression is seen. Some effects of pethidine are apparent 24–48 hours postpartum, and subtle differences, e.g. in feeding, may persist for up to weeks
Regional anaesthesia:	Lidocaine was suspected of impairing the ENNS in the 1970s (the 'alert but floppy baby') but this was not substantiated subsequently. There is no hard evidence of impairment after regional anaesthesia or analgesia for labour or Caesarean section with various local anaesthetics or opioids. Although some studies have claimed to find differences, the difficulty of using adequate controls and conflicting results from other studies make these uncertain
	Hypotension lasting less than 2–3 minutes has not been associated with demonstrable effects, although Apgar score, acid-base profiles and crude neurobehavioural scores have been found to be affected if hypotension is prolonged
	The place of regional anaesthesia when the fetus is compromised is still debated by anaesthetists and others, most anaesthetists supporting its use
General anaesthesia:	Its effects have been greater than those of regional anaesthetic techniques in most studies. Low concentrations of volatile agents are thought to have little effect

Key points

- Methods used to assess the neonate's state range from the very gross and simple to the complex and lengthy.
- The more complex the method used, the more subtle the changes found.
- Anaesthetic and analgesic drugs have all been implicated in affecting neurobehaviour to some degree; this is generally agreed for systemic opioids and general anaesthesia but less certain for regional anaesthetic techniques, as long as hypotension is mild and limited.
- In terms of neonatal neurobehaviour, regional anaesthesia for delivery of the severely compromised fetus is thought by most anaesthetists to have advantages over general anaesthesia but this is still disputed.

FURTHER READING
Littleford J. Effects on the fetus and newborn of maternal analgesia and anesthesia: a review. *Can J Anaesth* 2004; **51**: 586–609.

146 NEONATAL PHYSIOLOGY AND PHARMACOLOGY

The physiology of the neonate is best considered in relation to the various body systems. Some of these are considered elsewhere in this book but there follows a brief summary of the main points. Physiological factors that result in specific differences in drug handling by the neonate are also considered here. It should be remembered that functioning of the neonate's organ systems is closely related to the gestation at which it is born. Finally, factors that are important in the fetus may be equally important after birth; thus many of the following points refer to both the fetus and the neonate.

Circulatory system

In the fetus, oxygenated blood returning from the placenta is directed through the foramen ovale via the left atrium into the left ventricle, and thence preferentially to the brain. Deoxygenated blood from the brain passes via the right atrium and ventricle into the pulmonary artery; since the pulmonary vascular resistance is high, the blood passes through the ductus arteriosus into the aorta and thence via the two umbilical arteries (arising from the internal iliac arteries) to the placenta (Fig. 146.1). At birth, the systemic vascular resistance increases as the umbilical arteries close, whereas the pulmonary vascular resistance decreases as air is drawn into the lungs. Thus the circulation takes up the adult pattern, although the circulation remains transitional for about 2 weeks in term neonates, and fetal

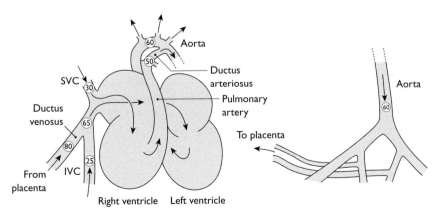

Fig. 146.1 Diagram of fetal circulation. IVC: inferior vena cava; SVC: superior vena cava. Arrows denote flow of blood. Figures refer to the approximate oxygen saturation. Reproduced with permission from Yentis, Hirsch & Smith: Anaesthesia and intensive care A-Z, 2nd edn, Butterworth Heinemann, 2000.

circulation may persist if pulmonary vascular resistance remains high (e.g. caused by hypoxaemia, acidosis, hypovolaemia and hypothermia). The neonate relies mainly on heart rate for maintenance of cardiac output, the stroke volume being relatively fixed.

Respiratory system

Two-thirds of the pulmonary fluid is expelled from the chest by compression during delivery (reduced in Caesarean section and if the neonate is small); remaining fluid is rapidly absorbed. Lung inflation is important to assist transition from the fetal to the adult circulation and to promote pulmonary surfactant production. Surfactant is required to enable alveolar expansion and is present in only small amounts up until about 34 weeks' gestation, although its production can be stimulated by maternal steroid therapy.

Fetal haemoglobin (containing α chains and γ chains) comprises about 80% of the circulating haemoglobin in the fetus. Its oxyhaemoglobin dissociation curve is shifted to the left compared with that of adult haemoglobin; thus transfer of oxygen from maternal to fetal blood is encouraged. Fetal haemoglobin normally persists for about 2–3 months after delivery, unless there is a haemoglobinopathy affecting adult haemoglobin.

The response of the neonate to hypoxia is discussed in Chapter 147, Neonatal resuscitation (p. 331).

Neurological system

The blood–brain barrier is generally accepted to be less complete in the neonate than in the adult, making the neonate more susceptible to depressant drugs, e.g. opioids. In premature babies, the fragile periventricular vessels are susceptible to fluctuations in arterial blood pressure and hypoxia, resulting in intraventricular haemorrhage.

Other systems

Heat production in the neonate is achieved by oxidation of brown fat, which results in increased oxygen requirements and may be inadequate if there has been growth retardation in utero. Thus a warm environment for delivery is especially important.

Pharmacology

Uptake of drugs by the fetus is considered in Chapter 16, Placental transfer (p. 39). The low plasma protein binding capacity of the fetus/neonate results in a greater amount of free drug in the plasma compared with that in the adult. Lipid-soluble drugs (e.g. anaesthetics) are extensively bound to fetal/neonatal tissues, offsetting this effect. Finally, fetal acidosis may result in the 'trapping' of drugs, which may persist postpartum if the neonate remains acidotic. The relative immaturity of both target organs (e.g. brain) and organs involved in metabolism (e.g. liver) make the neonate more susceptible to many drugs administered to the mother before delivery or directly to the neonate after delivery.

Key points

- Major circulatory and respiratory changes occur at birth.
- The neonate may exhibit the effects of intrapartum insults and remains susceptible to insults occurring postpartum.

147 NEONATAL RESUSCITATION

Published studies have reported some degree of resuscitation being required in up to 5–14% of neonates overall, although this may be higher in selected cases. Most neonates require assisted ventilation only. The need for resuscitation may often be predicted from the events and course of the pregnancy and labour (including the presence of meconium, the fetal heart rate and pH during labour and the mother's condition), although up to a third of cases occur after apparently normal labours. There has been a trend in recent years for paediatricians not to attend uncomplicated elective Caesarean sections, since surveys have suggested the requirement for neonatal resuscitation is low in such cases, especially where the indication for Caesarean section is previous operative delivery and when regional anaesthesia is used. In such situations, anaesthetists should not take on the *responsibility* of resuscitating the neonate since their primary responsibility is to care for the mother. However, all personnel in the delivery suite (including obstetric anaesthetists) should be competent at basic neonatal resuscitation.

Problems/special considerations

Cardiovascular
- The change from fetal to adult circulation normally accompanies delivery and the inspiration of air into the lungs. If there is poor lung inflation, high inflation pressures, hypercapnia, hypothermia or acidosis, the circulation (which remains transitional for about 2 weeks after birth in term neonates) may return to the fetal configuration.
- The neonate relies on a fast heart rate for cardiac output since stroke volume is relatively fixed. The neonatal heart responds to hypoxaemia with bradycardia, which in turn worsens oxygen delivery. The initial treatment is oxygenation.

Respiratory

- The squeezing of the chest during vaginal delivery helps to expel the fluid contained within the lungs in babies born this way. In babies born by Caesarean section, this effect is absent and respiratory support is more likely to be required, especially superimposed on the underlying reason for emergency operative delivery. Uterine contractions themselves help to expel fluid, and even a short labour may be beneficial.
- The first breath needs to overcome the forces tending to keep the alveoli collapsed, and thus requires great effort.
- If meconium is present, its dispersal throughout the lungs during resuscitation may result in the meconium aspiration syndrome.
- Hypoxaemia typically leads to vigorous respiratory efforts followed by a period of primary apnoea (accompanied by bradycardia), during which stimulation may provoke respiration. After a few gasps a period of terminal apnoea ensues during which active resuscitation is required. It is possible for both stages to occur in utero if the fetus is hypoxic.

Management options

Appropriate equipment includes an oxygen source, funnel, bag and facepiece, suction, laryngoscopes, tracheal tubes (sizes 2.5–3.5 mm, non-shouldered) and a radiant heater. The laryngeal mask airway has been used for neonatal resuscitation and has been suggested as being faster, more reliable and thus safer than tracheal tubes, although its use is not yet widespread.

Basic principles are as for adult resuscitation; particular aspects of neonatal resuscitation are shown in Table 147.1.

Specific points:

- Basic principles of the 'ABC' of resuscitation apply.
- Cardiac massage is performed either by encircling the baby's chest with the hands and compressing the sternum with the thumbs, or by using the index and ring fingers. The sternum should be depressed 1–2 cm. Compressions should occur at 120/minute, at a ratio of 3:1 with breaths.
- If controlled ventilation is required the first breath should be held for 3–5 seconds to help expand the alveoli, with subsequent breaths lasting for 0.5–1.0 second. A maximum of 30–35 cm H_2O should be administered. Vigorous oropharyngeal suction may cause apnoea.
- Intravenous access is usually obtained most easily with an umbilical venous catheter – the single umbilical vein is accompanied by two umbilical arteries, which aids its identification. The cannula should be flushed with saline after each drug is administered. The interossoeus route has also been used.
- High concentrations of bicarbonate have been associated with intraventricular haemorrhages.
- The neonate should be kept warm and dry throughout resuscitation.

Table 147.1. Neonatal cardiopulmonary resuscitation

Meconium absent	
Breathing/heart rate	Action
Regular breathing and heart rate > 100 beats/min	Observe baby
	Reassure mother
	Airway support + oxygen via funnel
	Gentle oropharyngeal suction
	If no response, ventilation via facemask until heart rate > 100 beats/min and breathing is regular
	Consider naloxone 100 μg/kg i.m. if maternal opioids given
Apnoea and heart rate < 100 beats/min, or no response to the above after a few minutes	Tracheal intubation and IPPV
	Cardiac massage if heart rate < 60 beats/min
	Intravenous cannulation and adrenaline 100 μg/kg if no response after 1 min (20–30 μg/kg for tracheal instillation)
	If no response after 1–2 min, consider 10–20 ml/kg volume expansion; further adrenaline (100 μg/kg – up to two doses); and 1–2 ml/kg sodium bicarbonate 4.2%
Meconium present	
Breathing/heart rate	Action
Vigorous breathing or crying	Gentle oronasal suction
Poor respiratory effort	Direct laryngoscopy and pharyngeal/laryngeal suction under direct vision
	Tracheal intubation if meconium seen below the cords; gentle suction and removal of meconium *before* IPPV unless heart rate < 60 beats/min

IPPV: Intermittent positive-pressure ventilation.

Key points

- Some degree of neonatal resuscitation is required in up to 5–14% of deliveries overall but the incidence is higher in selected cases.
- The anaesthetist's first duty is to the mother.
- It should be possible to predict two-thirds of cases in which neonatal resuscitation is required before delivery.
- Basic principles are similar to those of adult resuscitation but with specific differences.

FURTHER READING

International Liaison Committee on Resuscitation. International consensus on cardio
pulmonary resuscitation and emergency cardiovascular care science with treatment
recommendations. *Resuscitation* 2005; **67**: 293–303.

148 PERINATAL MORTALITY

Perinatal mortality rate (PMR) is defined as the number of stillbirths plus the
number of neonatal deaths within the first completed week of life, per 1000 total
live births. It was proposed by the World Health Organization in 1975 as an international definition of late fetal and early neonatal loss and is a measure of antepartum care and wellbeing, care during delivery and immediate care postpartum.
Perinatal mortality is thus generally accepted as a good indicator of general health
and healthcare provision across different countries. In the developed countries it is
about 6–12 per 1000 births, whereas in developing countries rates of up to 60 per
1000 births are reported, although many countries are unable to provide data.
In England and Wales it has fallen from 32.8 per 1000 live births in 1961 to 8.5 per
1000 live births in 2003. In some countries, infant mortality rate (IMR; the number of
deaths in the first completed year after delivery per 1000 total live births) is used as
the standard indicator; in the UK it was 5.3 in 2003 whereas in the developed
countries generally it is about 3–8.

Problems/special considerations

Apart from difficulties collecting data, the figures are susceptible to variations in
other definitions used; for example in the UK, an upward 'blip' in PMR was caused
in 1991 when the definition of a live birth was changed from 28 weeks' to 24 weeks'
gestation. Some of the definitions used are shown in Table 148.1.

Table 148.1. Terms and definitions pertaining to perinatal mortality in England and Wales

Live birth	Expulsion from the mother after 24 weeks' gestation and the presence of breathing or any other sign of life, e.g. movement, heartbeat, etc.
Stillbirth	Expulsion from the mother after 24 weeks' gestation without breathing or any other sign of life
Early neonatal death	Death within the first 7 completed days after delivery
Late neonatal death	Death after the first 7 days, but before the first 28 completed days after delivery
Neonatal death	Early + late neonatal deaths
Perinatal mortality rate	Number of stillbirths plus number of early neonatal deaths per 1000 total live births
Infant mortality rate	Number of deaths in the first completed year after delivery per 1000 total live births

Perinatal mortality has been found to increase with lower social class, age <20 or >30, parity <1 or >5, presence of medical conditions and poor management of labour. It has been estimated that application of what is already known about good and poor practice would achieve a greater reduction in perinatal mortality than any other single measure.

The annual Confidential Enquiry into Stillbirths and Deaths in Infancy (CESDI) reports on causes of perinatal death and areas of suboptimal care and has now joined with the Confidential Enquiries into Maternal Deaths to form the Confidential Enquiry into Maternal and Child Health (CEMACH). CESDI's recommendations include establishing strategies and protocols for improving communication, training and peripartum clinical practice, appropriate involvement of senior medical staff and improvements in neonatal resuscitation.

Key points

- Perinatal mortality rate equals the number of stillbirths and neonatal deaths within the first completed week of life, per 1000 total live births.
- It represents the quality of provision of general health care for a particular country, as well as specific maternity and neonatal care.
- In the UK, perinatal mortality was 8.5 in 2003.

FURTHER READING

Bell R, Parker L, MacPhail S, Wright C. Trends in the cause of late fetal death, 1982–2000. *Br J Obstet Gynaecol* 2004; **111**: 1400–7.

Guyer B, Martin JA, MacDorman MF, Anderson RN, Strobino DM. Annual summary of vital statistics –1996. *Pediatrics* 1997; **100**: 905–18.

Section 3 – Puerperium and after

149 DRUGS AND BREASTFEEDING

Mothers often ask their anaesthetist for information about breastfeeding after anaesthetic and surgical interventions. The majority of drugs administered to the mother enter her breast milk but many are present in pharmacologically insignificant amounts and do not therefore pose a risk to the baby. The amount of drug that a breastfed baby receives is dependent on the concentration of drug in the milk and the volume of milk taken by the baby. In the first few days following delivery, the baby receives colostrum and then very small volumes of milk, so that any drug exposure is likely to be minimal. It is, however, common sense to administer drugs to the breastfeeding mother only if they are considered essential.

The *British National Formulary* (BNF) contains a comprehensive list of drugs that are known to be present in breast milk following maternal administration, but also points out that in many cases there are insufficient data to enable accurate information to be provided.

Breastfeeding and anaesthesia

Production of breast milk is dependent on adequate maternal hydration and regular stimulation (either by the baby feeding or by the mother expressing her milk). A mother scheduled for anaesthesia and surgery should be encouraged to feed her baby as near as possible to the planned time of surgery and also as soon as she feels able to postoperatively. In some cases it may be more appropriate for her to express milk in the early postoperative period.

Intravenous agents

Both thiopental and propofol are found in breast milk in insignificant amounts following maternal administration. Levels of volatile agent excreted into breast milk are also negligible (most information relates to halothane, but extrapolation of data based on pharmacokinetic information suggests that isoflurane, sevoflurane and desflurane would be present in breast milk in even lower concentrations). Neuromuscular blocking agents are large, water-soluble, ionised quaternary

Analgesia, Anaesthesia and Pregnancy: A Practical Guide Second Edition, ed. Steve Yentis, Anne May and Surbhi Malhotra. Published by Cambridge University Press. © Cambridge University Press 2007.

ammonium compounds and therefore are not excreted into breast milk in any measurable quantity.

Analgesics

Transfer of non-steroidal anti-inflammatory drugs and opioids into breast milk has been extensively studied, and neither type of analgesic is present in clinically important quantities. Therapeutic doses of morphine and diamorphine given for postoperative analgesia (either following Caesarean section or other surgical intervention) can be given to the mother as required. The BNF states that breast-feeding is not recommended for mothers who are addicted to opioids, although this may be controversial since the American Academy of Pediatrics considers that up to 20 mg methadone daily is compatible with breastfeeding.

Antiemetics

All the commonly used antiemetics carry a manufacturers 'use with caution' or 'use only if essential' warning.

Benzodiazepines

Prolonged administration of benzodiazepines should be avoided. Diazepam is found in clinically significant quantities in breast milk and may cause hypotonia and impaired suckling in the baby. However, use of a single dose of temazepam or lorazepam as a premedicant drug is not contraindicated. Similarly, use of midazolam for intravenous sedation or during general anaesthesia is considered safe.

Other drugs

Anticoagulants

Warfarin is now considered to be safe in breastfeeding mothers; there are currently insufficient data about low molecular weight heparins, which the manufacturers therefore advise should be avoided.

Antidepressants

The most recent Report on Confidential Enquiries into Maternal Deaths/Maternal and Child Health has highlighted the risk of postnatal depression and its potential to lead to postnatal psychosis and suicide. There are numerous case reports offering conflicting advice about the use of psychotropic drugs in lactating women. The tricyclic antidepressants amitriptyline, nortriptyline and desipramine are all excreted into breast milk, with the baby being exposed to approximately 1% of the maternal dose. This poses a theoretical risk for the infant, but there are no case reports of adverse effects, and the balance of risks is generally believed to favour continuing treatment of the mother and allowing breastfeeding. Information about the selective serotonin reuptake inhibitors (SSRIs) in lactation is limited. The drugs are excreted into breast milk, but there are no controlled studies investigating effects on the infant. The manufacturer's data sheet states that fluoxetine should not be given to nursing mothers.

Anticonvulsants

Epileptic mothers can be allowed to breastfeed; although the commonly used anticonvulsants are excreted into breast milk, there have not been any reported adverse effects in babies.

Antihypertensives

It is common for pre-eclamptic women to receive β-blocking drugs for several weeks following delivery. Atenolol is excreted in breast milk in measurable amounts, but there is no evidence that this is harmful to the infant.

Key points

- Most drugs are excreted into breast milk; information about the effect on the neonate is scarce.
- Commonly used anaesthetic and analgesic drugs can be safely used in breastfeeding mothers.

FURTHER READING

American Academy of Pediatrics Committee on Drugs. The transfer of drugs and other chemicals into human milk. *Pediatrics* 2001; **108**: 776–89.

Hale TW. Maternal medications during breast-feeding. *Clin Obstet Gynecol* 2004; **47**: 696–711.

150 FOLLOW-UP

Follow-up of mothers after obstetric analgesia and anaesthesia is important for the individual anaesthetist, the hospital and obstetric anaesthesia as a whole. In an ideal world all anaesthetists would aim to follow up their own patients. This ideal is often not practical; therefore follow-up has to become part of the routine of an obstetric anaesthetic service. At national and international levels, data collection would enable anaesthetists to assess risk and monitor standards of care. At present there are very few data available at national or international level, and this is an area that comes more closely under the remit of audit.

Problems/special considerations

Follow-up of women who have had analgesia or anaesthesia administered by the anaesthetist should ideally be carried out within 24 hours. However, it may be difficult to see all women before they are discharged from hospital. This early discharge to the community means that anaesthetists must rely on midwifery, obstetric and general practitioner colleagues to refer back any problems. Areas that anaesthetists might wish to follow up can be divided into:

- Anaesthetic interventions perceived to be uncomplicated
- Anaesthetic interventions where there was a problem.

Follow-up of the first group is important to ensure that women are satisfied with their treatment and, if not, why not. The follow-up interview gives the woman a chance to voice her opinion of the treatment she received. The anaesthetist should be responsive to criticisms of the service as a whole, since many women make their comments in order to help improve the service to others.

Suggested list of questions that may be asked at follow-up:

- *Relating to analgesia in labour:* Were you satisfied with the pain relief you received for the first and second stages of your labour? Were you able to mobilise during labour where appropriate? Has your sensation returned to normal? Have you a headache? Have you any comments about the care that you received?
- *Relating to regional anaesthesia:* Were you satisfied with the anaesthesia that you received? Did you feel any discomfort or pain at any time during the Caesarean section? Have you had good postoperative pain relief? Are you up and about? Are you able to pass urine? Has your sensation returned to normal? Have you a headache? Have you any comments about the treatment that you received?
- *Relating to general anaesthesia:* Did you have a good sleep? Do you remember going to sleep? Do you remember waking up? Do you remember dreaming or waking up during the operation? Do you have a sore throat, sore muscles or headache? Were you in pain when you woke up? Has the postoperative pain relief been adequate (at rest and on movement)? Have you had nausea or vomiting? Have you any comments about your treatment?

The most common problems associated with an anaesthetic intervention are:

- Difficulty in siting a regional analgesic
- Accidental dural puncture
- Paraesthesia during insertion of a spinal or epidural, and/or neurological symptoms afterwards
- Poor analgesia in labour (especially in the second stage if the epidural was inadequately topped up)
- Pain during Caesarean section or operative delivery.

Patients with the above problems should always be followed up, ideally by a consultant obstetric anaesthetist. Continuity of care is important for these patients, and early involvement of other specialists, when appropriate, should occur at an early stage. For example, neurological consultation should be sought when there is any doubt as to the cause of a headache or neurological deficit. Early involvement of a clinical psychologist with a special interest in post-traumatic stress disorder following childbirth (if available) is often useful when there has been a painful experience during delivery.

Communication with the women, their partners and the midwifery and obstetric staff is essential to ensure that any problems, however small, are dealt with quickly and comprehensively. All women who have had a problem should have the opportunity to see the consultant obstetric anaesthetist after discharge from hospital. A follow-up visit at around 6–8 weeks post-delivery is useful for both the women and the obstetric anaesthetist. This consultation allows the lines of communication to remain open and offers the opportunity for a frank and open dialogue about any problems.

Key points

- Follow-up is important in both straightforward and complicated cases.
- Follow-up does not end when the woman leaves hospital.
- Consultant anaesthetic involvement is important.
- Communication is vital between all the professional groups involved.

FURTHER READING

Peach M, Godkin R, Webster S. Complications of obstetric epidural analgesia and anaesthesia: a prospective analysis of 10 995 cases. *Int J Obstet Anesth* 1998; **7**: 5–11.

151 MATERNAL SATISFACTION

Maternal satisfaction has become a major outcome measure, mentioned in several important documents and strategies concerned with childbirth. This means that providers of health care must pay attention to mothers' expression of satisfaction with their care during and after pregnancy. Anaesthetists have an important role to play in maternal satisfaction, since for many women aspects of their analgesia and anaesthesia can have an enormous effect on how they view their overall experience, in some cases irrespective of what happened in other areas of their care. Conversely, mothers' rating of their satisfaction with analgesia or anaesthesia in general, and different techniques in particular, may be affected by several factors unrelated to the anaesthetic itself. Despite this, studies comparing different techniques often quote measures of global satisfaction as evidence that one technique is superior to another. Similarly, obstetric anaesthetists are encouraged to assess and audit maternal satisfaction with the obstetric anaesthetic service as a marker of quality of performance.

Problems/special considerations

Apart from the confounding effects of various unrelated factors described above, another difficulty relates to the measuring tool used to assess satisfaction.

Methods used have varied from simple 'satisfaction scales,' e.g. visual analogue scale or verbal rating scale, to complex evaluations of different modalities that combine to produce a positive experience of childbirth such as fulfilment (e.g. happiness), lack of distress (e.g. pleasure) and physical wellbeing (e.g. lack of pain). The simpler systems will always be more attractive to busy clinicians such as anaesthetists than the more complex and time-consuming ones, even though simple questions such as 'Are you satisfied?' or 'Rate your satisfaction on a scale of 1–10' are next to useless as objective outcome measures.

Studies suggest that factors associated with dissatisfaction include being excluded from one's care and decisions relating to it, poor communication and lack of information, bad outcome (although there may be strong satisfaction with the medical care if this is perceived to have been good) and being led to expect a particular event and then not experiencing it (e.g. receiving assurance that an epidural will be available but not receiving it because the anaesthetist is unavailable).

Despite initial assumptions that effective analgesia in labour automatically guarantees maternal satisfaction, this is not necessarily the case, and factors such as control and involvement in proceedings may be more important. This has led to the suggestion that satisfaction is increased when motor block is minimised by using low-dose epidural techniques.

Management options

Until more work is done on the interplay between specific factors that contribute to maternal satisfaction, obstetric anaesthetists have to fall back on the use of vague and non-specific methods of assessing it. It is probably more important to assess dissatisfaction, which may indicate deficiencies in service, but any single measure of satisfaction is only as good as the methods used to obtain it. It is also important to ensure that if a mother has had a bad experience in childbirth but the anaesthetic care has been good and appropriate, her adverse opinion should not extend to include the anaesthetist. Sometimes attempts to prevent this are futile, especially when the opinions of other professionals on the labour ward towards anaesthetists are themselves adverse.

Attention meanwhile should be paid to those factors that have been shown to be important in promoting maternal satisfaction, such as involving the mother in decisions, keeping her informed, being prompt and courteous and other desirable general professional attitudes. Similarly, any expression of dissatisfaction should be taken seriously and an attempt made (and recorded in the notes) to discuss the particulars of the case, perhaps by offering an appointment at a later date. Medicolegal experience supports this approach as one of the most important factors in preventing subsequent legal action.

Key points

- Maternal satisfaction is an increasingly recognised but poorly defined measure of quality of care.
- Involving women in their care, good communication and honesty are important factors in increasing maternal satisfaction.
- Women expressing dissatisfaction should be identified and offered the opportunity to discuss their care further with a senior member of staff.

FURTHER READING

Hodnett ED. Pain and women's satisfaction with the experience of childbirth: a systematic review. *Am J Obstet Gynecol* 2002; **186**: S160–72.

Hundley VA, Milne JM, Glazener CMA, Mollison J. Satisfaction and the three Cs: continuity, choice and control. Women's views from a randomised controlled trial of midwife-led care. *Br J Obstet Gynaecol* 1997; **104**: 1273–80.

Morgan PJ, Halpern S, Lo J. The development of a maternal satisfaction scale for caesarean section. *Int J Obstet Anesth* 1999; **8**: 165–70.

Robinson PN, Salmon P, Yentis SM. Maternal satisfaction. *Int J Obstet Anesth* 1998; **7**: 32–7.

Section 4 - Organisational aspects

152 ANTENATAL EDUCATION

Women preparing for childbirth make use of many sources of information. These will typically include discussion with other women, magazine articles, books and classes. Classes may be run by the GP practice or maternity unit, or by external bodies such as the National Childbirth Trust (NCT). Antenatal education is beneficial, since it has been shown that the well-informed mother will cope better with labour, but it is important that the information received by the mother should be accurate, well balanced and relevant to local conditions (there is, after all, little point in discussing the virtues of epidural analgesia if no such service is available in the local hospital).

Much of the information given to mothers in the antenatal period is outside the control of the anaesthetist and may well be inaccurate or misleading; it is therefore particularly important for the anaesthetist to seek every opportunity to get his/her message across.

Problems/special considerations

Retention of information

The middle of a painful labour is the wrong time to attempt to provide quite complex information about regional analgesia. In addition to the pain itself and the inevitable tension, the mother may well be under the influence of powerful sedative/analgesic drugs. Theoretically, the antenatal period is the ideal time to educate mothers about pain relief and anaesthesia for Caesarean section. Unfortunately, many studies have shown that the ability of patients to recall details of explanations is poor and that such information tends to be retained for the short term only. This problem is exacerbated by the finding that around 50% of primigravidae who have epidural analgesia in labour were not planning to use it; these women would be especially unlikely to recall information given in the antenatal period.

Analgesia, Anaesthesia and Pregnancy: A Practical Guide Second Edition, ed. Steve Yentis, Anne May and Surbhi Malhotra. Published by Cambridge University Press. © Cambridge University Press 2007.

Written information

Poor recall of verbal explanations implies that antenatal classes should be supplemented with written information that mothers can take home and read at leisure; audiotapes and videos can also be very helpful. When preparing these sources, it is important to target them at a relatively low level of comprehension; it is all too easy to slip into medical jargon and unnecessarily complicated language. Studies have shown that written information for patients should be set at a reading age of about 12 years. The needs of mothers whose first language is not English should also be considered, and the Obstetric Anaesthetists' Association (OAA) has several translations of its information for mothers available on its website.

Content

Mothers need balanced information to enable them to make rational decisions; this is an essential element of the principle of consent. Talks, leaflets, videos etc. need to present an unbiased view of the benefits and risks of the available alternatives and should be based on the best available evidence. Inevitably, material that is designed to inform a large number of women will be too complex for some and have insufficient detail for others; it is therefore essential that mothers should be able to discuss their concerns individually with an anaesthetist if necessary, and antenatal education should not be seen as a substitute for this facility.

Management options

Undertaking a regular antenatal class is a major (and almost certainly unpaid) commitment, often involving regular evening lectures. Equally, not every anaesthetist is suited to giving informal talks to large groups of mothers and fathers. In some circumstances, it is better to enlist the help of parentcraft teachers, who may be willing to put across the anaesthetist's message themselves. If this is to be done successfully, however, it is essential that the teachers fully understand and agree with the content and emphasis of the information. The anaesthetist should still attend the classes on a regular basis to ensure that the teacher is not going 'off-message', and must be available (not necessarily on the same day) to deal with any queries outside the teacher's experience. Audiovisual aids are useful, particularly as a prompt if the talk is delegated to someone else, but slides must be kept simple, jargon free and not gory.

The use of written/video material is worth while, but preparation to an acceptable standard is more difficult than might be imagined. Many hospitals have departments dedicated to provision of patient information, and their help should be sought at an early stage. Presentation in an attractive format is also important, and this will almost certainly require professional input. Production of high-quality leaflets is not cheap, and it is tempting to seek sponsorship from a company with a commercial interest in pregnancy or labour; however, many midwives are reluctant to distribute information that appears to endorse products, and their views should be sought before embarking on such a course. In general, the cooperation of midwifery staff is important in ensuring that the target audience is reached and they should therefore be involved at the preparation stage.

It is important to remember that antenatal education often misses the most socially deprived – and hence high-risk – mothers. The extent of this problem may be assessed by discussion with local community midwives, who may be willing to establish 'outreach' clinics for this vulnerable group.

Several national organisations have produced leaflets and videos about pain relief in labour, including the OAA. These provide an attractive way of informing mothers in the antenatal period, but care should be taken if using such material to ensure that the information given reflects local practice and experience.

Key points

- Antenatal education allows explanation of key facts in a low-stress environment.
- Retention of information given in the antenatal period is poor.
- Information should be accurate, locally relevant and carefully targeted.
- Leaflets/videos are useful supplements, but may be difficult to prepare.

FURTHER READING

Bethune L, Harper N, Lucas DN, *et al.* Complications of obstetric regional analgesia – how much information is enough? *Int J Obstet Anesth* 2004; **13**: 30–4.

Stewart A, Sodhi V, Harper N, Yentis SM. Assessment of the effect upon maternal knowledge of an information leaflet about pain relief in labour. *Anaesthesia* 2003; **58**: 1015–18.

153   AUDIT

Medical audit is a process by which certain aspects of practice are assessed and compared with predefined targets. If those targets are not met then the reasons for not meeting them are analysed and addressed; subsequent audits can be used to confirm that the situation has improved (thus completing the audit 'loop'). Audit should be distinguished from research, which seeks to determine what the targets should be; e.g. research might suggest that drug A is best for uterine relaxation in premature labour whereas audit determines whether drug A is in fact being used appropriately in a particular unit.

Audit is widely supported as a means of encouraging evidence-based medicine and improving standards of care.

Problems/special considerations

The best known and oldest obstetric audit is the Report on Confidential Enquiries into Maternal Deaths/Maternal and Child Health, in which obstetric deaths are analysed, their causes determined and management compared against 'best practice', and recommendations made about standards of care in maternity units. Anaesthetic aspects are considered by specific anaesthetic assessors. Other than this, there is no comprehensive national obstetric anaesthetic audit system, although a few exist at local level (usually involving computers). This causes problems with estimating true incidences of adverse outcomes, since the denominators are rarely known (e.g. the number of general anaesthetic Caesarean sections in the UK), although there have been recent attempts by the Royal College of Obstetricians and Gynaecologists (and more recently, by anaesthetic organisations, particularly the Obstetric Anaesthetists' Association) to collect these basic data.

At unit level, rates of epidurals in labour, inadvertent dural punctures, anaesthesia for Caesarean section and complications are commonly recorded. Whether this information is used for true audit as defined above is uncertain. In addition, definitions of these various terms may not be uniform amongst units (for example, should 'epidural rate' include spinals/combined spinal–epidurals, and should the denominator be the number of women delivering, the number of women *in labour*, the number of *babies* delivered, etc?). Finally, the real impact of sometimes expensive audit on actual outcome of care has been repeatedly questioned.

It is important to perform audit with specific aims, rather than simply collect data for its own sake. Simple audit can easily be performed for particular aspects of care, e.g. to assess whether antacid prophylaxis is being given to all patients before elective Caesarean section or to labouring mothers in high-risk groups, or whether appropriate investigations are being performed in pre-eclamptic patients before regional analgesia. Administrative aspects can also be audited, e.g. response times of anaesthetists on call or provision of adequate teaching on the labour ward. The value of an audit is increased by concentrating on objective data, e.g. the measure of satisfaction is commonly done following obstetric anaesthesia, but data derived from vague satisfaction scales may be a poor reflection of quality of service.

Finally, if the data are unreliable the audit is worthless; thus each project should be planned carefully to ensure that high quality data are collected. During each cycle, the audit can itself be audited by sampling the data collected and checking it for accuracy and completeness.

Key points

- Audit comprises:
  1. Assessment of practice
  2. Comparison against 'best practice'
  3. Analysis of any shortcoming
  4. Correction of deficient practice
  5. Repeating the assessment.

FURTHER READING

Holdcroft A, Verma R, Chapple J, *et al.* Towards effective obstetric anaesthetic audit in the UK. *Int J Obstet Anesth* 1999; **8**: 37–42.

154 LABOUR WARD ORGANISATION

Unplanned situations and emergencies inevitably arise in the best-managed obstetric units, but good organisation should be able to reduce these to a minimum. Anaesthetists are present in most labour wards for a majority of the working week, are involved in the care of the complex cases that test the organisational structure, and are accustomed to communicating with other medical and non-medical staff. They are therefore ideally suited to help in the planning of the various aspects of labour ward organisation.

Problems/special considerations

The labour ward is a potential hot-bed of organisational problems. Workload may vary suddenly and dramatically, and the urgent nature of many admissions makes forward planning very difficult. A variety of specialists are intimately involved with the care of the patients, and conflicts, although regrettable, are inevitable. Priorities are often difficult to establish, and prolonged periods of routine work may be suddenly interrupted by an extreme emergency. All of this makes careful organisation essential but very difficult.

Maternity care is by far the largest source of medicolegal litigation in Europe and the USA, and analysis of claims against obstetric anaesthetists implicates communication and other organisational factors in over 40% of cases. For example, a common problem is failure to notify the anaesthetist of an impending Caesarean section until the last minute, resulting in inappropriate anaesthetic decisions or excessive delay.

In many labour wards in the UK and elsewhere, midwives are taking an increasing role as lead clinicians, and so-called 'low-risk' mothers are frequently cared for solely by a midwife. This situation, although not hazardous in itself, calls for careful guidelines to ensure early communication of potential problems to relevant medical staff. The problem can be exacerbated if independent practitioners are allowed to admit their clients to the labour ward.

Although the role of the anaesthetist is more widely appreciated by midwives and obstetricians than in the past, there is still a tendency in some units to regard him/her as an 'outsider', only to be summoned when required. This attitude fosters poor communication and should be discouraged.

Management options

There should be a consultant anaesthetist responsible for the provision of the obstetric anaesthetic service, who should act as a liaison officer between the midwives and obstetricians. A labour ward working party or equivalent, meeting on a regular basis, is an ideal forum in which to raise concerns and maintain communication, and there must be an anaesthetist on this body.

Guidelines and protocols should be drawn up to cover routine care, management of difficult cases etc. and must be agreed by all parties involved. These guidelines should be updated frequently, be readily available on the labour ward and be distributed to all new staff, who should undergo a formal familiarisation programme before being allowed 'on-call'. Standards laid down in guidelines should be the subject of regular audit. Independent practitioners who require admitting rights must also agree to abide by the unit guidelines.

A formal scheme for reporting all critical incidents and 'near-misses' must be in place, and a blame-free culture established to encourage staff to utilise the system. Regular multidisciplinary morbidity meetings are useful to identify potential organisational problems. Information from these should pass to a risk management committee (also multidisciplinary), responsible for ensuring good practice and minimising risk to patients.

Good communication is the most important factor in a well-managed labour ward. A system should be in place to ensure that potentially difficult patients are referred to an anaesthetist early in the antenatal period, and that the anaesthetist is also notified when they are admitted. The anaesthetist should be familiar with all the patients on labour ward and this is best achieved by participating in joint ward rounds with the obstetricians and midwives. The duty anaesthetist must be rapidly contactable at all times; 'bleep' systems should not be relied upon as a sole means of contact. The names and methods of contacting consultant staff should be visible at the central desk. In general, anaesthetists should ensure that they are regarded as part of the 'team', rather than someone to be called when the situation is desperate.

Extreme emergencies such as cardiorespiratory arrest are very uncommon on the labour ward, but a successful outcome depends on a rapid, efficient response and this can be threatened by the very rarity of such events. The whereabouts of resuscitation equipment and drugs must, of course, be known to all staff, and regular 'drills' for emergencies such as maternal collapse and massive antepartum haemorrhage should be carried out to ensure that the system works smoothly.

Detailed guidelines covering the above points, and more, have been published by the Obstetric Anaesthetists' Association/Association of Anaesthetists of Great Britain and Ireland, and the Royal Colleges of Midwives and of Obstetricians and Gynaecologists. These documents serve as useful reminders of the various aspects of labour ward organisation that need attention, and also serve as tools for ongoing audit.

Key points

- Poor organisation results in unnecessarily hasty, and sometimes incorrect, decision making.
- Anaesthetists should be involved in labour ward management.
- Good, early communication will help prevent many disasters.

FURTHER READING

Obstetric Anaesthetists' Association/Association of Anaesthetists of Great Britain and Ireland. *Guidelines for Obstetric Anaesthetic Services*, 2nd edn. London: AAGBI, 2005.

Royal College of Midwives, Royal College of Obstetricians and Gynaecologists. *Towards Safer Childbirth – Minimum Standards for the Organisation of Labour Wards*. London: RCOG, 1999.

155   MIDWIFERY TRAINING

Obstetric anaesthetists are part of the delivery suite team. This involves working closely with midwives who are often the lead professionals caring for the pregnant woman. It is therefore important to understand the training that midwives have had and for senior anaesthetists to take responsibility for teaching obstetric analgesia and anaesthesia to midwives.

Problems/special considerations

Until recently, midwifery training in the UK could only be started after basic training in nursing, and most nurses who embarked on midwifery training had already had several years of general nursing experience. However, direct entry into midwifery training is now common, and there are now many midwives who are not Registered Nurses.

Midwifery training usually requires the following topics to be covered:

- Biological sciences, applied sociology and psychology, and aspects of professional practice
- Pain in labour, the pain pathways involved, and pain relief (including both non-pharmacological and pharmacological methods)
- Anaesthesia; this includes both regional and general anaesthesia in pregnancy.

These modules do not have to be taught by obstetric anaesthetists, although in most training schools there is a good relationship between the midwifery tutors and obstetric anaesthetists, who may as a result be involved in many hours of teaching. This relationship has led to increasing awareness that anaesthetists are involved with the sick maternity patient and that they should be involved in teaching both high-dependency care and the recognition of clinical risk factors. Teaching of these skills is particularly important for the direct-entry midwives and has led to the following topics often being taught by obstetric anaesthetists:

- Postoperative and recovery skills
- Risk factors associated with women who have medical problems
- Care of the critically ill woman, e.g. high-dependency care for women who have pre-eclampsia or haemorrhage.

This extension of the teaching role of the obstetric anaesthetist may require around 18 hours of teaching to be given to each group of students. The students who have general nursing qualifications will require less time than the direct-entry students.

Each training school has different courses that may culminate in a degree or diploma qualification. The length of training can vary between three and four years (shorter if the student is already qualified as a nurse), and the structure of the courses varies considerably, as does the obstetric anaesthetic involvement.

In order to practise, midwives must be registered with the Nursing and Midwifery Council, which maintains a register. To remain registered they must maintain a professional portfolio as evidence of their keeping up to date, and notify the Council annually of their intention to practise. Part of midwives' continuing professional development/training will include the practical management of epidural analgesia. The ability to administer epidural top-ups requires additional in-service teaching, which is usually done on the delivery suite. A certificate is issued to the midwife on completing the training satisfactorily. The exact requirements of the training differ depending on local practice and may require an update of resuscitation skills.

Anaesthetists are often involved in other areas of professional development, e.g. intravenous cannulation, resuscitation (adult and neonatal) and specific high-dependency training.

Key points

- It is important that obstetric anaesthetists are involved in midwifery training.
- Midwives require instruction during their midwifery training as well as continuous education and maintenance of skills once qualified.

156 CONSENT

Consent for treatment is comprised of a number of components:
- Provision of adequate information to, and its understanding by, the patient
- The ability of the individual to assimilate this information, weigh up the alternatives and consequences, and come to a decision (in ethical and legal parlance, 'capacity' and 'competence' respectively)
- Allowing adequate time for the process
- Voluntariness, i.e. no coercion by others.

Consent may be implied or expressed. Implied consent is usually assumed when a patient cooperates in allowing a minor procedure, such as venepuncture, to take place. The maintenance of a suitable posture for, say, epidural analgesia, might be taken to imply consent to continue with the procedure, but it would be unwise to rely on this as carte blanche without regularly checking with the patient.

There is no legal difference between written and verbal consent. The only advantage of the latter is that it provides concrete evidence that consent was given if a dispute arises.

Failure to obtain consent before performing a procedure could invite an action against the anaesthetist for battery – the unlawful infliction of force upon another person. In practice, this is rarely, if ever, an issue in claims against doctors. Far more likely is the claim that a lack of informed consent resulted in a complication (if the patient had only been told of the risk, she would not have undergone the procedure) – i.e. a claim of negligence. A recent House of Lords judgment means that a doctor may now be found negligent with respect to provision of adequate information to the patient even if this failure had no effect on the patient's decision to undergo treatment.

The amount of information that a doctor must impart to a patient to aid her in making a decision is not clearly established. It is generally accepted that the 'Bolam' principle applies here as in other issues of medical negligence, i.e. that an action – in this case the failure to mention a complication – is not negligent if it can be shown that the doctor has acted in accordance with a responsible body of medical persons skilled in that particular art. However, this principle, which essentially allows the profession to set its own standards, has increasingly been challenged when applied to informed consent, and guidance now is that each patient should be given the information that she herself would want, not what the treating doctor thinks she needs.

Problems/special considerations

The principles of consent to treatment in obstetric anaesthesia are essentially no different from those in any other field, the main distinction being that, in the often fraught circumstances that surround labour and delivery, they may be more difficult to apply:

- Women in labour are usually suffering pain; they may be exhausted and in considerable distress, and may be under the influence of powerful analgesic drugs. They are hardly in a position to be able to assess critically a list of risks and benefits when deciding whether to have epidural analgesia. Prior information about epidural analgesia – e.g. in the antenatal clinic – would improve matters, but it should be borne in mind that up to half of primigravidae who end up with an epidural were not intending to have one beforehand.
- The presence of the fetus does not interfere with the patient's right to make an autonomous decision about her own care, even if the decision taken will compromise the wellbeing of her unborn child. It is, of course, still very important that the risks and benefits to the fetus are also explained to the mother when seeking consent to a particular course of action.
- Consent is ultimately a matter between the anaesthetist and the patient. However, the partner's views should not be dismissed summarily; he is an important participant in the birth process and should be encouraged to listen to the anaesthetist's explanation and accept the woman's decision.

- Patients whose first language is not English are as entitled as any others to an adequate explanation in their own language. The partner may act as translator in an emergency, but this is a very poor substitute for using an official interpreter. In hospitals where a substantial proportion of patients are from ethnic minorities, suitable interpreters should be made available at all times.

In difficult cases, it is wise to make sure that a witness (usually the midwife) is present, and that all present agree on what has been said and decided.

Management options

Good antenatal education about pain relief and anaesthesia, supported by booklets and/or videos, is an important part of the obstetric anaesthetist's job, and it is best not delegated to midwives unless the information that they disseminate is scrupulously checked.

Signed consent for epidural analgesia in labour is not currently considered necessary and in most units, verbal consent is taken only. What is important is to give an adequate explanation of the risks and benefits that are applicable to each particular woman making a decision in the prevailing circumstances. This will obviously vary according to the situation, but a note should always be made listing the matters discussed and identifying reasons why an explanation was brief or curtailed. If the procedure is difficult or prolonged, then verbal permission to continue must be sought at regular intervals.

For regional techniques, most obstetric anaesthetists would now consider, as a minimum, explanation of the risk of partial or complete failure of the technique, dural puncture and headache, motor block and neurological complications. An explanation of the risks of regional anaesthesia for Caesarean section should always include the possibility of discomfort, pain and conversion to general anaesthesia. Failure to do this has resulted in a recent rush of negligence suits against anaesthetists.

When offering anaesthetic options for elective Caesarean section, it is perfectly reasonable to stress the maternal advantages of regional block, but there is no argument at present for insisting on this when there are no contraindications to general anaesthesia. A patient undergoing emergency Caesarean section with a functioning epidural *in situ* is a different proposition entirely, and every effort should be made to encourage an epidural top-up, with refusal being carefully recorded in the notes.

Key points

- It is difficult to provide complex information to a woman in painful labour. Antenatal education makes this task much easier.
- The risks and benefits discussed with the patient should always be recorded.
- A pregnant woman's autonomy is not affected by the fact that she is carrying a fetus.

FURTHER READING

Association of Anaesthetists of Great Britain and Ireland. *Information and Consent for Anaesthesia*. London: AAGBI, 2005.

Bethune L, Harper N, Lucas DN, *et al.* Complications of obstetric regional analgesia: how much information is enough? *Int J Obstet Anesth* 2004; **13**: 30–4.

Hoehner PJ. Ethical aspects of informed consent in obstetric anesthesia-new challenges and solutions. *J Clin Anesth* 2003 Dec; **15**: 587–600.

Kelly GD, Blunt C, Moore PAS, Lewis M. Consent for regional anaesthesia in the United Kingdom: what is material risk? *Int J Obstet Anesth* 2004; **13**: 71–4.

Wheat K. Progress of the prudent patient: consent after Chester v Afshar. *Anaesthesia* 2005; **60**: 217–19.

White SM, Baldwin TJ. Consent for anaesthesia. *Anaesthesia* 2003; **58**: 760–74.

157   MEDICOLEGAL ASPECTS

There is a general trend in the UK towards patients seeking redress in the courts when they think that they have been harmed as a result of a negligent act on the part of their medical attendants. In 2004–05, the NHS Litigation Authority made payments in excess of £502,000,000 in respect of negligence claims, a 19% increase over the previous year. While all specialties are feeling the effects of litigation of this type, obstetrics and anaesthesia feature towards the top of the list, with birth-related brain injury accounting for 5% of all claims and 60% of all expenditure in 2002–03. It is therefore inevitable that the obstetric anaesthetist should be particularly exposed.

For a negligence claim to succeed, the patient has to demonstrate that the doctor had a duty of care towards her (normally not a matter for contention), that there was a failure of that duty of care (the standard applied here is that of the ordinary doctor professing skill in anaesthesia), and that she has suffered harm as a result. Until recently, the test for causation was that were it not for the failure of care, the harm would not have occurred. However, a recent judgment in the House of Lords relating to consent has established that, even were this not to apply, the doctor may still be found negligent.

Problems/special considerations

Consent

Consent is equally valid whether written or verbal, the only difference being that a record of the former is retained in the hospital notes as confirmation if a case comes to court after some years. Consent is only valid if it is informed, i.e. if the patient has been presented with enough information about the risks and benefits of the procedure to make a sensible choice. This can obviously be difficult in practice if a patient is in severe pain and under the influence of Entonox or opioids, as is often the case when epidural analgesia is needed in labour. It is generally agreed that provision of information in the antenatal period is best, although many women may not consider it applicable to them at this time.

Regional analgesia/anaesthesia

The extent of information required when seeking consent for regional analgesia/ anaesthesia is controversial, although most surveys suggest that some women would wish to know most, if not all, complications. Most obstetric anaesthetists would now consider, as a minimum, explanation of the risk of partial or complete failure of the technique, dural puncture and headache, motor block and neurological complications. Signed, written consent is not considered necessary, although a list of the pertinent aspects of the discussion should be recorded, and a note made if the patient's condition does not allow for a full explanation. Antenatal access to an anaesthetist should be available for women who have particular concerns.

Pain during Caesarean section

Pain felt during Caesarean delivery under spinal or epidural anaesthesia is the commonest source of successful litigation against UK obstetric anaesthetists. In practice, a pain-free procedure cannot be guaranteed, and the anaesthetist must mention this possibility when obtaining consent. The level of block must be carefully checked before starting the operation, and recorded, along with the sensory modality used. Any complaint of pain should be taken seriously, documented and treated.

Headache

Headache following inadvertent dural puncture is a common source of complaint. Dural tap is not, in itself, enough to demonstrate negligence, as long as it is correctly managed. This means that good analgesia should be established for labour and the patient followed up daily while in hospital. Any complaint of headache, neck pain or visual disturbances should be documented and definitive treatment, in the form of epidural blood patch, offered early. Any mother who has suffered a dural tap or postdural puncture headache should be encouraged to contact the hospital if there is a recurrence/worsening of symptoms. These patients should be routinely followed up at 6–10 weeks postpartum.

Backache

Claims are often made for backache after epidural analgesia, but few, if any, succeed. Prospective studies have shown that new, long-term backache is common following childbirth but is not related to whether or not regional analgesia has been used.

Management options

It is far easier to minimise the risk of litigation than to deal with it once it arises. Sensible guidelines for management of common obstetric anaesthetic situations are essential. Talking to patients and relatives and keeping them informed will ensure them of one's good intentions – very few patients institute proceedings against doctors who have communicated well. If the hospital has an efficient risk-management procedure with a rapid response to complaints, then patients, most of whom only want an explanation of what went wrong and an apology, will often be content without needing to take more formal action. Complaints from mothers or their partners, however informal, must be handled at a senior level.

If, despite these precautions, legal action ensues, then good record keeping will help the anaesthetist to recall what happened long after the case has faded from memory. Even if it was always an individual anaesthetist's routine practice to give a test dose after performing an epidural, for example, it will be difficult to convince a judge of this fact without documentary evidence. The same applies to the explanations given when obtaining consent for a procedure. A case of negligence will often come down to the anaesthetist's recollection versus that of the patient – needless to say, she will remember the whole incident perfectly, while the anaesthetist may have performed 100 similar procedures since. The need for accurate records is particularly important when the complaint is of a subjective nature, such as pain or awareness during Caesarean section.

An accusation of negligence is a very painful and traumatic experience for a doctor, and it is important to seek support from peers and seniors, especially those who have experience of medicolegal practice.

Key points

- Negligence claims against obstetric anaesthetists are increasing.
- Good relations should be maintained with patients and their relatives.
- Any complaint should be dealt with promptly.
- Full records are the best defence and should include details of explanations before consent.

FURTHER READING

Wheat K. Progress of the prudent patient: consent after Chester v Afshar. *Anaesthesia* 2005; **60**: 217–19.

White SM, Baldwin TJ. Consent for anaesthesia *Anaesthesia* 2003; **58**: 760–74.

158 RECORD KEEPING

The increase in negligence litigation against doctors in general, and obstetric anaesthetists in particular, has led to increased concerns about the standard of record keeping in hospitals. Many hospitals now have clinical risk managers, and one of the main tasks of these individuals is to ensure that records are clear, complete and retrievable. Many practitioners criticise the current medicolegal climate as leading to the practice of 'defensive medicine', but in the area of record keeping at least, the benefits for practitioner and patient alike are clear – there is no doubt that record keeping has often been poor in the past and that this has led to delays, unnecessary repetition of investigations and breakdowns in communication.

Problems/special considerations

Legibility

Although it is not always easy to maintain good legibility in the heat of the moment, every effort should be made to ensure that entries in the notes, and particularly signatures, can be read. While most doctors can read their own handwriting, this is not always true 20 years later, and it should be borne in mind that the interpretation will often be made by someone other than the writer. Each signature in the notes should be followed by the author's name in capital letters.

Hospitals rarely release original notes, and solicitors usually receive a photo-copied bundle of records, often prepared in haste by the most junior office assistant. Therefore, black ink (it photocopies better) should be used, and notes should not be written in the extremes of the margin (often missed in the photocopying process).

Contemporaneity

The courts appreciate that it is often impossible to deal with a crisis and keep good, contemporaneous records. It is perfectly in order, for example, to copy a series of blood pressure results from the monitor 'trends' screen into the record after an operation. Similarly, it is quite reasonable to sit down after a dangerous situation has been stabilised and make a retrospective record of what happened – in this instance, however, the time at which the record was written should be included in the entry. It is even acceptable to go back and alter or add notes some time after the event – as long as the alterations are honest – but it must be made very clear in the notes that these are later additions. In general, complex notes should be made as soon as possible after the event, while the memory is fresh.

Completeness

While it may be one's standard practice to warn of the risk of headache before siting an epidural or to assess the level of block after instituting spinal anaesthesia for Caesarean section, it is prudent to note that this has been done in each indi-vidual case. An anaesthetist's actions may be queried many years after the event, by which time he/she will have no recollection of the individual case; the patient, on the contrary, will remember it as if it were yesterday. In this situation, the defence that something must have been done because it was one's routine practice always to do so does not carry much weight if there is no mention of it in the notes. Reasons for making clinical decisions – such as withholding a blood patch for a postdural puncture headache because it seems to be improving – should always be carefully noted, especially when the decision deviates from standard guidelines. Finally, all entries should be dated, timed and signed legibly.

The maintenance of complete records can be encouraged by developing forms with prompts for commonly omitted data, such as level of block and mode of testing after regional anaesthesia. Good record keeping can also be encouraged by stressing its value in departmental guidelines. One of the most effective methods for ensuring standards is to incorporate a review of clinical records into the audit programme.

Retrievability

The best records in the world will be of no help if they cannot be found. Anaesthetic notes, especially epidural forms, are often made on sheets that do not form part of the main record. There must be a system in place for incorporating these into the bound folder, preferably not by just inserting them into a pocket in the back.

Obstetric litigation may arise up to 21 years after the birth of the child. Maternity records must be kept for at least this long, and this often causes considerable logistic problems, as does the difficulty in tracing the practitioners involved after such a long period.

Key points

- Notes should be written clearly and legibly in black ink.
- The date, time and the author's name should be included.
- Even if a practice is routine, details should be noted.

159   MINIMUM STANDARDS, GUIDELINES AND PROTOCOLS

Recent years have seen a proliferation of documents aimed at standardising and improving medical care. These are variously known as standards, guidelines and protocols and are developed at local, national and even international level. There are no firm, accepted definitions of these terms, and in practice, they are often used interchangeably. However, the term 'minimum standards' tends to be used for establishing general standards of services/care to which practitioners/ units should aspire, while 'protocols' tends to refer to specific management of a particular condition or group of condition. 'Guidelines' is commonly used in both contexts.

Such documents are increasingly used throughout medicine since they are seen as an efficient way of maintaining good practice, although they may have some disadvantages (Table 159.1). They are generally seen as an important part of risk management.

Table 159.1. Advantages and disadvantages of minimum standards, guidelines and protocols

Advantages	Disadvantages
Relating to general services/standards	
• Can support local departments/units in their argument for adequate resources/facilities	• Require continuous updating and removal when obsolete
• Encourage practitioners/units to examine their own practice and establish good risk management procedures	• Lay the organisation or individuals open to potential criticism if not adhered to or if badly written
• Represent an overview from established authorities	• May be ignored if the targets set are seen as unduly unrealistic
Relating to management of specific conditions	
• Increase uniformity of practice, especially where there is a large turnover of staff	• May restrict clinical freedom
• Allow better adherence to evidence-based medicine	• May result in blind adherence to a set management path even though it may be inappropriate in certain circumstances
• Improve management of rare but serious conditions, e.g. anaphylaxis, major haemorrhage	• May remove the incentive to 'think for oneself'
• Can be used for teaching and training of staff	• Require continuous updating and removal when obsolete
• May reduce the risk of medicolegal claims	• Lay the organisation or individuals open to potential criticism if not adhered to or if badly written
• Required by most accreditation/assessment authorities as a indicator of good risk management	• Rely on consensus; if opinions vary widely the resultant protocol may be too loose to be useful

Current national standards and guidelines

In the UK, the Association of Anaesthetists of Great Britain and Ireland has promulgated a series of standards and guidelines over the past 15–20 years. In the field of obstetric anaesthesia, the Obstetric Anaesthetists' Association (OAA) produced its *Recommended Minimum Standards for Obstetric Anaesthesia Services* in 1994. In 1998, both organisations jointly produced *Guidelines for Obstetric Anaesthesia Services*, which were updated in 2005. This important document specifies recommendations for staffing levels; acceptable response times; monitoring during regional analgesia and Caesarean section; theatre, recovery, high-dependency and intensive care unit facilities; availability of blood; consent; support services; assistance and departmental guidelines. In addition, it has a section on professional relationships with midwives and obstetricians.

In 1999, the Royal Colleges of Midwives and Obstetricians and Gynaecologists published *Towards Safer Childbirth – Minimum Standards for the Organisation of Labour Wards*, setting out recommendations for organisational aspects of maternity services and risk management (due for revision 2007).

In the USA, the American Society of Anesthesiologists produced its *Guidelines for Regional Anesthesia in Obstetrics* in 1988 and last amended them in 2000. *Practice Guidelines for Obstetrical Anesthesia*, the report by the ASA's Task Force on Obstetrical Anesthesia, was produced in 1999 and revised in 2006, covering more aspects of obstetric anaesthetic practice. ASA published a joint statement with the American College of Obstetricians and Gynecologists, Optimal Goals for Anesthesia Care in Obstetrics, in 2000.

Local protocols and guidelines

It is important that these are written clearly and unambiguously. Once a protocol has been written, it becomes an important legal document (e.g. in future claims that negligence occurred) even if it has not yet been formally introduced, since merely by existing it demonstrates that any other management is suboptimal. This potential exposure to criticism and possibly legal action has deterred some clinicians from utilising protocols more widely.

Each version of a protocol should be dated and previous ones removed in order to maintain consistency throughout the unit. Obsolete ones should be stored since subsequent legal actions may refer to guidelines that were in force at the time of the supposed mismanagement.

Although there have been calls for national protocols that can be used by all units, most prefer to alter basic schemes to suit the local circumstances.

Writing a protocol requires the clinical problem or procedure to be carefully defined at the start. It is important that protocols are written by multidisciplinary groups and that all individuals involved are consulted before their introduction, since the protocols must be willingly followed by all clinicians unless specific exclusion criteria are met. Management of cases meeting exclusion criteria should also be covered. It is equally important that adherence to the protocol is audited to ensure consistency of management.

Medicolegal considerations

As a method of protecting the practitioner from legal actions for negligence, documents of this type are obviously a two-edged sword, since they could be a useful weapon for lawyers when the stated standards have not been achieved.

In practice, however, standards and guidelines have not been afforded a great deal of weight in courts of law in the UK or USA. This is partly because, although they may reflect the views of a group of senior and respected practitioners, they are rarely firmly based on good scientific evidence, and there is often an equally respectable opinion that would support a different course of action or standard of care. Furthermore, since such documents and their authors cannot be cross-examined in court, greater weight is often attached to the evidence given directly by expert witnesses.

Key points

- Minimum standard documents provide a useful reference when developing local protocols and are an impetus to improving and maintaining the quality of medical care.
- Local protocols and guidelines can improve clinical management and form an important part of risk management.
- Many potential problems can be avoided by careful writing and achieving consensus.
- Each copy should be dated, and obsolete versions removed from all clinical sites and kept for future reference.

FURTHER READING

Obstetric Anaesthetists' Association/Association of Anaesthetists of Great Britain and Ireland. *Guidelines for Obstetric Anaesthetic Services,* 2nd edn. London: AAGBI, 2005.

Practice guidelines for obstetrical anesthesia: a report by the American Society of Anesthesiologists Task Force on Obstetrical Anesthesia. *Anesthesiology* 1999; **90**: 600–11.

Royal College of Midwives, Royal College of Obstetricians and Gynaecologists. *Towards Safer Childbirth – Minimum Standards for the Organisation of Labour Wards.* London: RCOG, 1999.

---

160   RISK MANAGEMENT

Risk management is a process by which adverse outcomes are minimised by analysing their causes and instituting preventative steps, thus reducing both the chance of an adverse event occurring and its cost (both clinical and financial) should it occur. Although it may involve audit, the emphasis is based more on the analysis of individual real or potential adverse events rather than assessment of standards of practice generally. This approach is widely used throughout (and outside) health care to reduce risk and also liability.

Problems/special considerations

- Traditionally, anaesthetic risk has been seen as individual based (e.g. arising from human error), but recent emphasis has focused on risk being operating room based (arising from the interaction between anaesthetists and their working environment, in this case the labour ward) and most recently system based (human actions superimposed on inherent flaws in a system or process). Examples of system-based errors might include the patient with pre-eclampsia who presents unbooked late in pregnancy, requires emergency Caesarean section but is not given antacid prophylaxis because her drug chart is missing; she is anaesthetised by a junior trainee, aspirates on induction and is transferred to another hospital because of a shortage of intensive care beds.

- Important steps in the development of a risk management programme include:
  - Analysis of risks (e.g. morbidity and mortality meetings, critical incident reporting schemes)
  - Prevention of risks associated with routine activities (e.g. proper training and supervision, provision of trained anaesthetic assistants)
  - Avoidance of particularly high-risk practices (e.g. use of regional anaesthesia in preference to general anaesthesia for Caesarean section)
  - Minimising the severity of adverse events should they occur (e.g. having an antacid prophylaxis protocol in place)
  - Risk financing (e.g. indemnity)
  - Having a system in place for dealing with disasters and complaints: this may reduce both psychological sequelae and legal proceedings.

  Such a programme has implications for training, purchase and upkeep of equipment and other potentially costly processes but should ultimately reduce costs related to legal actions.
- Relatively simple measures can be taken to reduce the risks attached to specific activities, such as analysing a single procedure (e.g. Caesarean section) at all its stages or focusing on a specific complication (e.g. dural tap) and working back. A climate in which mistakes and critical incidents can be openly discussed without fear of retribution is important. Once a risk management programme is instituted, specific audits can then be performed to highlight areas where inadequacies still exist. Protocols are generally seen as a way of reducing risk if they are widely circulated and followed (itself a worthy subject of audit). Wider use of critical incident reporting schemes has been suggested as a more effective means of improving service than traditional reliance on outcome studies (e.g. looking at mortality), firstly because serious adverse outcomes are rare and secondly because a proactive approach is inherently more attractive than a reactive one.

Key points

- Risk may involve human actions and/or an underlying flawed system.
- Management includes:
  - Analysis
  - Reduction of risk attached to routine activities
  - Avoidance of high-risk activities
  - Damage limitation
  - Risk financing.

FURTHER READING

Holden DA, Quin M, Holden DP. Clinical risk management in obstetrics. *Curr Opin Obstet Gynecol* 2004; **16**: 137–42.

Luckas M, Walkinshaw S. Risk management on the labour ward. *Hosp Med* 2001; **62**: 751–6.

161 POST-CRISIS MANAGEMENT

Obstetric anaesthesia is a particularly stressful subspecialty of anaesthesia. It is important that all staff are aware that there are times when colleagues may need someone to talk to and they may need support in communicating with the patient and other colleagues. It is also clear that proper debriefing after catastrophes is an important part of risk management.

A crisis may be precipitated by a variety of factors, some obvious and others less obvious (Table 161.1).

Problems/special considerations

The reasons for the stress are many:

- The anaesthetist is looking after two people – the mother and the baby – during an important life event. There is therefore much at stake should things go wrong.
- Both mother and fetus are physiologically stressed and thus have less reserve than healthy patients. When adverse events occur, they often do so rapidly and without

Table 161.1. Causes of major stress when support and counselling of colleagues may be required

Serious adverse outcome	Maternal death or severe impairment
	Fetal death or severe impairment
Unexpected crisis	Anaphylaxis
	Failed or difficult tracheal intubation
	Shoulder dystocia
	Sudden severe maternal haemorrhage
	Maternal cardiac arrest
Complication of technique	Accidental dural puncture
	Neurological deficit following regional analgesia and anaesthesia
Failure of technique	Awareness during general anaesthesia for Caesarean section
	Pain during regional anaesthesia for Caesarean section
	Failed regional analgesia for labour
Human error	Giving the wrong drug or blood
	Not checking a blood result
Other	Letter of complaint from patient or solicitor
	Formal complaint from other hospital staff
	Violence from patient or relative/partner
	Coincidental professional or personal crisis

warning, with little time to treat them before irreparable damage occurs. Obstetrics thus represents a truly 'high-risk' area of medical practice.

- Pregnancy is perceived as a normal physiological function in which the outcome should be safe and happy. The public expectations are very high and it is inevitable that these high expectations may sometimes not be met.
- It is obvious that a maternal death will be a very traumatic event, but less obvious that a junior anaesthetist will be very upset by causing an accidental dural puncture. Because maternity units are often very busy places and turnover of staff is high, there may not be a suitable opportunity to discuss potential problems with colleagues.
- Maternity units are areas where different professional groups (anaesthetists, obstetricians and midwives) work closely together, with sometimes different priorities. Communication may be less than ideal.

Management options

Failure of communication is one of the main reasons for complaint, and it is important that the anaesthetist continually informs the patient and her relatives when there are problems.

Communication between staff is also crucial. Trainees must always feel able to discuss a problem with their senior colleagues, without embarrassment, and must feel that they, as a trainee, are part of the team whose aim is a high standard of care to all the women.

It is important that there is regular multidisciplinary discussion and that staff do not automatically blame each other when outcomes are bad. Senior staff of all disciplines should ensure that each major catastrophe is fully discussed in an open fashion, and that all staff involved with the case have a chance to discuss it. Counselling should be made available if required by any staff.

When any member of staff is worried that there has been a problem, it is often helpful to seek advice from their medical protection organisation. It is also useful to go back to the medical record and, where appropriate, expand the account of the events and keep a full copy for personal use.

Post-crisis management also includes identification of any legal and/or financial threats to the hospital and taking steps to avoid or reduce them.

Key points

- All staff are vulnerable to experiencing a catastrophe in the maternity unit.
- Communication with all levels of staff and a non-judgemental approach are essential.
- All members of staff involved in a catastrophe should be offered support and, if necessary, counselling.

162   RESEARCH ON LABOUR WARD

Research involving pregnant women has particular ethical and practical considerations. Perhaps partly because of this, much of obstetric and anaesthetic practice on the labour ward has traditionally been based on tradition and dogma, with either little evidence available or little attention paid to what evidence there is. Fortunately there has been increasing reliance on published studies in guiding management, although in the quest for 'evidence-based' decisions it is often forgotten that the best evidence there is may be far from perfect, i.e. the ideal randomised controlled trial (RCT) has not been done. For example, the question of whether loss of resistance to air is indeed associated with a greater incidence of accidental dural tap than loss of resistance to saline would require a huge study, which would involve more centres and take more time than is practicable. In this situation one is left with methodologically weak studies (e.g. retrospective reviews) which may suggest a causal link but no more.

In the generally quoted hierarchy of evidence, the best of all is the systematic review, in which all known RCTs are screened for correct methodology and the results pooled to increase power. Next, prospective RCTs themselves are still considered the gold standard for comparing different treatments or courses of management (particularly relevant to obstetric anaesthetic practice) if of adequate size; in descending order come non-randomised, single group, cohort or case–control studies; non-experimental studies; and finally case reports and 'expert' opinions.

Problems/special considerations

- Ethical issues are related to the special vulnerability of pregnant women who are going through an intensely emotional time; the increasing involvement of mothers in decisions affecting their pregnancy and thus exposure of them to many potentially difficult choices already; the fact that many drugs in current obstetric anaesthetic practice are not licensed for use in pregnancy (largely related to the cost to manufacturers of separate trials in this group); and to the often uncertain effects of experimental drugs and procedures on the pregnancy, labour or fetus.

- The care of pregnant women has traditionally been something of a battleground between various medical and non-medical staff, and the risk that a well-intentioned study may be viewed as an intrusion into a normal process should not be taken lightly. Courtesy dictates that the obstetrician under whose care potential subjects are should be informed of the study protocol. The situation of independent midwives caring for women with epidurals without the input of an obstetrician is already a controversial one and there may be conflict if such mothers are approached for enrolment into an anaesthetic study.

- The issue of consent may be cause for discussion. It has been argued that a labouring woman is unable to give truly informed consent for inclusion in a study (or even for a procedure such as an epidural) because of the pain and distress she may be suffering, especially if drugs such as pethidine have been given. This makes studies of epidural techniques especially difficult, since it may not be possible to identify in advance women who might go on to request epidural analgesia. An especially controversial area concerns the calls for randomised studies of epidural versus non-epidural analgesia, in order to assess side effects in particular; some would consider it unethical to withhold the only really effective form of analgesia from mothers, whereas others claim it is unethical not to do so if it is the only way of properly evaluating the effects of epidurals.

- Practical difficulties of conducting obstetric anaesthetic studies relate to the obtaining of consent discussed above; the defining of a homogenous group of subjects (the 'standard primip' was suggested by Crawford over 25 years ago as suitable for the majority of studies; women in this category are aged 25, healthy, with a full-term normal singleton pregnancy and no malposition or malpresentation); the fact that labouring women in particular are demanding in terms of requesting information and determining their own management; and the largely unpredictable nature of the workload. In addition, since all subjects must have the right to withdraw from any study at any time without penalty, randomised studies may suffer from considerable drop-out rates (e.g. those studies of epidural versus non-epidural analgesia). Since a mother's situation may change suddenly during labour, this may further increase the drop-out rate. Finally, the records relating to the research may easily become lost amongst the voluminous paperwork that passes through the labour ward.

Management options

Apart from the considerations mentioned above, research methods are as for any other clinical situation. The practicalities of labour ward research preclude many topics from being suitable for study, even though they may be of interest and clinical value. Many potential or actual studies suffer from either too few subjects or too rare an outcome, or both; thus, for example, many complications that are relatively uncommon can only be meaningfully studied in multicentre trials (e.g. dural taps, neurological complications). Studies comparing different regional anaesthetic techniques are relatively easy to conduct in a single unit, since so many anaesthetic interventions involve regional techniques.

As for any project, an obstetric anaesthetic RCT requires appropriate consideration of the primary hypothesis (what question is the study asking – and is it worth asking?); the subjects to be studied (inclusion and exclusion criteria); the type of data collected (what is being measured and how); the methods of analysis (which statistical tests to use); and the overall power of the study (related to the number of subjects per group, the size of the difference between the groups and the statistical test used).

Finally, it should be remembered that a statistically significant result may not be *clinically* significant (e.g. a 30-second difference in onset of epidural block), and also that a statistically significant result found in a single study may still be a chance finding (albeit with a likelihood of less than 5% if a probability of 0.05 was taken to denote 'statistical significance'). Conversely, just because the evidence supporting a particular course of action or management may be overwhelming, it does not necessarily follow that clinicians will adhere to it.

Key points

- For research on the labour ward, basic ethical considerations apply.
- Subjects are especially vulnerable but may be especially demanding.
- Practical difficulties include obtaining consent and the unpredictability of labour.

FURTHER READING

Americal College of Obstetricians and Gynecologists. Ethical considerations in research involving women. *Obstet Gynecol* 2003; **102**: 1107–13.

Lupton MGF, Williams DJ. The ethics of research on pregnant women – is maternal consent sufficient? *Br J Obstet Gynaecol* 2004; **111**: 1307–12.

Yentis SM. Ethical guidance for research in obstetric anaesthesia. *Int J Obstet Anesth* 2001; **10**: 289–91.

163   OBSTETRIC ANAESTHETIC ORGANISATIONS

Several organisations and societies relevant to obstetric analgesia and anaesthesia exist. In the UK, there are many regional societies and groups, some involving non-anaesthetists as well as anaesthetists. National organisations exist in many countries but not all. There are no separate international organisations (the European Society of Obstetric Anesthesia (ESOA) was active for a few years in the late 1990s but is now inactive), although the European Society of Anaesthesiologists (ESA) has an Obstetric Committee. The Obstetric Anaesthetists' Association (OAA), which represents obstetric analgesia and anaesthesia in the UK, has many members from overseas.

Obstetric Anaesthetists' Association (OAA)

The OAA was formed in 1969 to promote the highest standards of anaesthetic practice in the care of the mother and baby and has an international membership in the order of 2000. It provides a focus for all anaesthetists who want to improve the care and safety of women in childbirth. The Association has charitable status, supports a research fellowship and offers annual research grants and bursaries. It also offers prizes for trainees for research presented at the annual scientific meeting.

The OAA holds three main meetings a year: in March, a one-day meeting in London on controversies in obstetric anaesthesia; in the spring, a 2-day meeting at different venues in the UK on current research and practice (the Association's Annual General Meeting is held at this meeting); and in late autumn, a 3-day course in London presenting the latest academic and clinical views on modern obstetric anaesthesia and analgesia. Further smaller refresher courses and meetings on various topics are also held.

The *International Journal of Obstetric Anesthesia (IJOA)* is the official Journal of the OAA, carries OAA notices, and is included in the annual subscription. The OAA also supplies educational videos and publications; details are available from:

Obstetric Anaesthetists' Association
PO Box 3219
London SW13 9XR, UK
Tel: +44 020 8741 1311; fax: +44 020 8741 0611.
Email: secretariat@oaa-anaes.ac.uk
Website: www.oaa-anaes.ac.uk

Society for Obstetric Anesthesia and Perinatology (SOAP)

Outside Britain, SOAP is the biggest and most active group for obstetric anaesthetists. It was founded in the USA in 1968 to provide a forum for discussion of problems unique to the peripartum period. SOAP is comprised of anaesthetists, obstetricians, paediatricians and basic scientists who share an interest in the care of the pregnant patient and the neonate; membership currently numbers approximately 1000.

The mission of the society is to promote excellence in research and practice of obstetric anaesthesia and perinatology. Through its newsletter, internet site and annual meetings, SOAP allows practitioners of several specialties to meet and discuss clinical practice, basic and clinical research and practical professional concerns. SOAP has a travelling scholarship programme, allowing overseas anaesthetists from developing countries to travel to the annual meeting and to spend one week at a centre of excellence in the USA. The society awards an annual research fellowship and a smaller research starter grant is also offered. The address of SOAP is:

Society for Obstetric Anesthesia and Perinatology
2 Summit Park Drive, #140
Cleveland, OH 44131-2571
Phone: 216-447-7863
Fax: 216-642-1127
Email: soaphq@soap.org
Website: www.soap.org

164 VITAL STATISTICS

In the UK, figures are collected by three main mechanisms: statutory reporting schemes (e.g. registration of births to the Office of National Statistics (ONS) by the parents; birth notification to the Director of Public Health by midwives or medical staff; reporting of congenital abnormalities to ONS); non-statutory but obligatory schemes (e.g. those organised for accreditation and training by the Royal Colleges; the Confidential Enquiries into Maternal and Child Health); and specific projects, which may or may not be supported by national or professional bodies (e.g. surveys carried out by the Audit Commission or National Birthday Trust; hospital- or department-based projects; Obstetric Anaesthetists' Association or Association of Anaesthetists projects).

Anaesthetists may be involved in some of the above schemes and the information gained may be of interest to obstetric anaesthestists in particular. There may be considerable overlap between the information gained for public health or political purposes and that gained for research or audit purposes; there may also be conflicting interests of the bodies supporting them. Specific schemes related to obstetric anaesthesia are few and far between.

Some of the national figures from recent years are provided in Table 164.1.

Problems/special considerations

As with all large information-gathering schemes, there may be inaccuracies in the figures collected, which in turn can be interpreted in different ways. It is also generally easier to collect information about outcome events than about

Table 164.1. UK maternity statistics (per year). Figures are from Confidential Enquiries into Maternal and Child Health and/or Department of Health statistics

Total no. live and stillbirths (NHS)	~584 000 in 2004–5 (680 000–790 000 over past 20 years)
Fertility rate	60–4 per 1000 women aged 15–44 over past 20 years (was around 90 in the late 1950s–early 1960s)
Total no. pregnancies (estimated)	900 000–1 000 000
Legal abortions	~175 000
Mothers <20 or ≥35 years old	7–9% each
Gestation <37 weeks or >41 weeks	7% and 4% respectively in 2004–5
Caesarean section rate (England)	23% in 2004–5 (<3% in the 1950s, 10–11% in the 1980s and 15.5% in 1994–5); emergency rate 12% and elective rate 11%
General anaesthesia for Caesarean section	6-7% in 2003–4 (>50% in 1989–90)
Forceps or ventouse delivery (England)	10–11%
Induction rates (England)	17–20%
Epidural rate in labour	21–28%

denominators, e.g. the total number of births is known but the total number of pregnancies is not (it is estimated from the number of births, the number of ectopic pregnancies and the number of legal and spontaneous abortions from hospital data systems and morbidity reports). There may also be discrepancies between data collected for the UK and its composite parts. There are also considerable differences between the ability to collect information, and thus contribute to the various reporting schemes, of the approximately 320 National Health Service and independent units in the UK in which babies are born. Finally, centrally collected and administered schemes invariably report several years after the period of interest.

Key points

- Collection of maternity and related data may be a statutory requirement, an obligatory professional requirement or a non-obligatory but desirable practice.
- A number of national data collection schemes produce reports of interest to anaesthetists.
- Intervention rates are increasing steadily.

FURTHER READING

Garcia J, *et al. First class delivery*. London: Audit Commission, 1998.
NHS *Maternity Statistics*, England: 2004–5. London: Dept of Health, 2006.

165   HISTORICAL ASPECTS OF OBSTETRIC ANALGESIA AND ANAESTHESIA

Knowledge of the major developments in obstetric anaesthesia and analgesia helps to put modern obstetric practice into context. The following brief summary outlines some of these developments and also those in general anaesthetic practice who have had profound effects on the subspecialty.

General

- Ancient methods of pain relief included various plant-derived sedatives, acupuncture and physical methods such as binding.
- 1933: Grantly Dick-Read, English obstetrician, published his book *Natural Childbirth*, followed in 1944 by *Childbirth Without Fear*. He proposed a link between fear, tension and pain, suggesting that the cycle could be broken by abolishing fear.
- 1952–4: the period covered by the first Report on Confidential Enquiries into Maternal Deaths, published by the Department of Health.

- 1953: Virginia Apgar, anesthesiologist at Columbia University, described her scoring system for assessing neonates.
- 1958: Ferdinand Lamaze, French obstetrician, published his book *Painless Childbirth*, in which he suggested that pain was a conditioned reflex triggered by uterine contractions, and that a period of unconditioning followed by reconditioning (psychoprophylaxis) could reduce pain.
- 1975: F. Leboyer, French obstetrician, published *Birth Without Violence*, in which he advocated delivery in a quiet, darkened room, with minimal stimulation.
- 1993: the Department of Health's Expert Maternity Group published its report *Changing Childbirth* (the Cumberledge Report), which placed the expectant mother at the centre of care, emphasising her right to choose and signalling a formal move away from the traditional paternalistic 'medical' approach.

Systemic analgesia

- 1902: morphine and hyoscine first used in labour.
- 1940: pethidine first used in labour.
- 1950: pethidine approved by the Central Midwives Board.

Inhalational analgesia

- 1847: James Young Simpson, Professor of Midwifery at Edinburgh University, administered the first obstetric general anaesthetic using ether. Considerable opposition came from religious leaders for going against the Bible and from medical authorities for compromising safety. Simpson went on to advocate chloroform in preference to ether, having used it the same year. He was a major influence in British obstetrics and also designed obstetric forceps, which bear his name.
- 1853: John Snow, London physician, generally considered the father of British anaesthesia, delivered Queen Victoria's eighth child (Prince Leopold) under chloroform, putting an end to the above objections. Snow is also famous for his part in ending the London cholera epidemic of 1854.
- 1881: Stanislav Klikovitch, Russian physician working in St Petersburg, described the use of nitrous oxide (80% with 20% oxygen) for labour, noting its lack of effect on the uterus and the requirement for inhalation before each contraction started.
- 1936: Minnitt's nitrous oxide/air apparatus approved by the Central Midwives Board.
- 1961: Michael Tunstall, Aberdeen anaesthetist, described the use of premixed nitrous oxide and oxygen in labour. The mixture was marketed 2 years later in the UK as Entonox. Tunstall also described the isolated forearm technique for detecting awareness, developed the Entonox demand valve (from diving equipment) and advocated the 'failed intubation drill' in obstetrics.

Regional analgesia

- 1884: Carl Koller, German ophthalmologist, used cocaine for eye surgery.
- 1885: James Leonard Corning, New York neurologist, produced spinal and epidural blockade in dogs.
- 1899: August Bier, German surgeon, used spinal anaesthesia for surgery. Bier described postdural puncture headache for the first time.
- 1901: Jean-Athanase Sicard and Fernand Cathelin, French neurologist and urologist respectively, introduced caudal analgesia.
- 1921: Fidel Pages, Spanish surgeon, used lumbar epidural blockade for surgery.
- 1931: Eugen Bogdan Aburel, Romanian obstetrician, described continuous caudal plus lumboaortic plexus blocks in labour.
- 1933: John Cleland, American obstetrician, described paravertebral block in labour.
- 1942: Robert Hingson, American obstetrician, described continuous caudals in labour.
- 1949: Cleland described continuous lumbar epidural block in labour.
- British pioneers: Andrew Doughty (Kingston; 1960s–70s); J. Selwyn Crawford (Birmingham; 1960s–80s); Donald Moir (Glasgow; 1960s–80s); Barbara Morgan (Queen Charlotte's, London; 1980s–90s).
- More recent developments:
  (i) Pencil-point spinal needles first described in 1920s but advances in their manufacture resulted in their wide availability in the late 1980s/early 1990s.
  (ii) Combined spinal–epidural technique first described in the UK in 1981–2; popularised in obstetrics in the 1990s; 'mobile epidural' combined spinal–epidural technique popularised at Queen Charlotte's by Barbara Morgan.
  (iii) Microfine spinal catheters used in the late 1980s/early 1990s; withdrawn in the USA by the Food and Drug Administration in 1992.
  (iv) Patient-controlled epidural analgesia used in the 1990s.

General anaesthesia for Caesarean section

- 1945: Curtis Mendelson, American obstetrician, described the syndrome of acid aspiration both clinically and experimentally, distinguishing it from upper airway obstruction caused by inhalation of large pieces of food.
- 1961: Brian Sellick, London anaesthetist, described cricoid pressure as a means of preventing aspiration of gastric contents.
- 1960s: the problem of intraoperative awareness became topical, with up to 9% of mothers who received thiopental, nitrous oxide and neuromuscular blockade remembering intraoperative events. Donald Moir, Glasgow anaesthetist, described a technique of halothane 0.5% with 50:50 nitrous oxide:oxygen in 1970, with no recall. Tunstall described the isolated forearm technique as a means of monitoring consciousness during general anaesthesia, in 1979.

Index

Note: page numbers in *italics* refer to figures and tables